HERBAL MEDICINE, HEALING & CANCER

HERBAL MEDICINE, HEALING & CANCER

A Comprehensive Program for Prevention and Treatment

DONALD R. YANCE, JR., C.N., M.H., A.HG.,

WITH ARLENE VALENTINE

FOREWORD BY JOEL M. EVANS, M.D.

Library of Congress Cataloging-in-Publication Data

Yance, Donald.
    Herbal medicine, healing & cancer / by Donald R. Yance ; with Arlene Valentine.
      p.   cm.
    Includes bibliographical references and index.
    ISBN 0-87983-968-6
    1. Herbs—Therapeutic use. 2. Cancer—Alternative treatment. I. Valentine, Arlene.
II. Title. III. Title: Herbal medicine, healing, and cancer.
    RC271.H47Y36   1999
    616.99'4061—dc21   99-35821
                                                 CIP

Published by Keats Publishing, a division of NTC/Contemporary Publishing Group, Inc.
4255 West Touhy Avenue, Lincolnwood (Chicago), Illinois 60646-1975 U.S.A.

Interior design by Andrea Reider
Cover design by Monica Baziuk

Printed in the United States of America
International Standard Book Number: 0-87983-968-6
        03 04 LB 18 17 16 15 14 13 12 11
10 9 8 7 6 5

To all the people with cancer
with whom I have worked over the years.
They have taught me so much about healing,
and their spirits continue to inspire me.

Contents

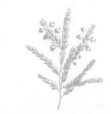

Foreword

Herbs heal.

Why is it that stating such a simple truth elicits responses as passionate as the most controversial religious, social, or political issue? The answer lies in the importance of health and healing to society. In all cultures, the ability to cure the sick was considered a special gift of honor. Historically, it was bestowed upon those deemed to have a special closeness to God or the spirit world, such as religious officials, tribal medicine men, or witch doctors, who could make use of an intuitive connection to help people heal. More recently, a different quality—a superior intellect as demonstrated by academic achievement—became a highly valued prerequisite required by our culture for entrance into the healing profession.

With some of the most prestigious members of society involved in the noble cause of healing, it became natural for people to transfer the "power to heal" from themselves and the spiritual world to the intellectuals who proclaimed they had the "knowledge to heal." The notable exception to these modern-day practitioners are the many healers of indigenous cultures who continue to utilize the power of their spiritual beliefs.

Ultimately, those with the intellectual "knowledge to heal" became quite comfortable with, and even addicted to, the power that society had given to them. Thanks to unrelenting self-promoting and fear-inducing proclamations by the medical establishment, such as the infamous Flexner Report, most schools of nonallopathic healing, such as colleges of homeopathy or Eclectic medicine, were forced to close their doors. Individuals then soon lost faith in any nonscientifically proven method of healing. Unfortunately, this fate befell all non-Western, nontechnologic healing modalities no matter how strongly validated by history or culture, whether it be spirituality and prayer, acupuncture, or, what is especially germane here, the medicinal properties of plants.

That is why *Herbal Medicine, Healing & Cancer* is such a seminal work. After all, knowledge is power. By educating the reader in such a profound and thoughtful way, Donald Yance takes the "power to heal" away from the institution of medicine and returns it back to its rightful owner, the unbeatable, historically proven trio of nature, spirit, and the individual.

In this book we learn about the beauty of the forest and the chemical composition of herbs and can't help but compare that to the beauty and composition of the human body. We learn about the interactions of aromatic oils and active phytochemicals that mimic the interactions between and amongst our cells and organs. We are awestruck as the author paints a picture of a divinely designed plant world so complex that it is filled with compounds that interact perfectly and precisely with the proteins and enzymes in our bodies. We are humbled as we realize that we are only just beginning to understand the magnitude of the healing potential of nature.

The thoughtful organization of this book makes it useful to many different audiences: medical doctors interested in expanding their horizons; naturopathic physicians, herbalists, or nutritionists seeking to enhance their existing knowledge; or the layperson, either with cancer or a caregiver to a cancer patient, who can learn the process of designing a unique, individualized treatment plan.

Donnie, as he likes to be called, is a certified nutritionist and master herbalist who has successfully treated scores of cancer patients. He has advised doctors and lectured at hospitals on natural medicine. In this book, Donnie achieves the lofty goal of transferring his extensive knowledge about herbs and healing to the reader in a way that is easily understood regardless of one's pre-existing knowledge of botanicals.

The book begins with a description of Donnie's holistic approach, followed by a thorough explanation of what we know scientifically about cancer and herbal medicine. We are then treated to the latest information on diet, herbs, and supplements. Finally, Donnie tells us about specific treatment regimens and gives sample protocols.

Donnie has been one of my teachers on my journey to starting a holistic women's center and has cared for me personally. Writing this foreword is but a small token of my heartfelt appreciation.

After finishing this comprehensive treatise on herbal medicine, healing, and cancer, you can be assured that you too will have acquired one very passionate, steadfast, almost religious conviction . . .

Herbs heal.

—JOEL M. EVANS, M.D.
Founder and Director,
The Center for Women's Health,
Darien, Connecticut

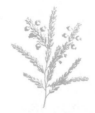

Acknowledgments

To my wife and daughter for their loving support and patience in allowing me time away from them to write;

To Arlene Valentine for her help, input, support, and love, without which I could not have accomplished this goal;

To my editor, Phyllis Herman, for her understanding and skill and my copyeditor, Anne Harris, for her focus and expertise;

To Ellen Meyer and Ellen McCarthy for their help in editing my early work, long before it evolved into this book;

To Garret Miller and Father Phillip O'Shea for their inspiration, motivation, and lessons about life;

To the great jazz musicians, particularly Bill Evans and John Coltrane, for their beautiful music that taught me how to improvise, create, express, and listen—all of which I exercise in the art of healing;

To my mother and father, who first taught me to listen;

To all my herbal colleagues, teachers, healers, and visionaries who teach and inspire me daily;

To the Eclectic and Physiomedical physicians, particularly Eli Jones, John Scudder, and J.M. Thurston, whose work continues to teach me the healing ways of the American school of herbal medicine;

To all the grandmothers and grandfathers who, with humility and respect, have been the true healers of herbal medicine, empowering me with the wisdom, the tools, and the God-given right to heal with herbs;

To St. Francis of Assisi, whose example has taught me that love of nature and humanity are not separate, but one in the face of God;

And finally, I thank the Lord, who has given me the strength, courage, and ability to write this book.

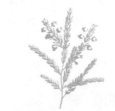

Introduction

Wherever the art of medicine is loved, there also is love of humanity.

—*Hippocrates*

Herbal Medicine, Healing & Cancer focuses on the many ways that natural forms of healing can treat or prevent cancer. Herbs, vitamins and other micronutrients, proper diet, and other health-enhancing modalities can all be used with or without conventional therapies in the healing process. These nontoxic therapies can also inhibit cancer recurrence as well as second-line cancers caused by chemotherapy or radiation therapy.

Another essential aspect of healing—one that I utilize both in my practice and in my personal life—is prayer and spirituality. I do not believe in preaching about my spiritual beliefs, but will, at times, share my feelings about the importance of God in my life. I pray in silence for each and every patient I see. Body and spirit, humanity and nature—these are not separate entities but one entity, and when they are brought together and nurtured they enable healing to happen. Approaching healing in this way allows for a certain aspect of mystery in the healing process, which we, with all of our modern technology and need to be in control, often ignore.

Although this book contains numerous references to medical research studies, it is based primarily on my own firsthand experiences in helping people who are dealing with cancer.

I am frequently asked what really heals cancer. Frankly, I don't know whether it's the herbs, the nutritional supplements, changes in diet or lifestyle, changes in mind and spirit, or even some conventional protocols. Perhaps it's a combination of all these things. I do know, however, that just as each herb is a complex entity, so too is each individual. Thus, healing with herbs brings us into a realm where physical explanations are not always as clear and scientific as we would like. The synergy that takes place between the body's own innate tendency to heal and the herbs that aid in that process is, in some ways, a mystery even though the healing itself is indisputably real.

Whatever the reason, I am simply overjoyed when a healing happens. I am thankful and believe it to be a miracle from God.

I believe if we truly want to heal people, we need to cut through, not eliminate, a lot of modern science. At the same time, we need to restore some important basics like compassion, humility, and respect for each individual's uniqueness. Doctors (as well as the entire technology-driven medical establishment) need to look at patients as human beings, not objects; individuals, not cases; creative eccentrics, not benumbed normals. Unfortunately, in spite of all its advances, modern medicine as it is practiced today is leaving its mark on human life in the shallowest of ways.

I believe that the human body has an amazing ability to maintain homeostasis if we provide the proper environment for it to do so. I also believe that an overwhelming amount of stress underlies most chronic illness, and that patients need to address the issues of stress in their lives for true healing to take place. Conventional medicine, on the other hand, preaches that only medical interventions and modern drugs will lead to healing. It also holds that the body's healing responses to illness must be treated and suppressed.

It is standard procedure, for instance, to suppress the body's curative powers by using Tylenol to lower a fever or to relieve the aches and pains often caused by interferon production when one is ill. Is this helping or making matters worse? I believe, as all traditional healers have known for thousands of years, that a fever is the body's healing reaction to an infectious organism and that, instead of being suppressed, it should be worked with to allow the body to disperse the heat by sweating. When a patient is taking interferon, for example, I would recommend drinking a diaphoretic tea and taking an Epsom salt bath before bed at least three nights a week. The diaphoretic tea would be made with herbs like boneset, yarrow, elder, peppermint, and ginger. This not only relieves the achiness and flulike symptoms that interferon brings with it, it actually helps the interferon to be more effective.

Often, when a person is first diagnosed with cancer and decides to follow a standard form of therapy in hopes of a cure, he can be successful at putting the cancer into remission, but what about the future? There are a few very important questions that need to be asked:

1. Does the patient have choices or is the decision-making process in the hands of others?

2. What are his or her chances for a cure?

3. How long will the remission last?

4. How successful will the next treatment(s) be? Although treatment may cause tumor regression or inhibit further tumor growth, will the treatment ultimately provide longer life and/or better quality of life?

5. Can holistic complementary therapies be integrated into a comprehensive approach or would holistic treatments alone be better in this situation?

6. Is there anything that can be done to inhibit the cancer from returning or to prevent another cancer from forming?

7. If the doctor says the patient is just wasting time and money with an organic diet and medicinal herbs, should the patient abandon responsibility for her long-term health and well-being?

For many people, serious problems and conflicts arise when their conventional doctor disapproves of their interest in natural therapies. However, I have worked with thousands of people who have cancer and have learned that those who include herbs, good nutrition, and other nontoxic approaches in their treatment are able to reduce the likelihood of recurrences, enhance any conventional therapies that they are undergoing, and lessen their side effects. My approach has been used as the primary treatment for healing as well as a complementary addition to conventional treatment. Believe it or not, many of the people I work with actually tell me that having cancer has been a blessing in their lives as their values change, relationships improve, and they begin to live life with joy rather than with fear.

I don't believe we were meant to live as far removed from nature as we do today, and we do so at our peril. Surely, God did not create us to lead lives spent in front of computer screens and TVs while eating processed foods and then try to correct our mistakes by ingesting high-tech medicines. We need to reconsider why we are here and to honor our connection with each other, with God, and with nature. We are naturally healed by these connections, and it is vital to include them in our lives. One of my favorite prescriptions for patients is to go home and grow a garden—as the garden grows, so does the gardener!

Drawing on my twelve years of experience in working with cancer patients, I have included in this book only proven and safe remedies for the prevention and treatment of this dread disease. I offer suggestions for treating not only common problems caused by the cancer itself, but also the life-disrupting side effects of conventional treatments such as chemotherapy, radiation, interferon, or other forms of therapy.

As chapter 2 explains, cancer is a multistage process of initiation, promotion, and progression that can be influenced by both permissive and protective factors—choices under our control that may either cause a tumor to grow or stop it in its tracks. Cancer is not a single disease but many diseases, all of which involve many factors. It is characterized by the properties of unregulated growth, invasion, and metastasis. Distant cells and molecular processes are associated with each of these events.

Nutritional factors, for example, may account for up to 70 percent of avoidable cancer mortality in this country, according to an eye-opening report in a 1992 issue of *Oncology*.[1] With a statistic like this one, it is time to look at herbs, diet, nutrition, and natural healing modalities as normal and life-affirming, not as "alternative" choices. Herbal medicine is one of the main pieces of the pie in my approach to cancer and it is therefore the main focus of this book. Currently, herbal medicine is getting a great deal of long-overdue attention from clinicians and researchers. Studies have shown that herbs can strengthen the immune system, reduce inflammation, inhibit mutations, and battle cancer by supporting the function of the immune system, including the enhancement of T-cells, natural killer-cells, and interferon, as well as by activating macrophages. Herbs contain many more powerful cell-protective factors than vitamins or minerals. They can lessen and relieve the side effects of chemotherapy and radiation as well as inhibit infections. Amazingly, they can also enhance the cytotoxic effects of many conventional therapies.

As a holistic clinician, I view each one of my clients as a whole person. I combine physical, mental, and spiritual aspects of healing in my practice. These aspects are interrelated and should not be separated. I believe that medicine and health care should be an integrated system that encompasses a variety of medical techniques, philosophies, and practices. I focus on healing first, and the mechanics of "curing" afterward. Healing is transformational; it transcends the physical and actively involves the emotional and spiritual. Healing imbues the whole being; it grows, gives meaning to life, provides peace, and makes room for love.

Although I have successfully treated many people with cancer by solely using herbs, diet, and other natural therapies, most of the people I treat for cancer have used these approaches in conjunction with conventional therapies. This is beginning to change as more and more people consider me their primary practitioner and natural therapies their primary treatment. In many cancers (and for certain people), I am confident that natural modalities can be more effective than a combination approach; however, in some cases I am not so sure; in still others, I truly believe a combined effort is best.

Each type of cancer is different, and each person's individual case is unique. Those who choose to use the conventional treatments recommended by their oncologists should not be discouraged from pursuing natural treatments as well. Better results will be achieved if the methods are combined because the expertise of both the oncologist and the holistic practitioner will govern the protocols. With proper nutritional support that includes specific herbal therapies, the side effects of conventional cancer therapies can be reduced, and cure rates can increase dramatically.

My goal is to help those afflicted with cancer by using the most effective treatments available. Proper diet and herbs help to create the right conditions for maximum healing, and that can only be beneficial no matter what other course of therapy is followed, if any. At the same time, my intention is to offer guidance and information to practitioners who work with cancer patients.

Many people are now getting their information about cancer treatment through the Internet. While this can be helpful, one problem with Internet information is the lack of regulation. One needs to be very cautious about the source of information as well as its validity.

Another problem is that the medical establishment insists that the truth about herbal and nutritional medicine can be learned only through double-blind studies. I feel that most doctors and researchers are confused about nutrition and ill-equipped to explain the workings of herbs. Because science isolates and looks at just one element of a food or an herb independent of its other components in order to analyze its benefits, we may wind up with studies that tell us how bad it is for us only to have the information reversed at a later time when other components of the same food or herb are studied. Nature has spirit, a vital force that imbues foods and herbs as well as each one of us; in addition, nature has an intelligence and inherent wisdom that science has apparently lost. In healing with herbs, one treats people, not their disease.

Today, because modern medicine is failing to fully heal those with serious ailments, many people are turning to natural and traditional healing methods. Throughout this book, I will share with you my knowledge, wisdom, and experience in the use of herbs, nutrition, diet, health education, and counseling for the prevention and treatment of cancer. I deeply believe in the value of a life lived simply and fully in harmony with nature, nourished with the bounty that God has provided. My prayer is that this book be a blessing and a true healing guide for all who read it.

1

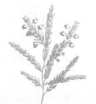

My Personal Philosophy of Healing

Where there is faith, there is love. Where there is love,
there is peace. Where there is peace, there is God. Where
there is God, there is no need.

—Anonymous

O f the many individuals who have influenced my philosophy of healing, no one has inspired me more than the thirteenth-century saint, Francis of Assisi, founder of the Franciscan order of monks. The son of a wealthy Italian merchant, St. Francis renounced a life of privilege and pleasure-seeking after a religious conversion, and took up a life of prayer and selfless service to the poor. Esteemed to this day for his deep love of nature and all of God's creatures—even the humblest among them—St. Francis felt called to serve God in many ways, including caring for the sick, particularly lepers, whom he had despised prior to his conversion.

1

Moved by St. Francis's life, I became a member of the secular Franciscan order in 1983. This lay group of men and women is dedicated to serving God and humanity without striving for material wealth or power but as brothers and sisters to all people. As I go about my daily work, it is the example of St. Francis that inspires me to be a compassionate, focused, and attentive listener so I can truly understand my clients and be present to their needs.

My first exposure to the world of natural healing began in the late 1970s while working in a small health food store in Stamford, Connecticut. Here I quickly became fascinated by natural foods, nutritional supplements, and the healing power of herbs. Around this time I was still seeking my life's path—one that would nourish my soul—when my cousin sent me the classic herbal book *Back to Eden* by Jethro Kloss. I read the book from cover to cover several times, thus beginning my herbal studies. I was impressed by several references to the Bible that helped me to see herbs in a spiritual light, and it was then that I undertook what has become a lifelong investigation into the world of natural healing.

Subsequently, I graduated from the National Institute of Nutritional Education and the Sequoya College of Herbology. Along with a friend, I eventually owned and operated a large health food store in Westport, Connecticut, that focused on organic foods and herbal medicines as well as nutritional supplements. This is where I began a private practice that offered people guidance in the areas of nutrition and herbal medicine.

Today, as a master clinical herbalist, certified nutritionist, aromatherapist, and secular Franciscan, I continue that work with a deep sense of mission to help people afflicted with chronic illnesses such as cancer. I offer my clients guidelines and support in the areas of diet, nutritional supplements, herbs, and lifestyle at a clinic and wellness center I opened in 1994. Located in Fairfield, Connecticut, it is called WellSprings Center for Natural Healing (WellSprings East). It includes an apothecary and herbal dispensary and is now staffed by three full-time and three part-time clinicians besides myself.

Thanks to the efforts and contributions of many, a second center, WellSprings West, has recently opened in Ashland, Oregon, and plans for a larger retreat center in Ashland are underway. My mission in founding WellSprings (a nonprofit corporation) was to create a healing retreat center that would offer a holistic approach to health by utilizing herbal medicines, nutrition, and other healing modalities for disease prevention and treatment and for wellness promotion. This planned center, with its hot water artesian springs and ornamental, culinary, herb, and staple food gardens, will provide a sanctuary for healing in body, mind, and spirit. When complete, WellSprings West will offer clinical treatment and support services, including hydrotherapy, acupuncture, and yoga; state-of-the-art research, development, and validation of complementary medical practices; and comprehensive educational programs, classes, lectures, and seminars. Like WellSprings East, it will also include an apothecary and herbal dispensary.

In my practice, I see a wide variety of individuals and a wide variety of illnesses, including diverse forms of cancer. In fact, nearly half of my practice at this time is devoted to clients dealing with this disease. They range from people with a genetic predisposition to cancer who are focusing on prevention to those diagnosed as terminal and for whom all other treatments have failed. Though I do not have all the answers, I am making progress every day in guiding these patients to wellness. I feel passionately devoted to this work, and I pray daily for the well-being of my clients and for the strength and wisdom to guide them in their healing process.

THE WISDOM OF *CHI*, THE VITAL LIFE FORCE

In terms of biological and cellular functions, twentieth-century medicine can brilliantly describe cancer's process from oncogenes to tumor-suppressor genes, to growth factors and specific cell receptors. However, although conventional medicine understands that malignant cells function in a chaotic fashion, it ignores that which imposes order in a healthy organism.

This is not the case with traditional healing systems. Traditional Chinese Medicine (TCM), for example, tells us order is imposed by *chi*, the vital energy or life force present in and activating all creation. India's medical system, Ayurveda, calls this life force *prana*. Japanese medicine calls it *ki*. All traditional healing systems recognize this life force as an invisible intelligence that "knows" how to direct and regulate all the body's autonomic functions, such as respiration, circulation, digestion, elimination, infection-fighting processes, and so forth. The traditional systems attribute any breakdown in health directly to an imbalance in the life force, a condition that existed for some time before disease manifested.

Thus, the approach of the traditional healer in treating illness is very different from that of most twentieth-century physicians. The principal task is to identify imbalances or blocks in the life force and correct them by applying the appropriate remedy rather than to treat specific symptoms or organic disturbances. When blocks and imbalances in the life force are eliminated, the traditional healer believes that the renewed life force itself will restore the body to health and resolve any symptoms of illness. The traditional healer also recognizes that any impairment in the life force affects not only the body, but the mind, emotions, and spirit as well, so it is essential when determining how to treat a client to get to know that person as an individual. This approach also contrasts with modern medicine, which generally has a "one-size-fits-all" treatment for a specific illness regardless of the individual being treated.

Like the traditional healers of old, I see my clients as unique individuals, each possessing a vital life force, a soul, that yearns to be directed, guided, and enhanced. My approach to each is to offer herbs, nutritional supplements, lifestyle guidelines, prayer, and love specifically for that individual.

THE ROLE OF HERBS

I believe that herbal medicine, which has its roots in the ancient healing traditions, including TCM and Ayurveda, has much more to offer the sick than the trendy new medical techniques and practices being heralded in the media today. As an art and a science, it has remained a reliable healing modality for thousands of years because it supports the life force in a unique manner that is still, in some ways, a mystery. Herbs are effective because plants, like all living organisms, are imbued with the same vital, intelligent life force that animates the human body. When the right herb is selected as a remedy by an experienced practitioner, its vital life force works synergistically with that of the patient, thus bringing about deep healing at all levels. Technology allows us to research plant life in ways never before imagined. Nevertheless, we may never fully understand in a fully scientific way how it is that herbs heal any more than we understand exactly how the human body "knows" how to carry out its autonomic functions.

The spirit of herbalism is the foundation of my work. The mystery of the plant world has revealed a face of God that will forever touch me. As each day passes, I am drawn deeper into the world of aromatic oils, roots, leaves, barks, and flowers that so humbly exists for our food and medicine.

Two American systems of herbal medicine that evolved during the latter half of the nineteenth century have influenced me greatly. They are Eclecticism and Physiomedicalism, which, like all forms of traditional medicine, sought to promote healing and restore health by strengthening the body's vital force. In his book, *The Philosophy of Natural Therapeutics*, published in 1919, Henry Lindlahr described the principles underlying these systems particularly well— principles that I, too, apply in my practice. For example, he wrote that every living cell is endowed with an instinct for self-preservation that is sustained by the vital life force, and that any illness is activated by that force to cleanse the body when it is affected by harmful influences such as bacteria, viruses, stress, or air pollution. The healer, therefore, according to Lindlahr, should not eliminate such symptoms as diarrhea, fever, or sneezing, but rather assist the body's inborn quest for wholeness.

NATURAL APPROACHES TO HEALING CANCER

Another individual who has influenced my philosophy of healing is Eli Jones, an American Eclectic Physiomedical physician who practiced from the late nineteenth century into the twentieth century. In my opinion, the doctor most successful in treating cancer, Jones maintained that even cancer is only a local manifestation of a constitutional (or blood) disease affecting the whole organism. Therefore, the patient's general health must be restored before the cancer can begin to improve.

Jones took a holistic approach to healing cancer. "Worriment of the mind," he felt, was one of the leading causes of cancer and topped his list of impediments to healing. He believed good blood, which he equated with a strong constitution, could only be produced by good digestion (essential for the proper assimilation of nutrients and the elimination of toxins), pure food, pure water, and pure air. Jones used herbs, homeopathic remedies, hydrotherapy, and nutrition to improve his patients' digestion and their overall vitality while they were under treatment. No matter how sick his cancer patients were, he insisted that they go outside every day for air and exercise.

Jones was firmly against surgery, claiming that the knife irritates cancer and makes it grow faster; that surgery shocks the system and weakens vitality; and that surgery only removes a local problem and does not address the constitutional disorder. Jones had similar reservations about radiation treatments and recognized the hazards of giving poisonous remedies or highly toxic doses of medicine because he saw how these treatments weakened patients, preventing them from developing the robust health so necessary for fighting their cancer.

WHAT TRADITIONAL APPROACHES OFFER TODAY'S PHYSICIANS

"Seek to understand rather than to be understood" is part of a famous Franciscan prayer, sometimes called The Peace Prayer. Though time is in short supply today for just about any doctor, the only way to fully understand a patient's condition is to listen without checking a clock and without anticipation of results. This is also a highly effective way to learn about giving, loving, and, in the process, becoming a better healer.

Most physicians practicing medicine today make full use of the steadily increasing body of scientific medical knowledge, sophisticated diagnostic procedures, and pharmacology, but many, in their fascination with the latest scientific advances, including diagnostic hardware, blood testing, and the wide array of cytotoxic cancer treatments currently available, have forgotten that some of the most valuable healing experiences—for both patient and healer—come from the human interaction that takes place between the two.

Most doctors today are running busy practices—actually small businesses that have all the concerns of any modern business. Modern medicine as a business is first and foremost profit-oriented. This does not bode well for patients who hope for some quality private time with their doctors.

Some of today's physicians treat their patients like spiritless robots and rarely acknowledge that diet, lifestyle, and attitude can affect one's health. With their focus almost exclusively on symptoms, they don't see their patients as individuals and fail to take into account the subtle interplay of body, mind, emotions, and spirit unique to each individual. To make matters worse, many patients see a number of different doctors. Take the cancer patient, for example, who may see a general practitioner, a gynecologist or urologist, a surgeon, an oncologist, a radiologist, a psychiatrist, and so forth. Though these doctors may be tops in their fields, they don't always communicate with each other about their patients or consider anything about those patients beyond their presenting symptoms.

What's more, the treatments they inflict on their patients can be needlessly harsh, often doing more harm than good. For example:

- Most of today's oncologists believe that medicine is of no value unless it is a deadly poison strong enough to "kill" cancer cells. Unfortunately, such toxic medicines bring with them side effects that poison healthy cells too and often lead to new cancers or other diseases.

- Too many invasive medical procedures are being done in the name of medical science. Some of them are not needed, and some may actually cause cancer to spread. These include lymph node removal following breast surgery, "look-and-see" surgery (sometimes after ovarian cancer surgery and/or following chemotherapy to see if there is any remaining cancer), and removal of cancerous primary organs, such as the spleen when treating lymphomas or leukemias, for example.

Admittedly, despite these criticisms, great strides have been made in conventional medicine, and I believe there are many good doctors who want their patients to get well no matter what kind of treatment is ultimately responsible for their healing. What is unfortunate, however, is the number of conventional doctors who have no interest at all in the historic wisdom found in traditional herbal medicine and other natural healing modalities that have proven curative.

To truly create healing, conventional medicine must also consider the whole person when making a diagnosis, developing a treatment plan, and following the patient throughout the course of treatment. Cancer patients, in particular, will be the beneficiaries. There is much to gain by combining past wisdom with current technology, and I believe that the health care profession must begin to move in this direction. Many doctors have already done so.

For instance, the late Dr. Hans Nieper, an orthomolecular physician in Hanover, Germany, worked with cancer patients for over forty years, using both conventional and traditional therapies for his patients. Depending on the patient, Nieper's protocol included drugs as well as vitamins, minerals, plant and animal extracts, diet, and lifestyle changes.

Dr. Nieper's approach looks beyond outward signs of illness to correct imbalances in his patients' vital life force. I believe that since such imbalances are always the underlying cause of illness, correcting them should always be the first order of business for health care practitioners. When the life force is in balance, it can do its work in sustaining the body's inherent instinct for self-preservation. Healing comes from within. A true healer will merely assist as an individual moves toward a state of balance and optimum health.

HOW I WORK

When someone comes to see me for the first time, I treat that person as a unique individual. I take the client's case by listening closely and jotting down some notes as I learn about any physical, emotional, mental, and spiritual problems. Here and there, I might prod with gentle questioning if I feel that important information is missing. I might order specific blood work, for example, to check the thyroid function or DHEA level in a woman with breast cancer, or to check for high platelet or fibrinogen levels that are cause for concern because they may indicate blood clots and tumor invasion. I review all medical reports from the client's conventional physicians.

Diet is an area that requires special consideration. A high-energy type-A person has different dietary needs than a calm, laid-back type-B individual. A highly trained athlete has different needs than a person with a sedentary lifestyle. A person living in a cold climate has different needs than a person in a tropical climate. There are as many variables as there are individuals. Some patients do better with more cooked food than raw; some need a moderate intake of dairy and meat, while others require a strict vegetarian diet for optimum well-being. Dietary needs change when individuals are undergoing chemotherapy and radiation therapy and then change again when these therapies are completed. For me, it is also important that people are happy with their diets. What good is a healthy diet if it becomes a source of conflict to the individual? Enjoying food and the process of nourishing oneself should be a very natural and fulfilling part of daily life. Unfortunately, for too many people, choosing healthy foods has become just another depressing chore fraught with anxiety and guilt. This is the challenge I face that makes what I do both difficult and fulfilling and why, in general, I give guidelines with some flexibility.

To successfully support and facilitate the healing of a person with cancer, I adapt my herbal and nutritional protocol to the following:

- Type of cancer
- Types of conventional treatment being received, if any
- Individual typology (temperament, organ problems, hereditary weaknesses, symptoms)
- Metabolic typing (based on a patient's endocrine system and whether the individual is a fast or slow oxidizer)

I look at the nervous, circulatory, and digestive systems and consider whether glands are under- or overactive. In particular, I have noticed that many people with cancer have underactive thyroid and/or adrenal glands.

In my work, it is important to use all available information, be intuitive, and avoid tunnel vision, i.e., using only one system to assess the client. My intention is to use information from any source that can help me to create the very best protocol for each individual.

Besides an appropriate medical approach, patients seek a hopeful prognosis and humane, caring treatment, and emotional support from their caregivers. Support groups with fellow patients also offer exceptional opportunities for nurturing and comfort. This is an area in mainstream medicine that needs improvement.

Many people with cancer feel they are treated disrespectfully by conventional (and sometimes nonconventional) doctors. People have described practitioners as arrogant, aloof, even cold, and have come away feeling discouraged and alone. To be rushed out of office appointments armed with the same drug and diagnostic test prescriptions that are uniformly presented to all cancer patients is demeaning. Patients need to be treated with respect, listened to, given adequate time to talk of fears and worries, and to feel confident about what treatments they will be receiving.

Each person with cancer views the situation in a different way. Some see it as a gift because it causes them to stop and evaluate what's really important in their lives; others are angry or feel helpless; still others feel cursed and wonder what they've done wrong. It's important to allow these feelings to surface and to discuss them. I can feel the benefit as I sit with people, particularly at initial consultations, and we take the time to talk about many things other than cancer. I dive into my clients' lives—into their hearts and souls, not just their pressing physical problems. I am not afraid to be involved, to love freely, to be helpful at each of the many levels at which healing takes place. We may never scientifically prove that happy people are much better able to overcome illness, but I see loneliness and sadness as epidemic illnesses in our society. Therefore, for me, friendship and love are essential to the healing process. Over time, my patients and I get to know each other. This is important for me in order to create an individual's protocol. Our time together also allows the client to feel more like a whole person and less like a disease.

To be successful in treating cancer patients, practitioners must have confidence in themselves and in their treatments. I read and study everything I can find on the subject of cancer, herbs, and nutrition, and I know that treating people with cancer is a lifetime commitment involving my heart, mind, and soul. Practitioners also need to be honest in evaluating the pros and cons of cytotoxic therapies. I see many toxic, sometimes barbaric, treatments that only add to the burden of suffering that a client is already enduring. While it is clear to me that in cases of fast-growing tumors, particularly childhood cancers, acute leukemias, Hodgkin's lymphoma, and testicular cancers, these treatments are highly effective and curative in many cases, we need to be more attuned to each individual situation and recommend treatments accordingly.

Each person is an individual and each healing program is unique to the patient's own situation. There is no single herb or vitamin combination that cures cancer. Each type of cancer and each individual requires a somewhat different protocol.

CLINICAL ASSESSMENT AND PHYSIOLOGICAL TYPOLOGY

These evaluations consider the various factors listed below:

- *The nervous system:* How is it affected by stress?
- *Personality:* How does it affect an individual's overall health status?
- *Heredity:* What patterns apply, if any?
- *Organs:* What organ system weaknesses have manifested?
- *Tongue diagnosis:* Provides information about the digestive function.
- *Pulse diagnosis:* This reflects the vital state, including the strength or weakness of the individual. The pulse of the cancer patient is often weak, yet quicker than normal.
- *Temperature:* It is important to note temperatures that are below the normal range of 97.8 to 98.6 degrees Fahrenheit.
- *Eye diagnosis:* This reflects the health of the blood and vital organs. All traditional systems of medicine use this assessment for evaluation.
- *Urine evaluation:* This is helpful in determining the constitutional health status of an individual.

When evaluating an individual, it is also essential to be able to differentiate between conditions that impede function and those that reflect the positive, eliminative, or reconstructive action by the vital force. The secret of good herbal and nutritional therapies is to recognize and draw upon the vital resources inherent in the unique constitution of each individual. Thus, a typological assessment is essential before deciding upon specific treatments.

Blood Chemistry

I also pay close attention to two important markers found in the blood chemistry: albumin and platelet levels. What I look for is an albumin level as high in the normal range as possible (4.5 to 5) and a platelet level in the low normal range (150 to 200).

Albumin is the most abundant protein found in the bloodstream, and optimal levels are vital to many of our body's important functions. Some of these vital functions include liver and kidney function; antioxidant functions within the blood and connective tissue; scavenging the stress hormone cortisol in the blood; removal of waste products from connective tissue; transportation of many vital nutrients throughout the body, including vitamins, minerals, and fatty acids; detoxification of heavy metals and chemicals, and protection of cellular oxidation of such metals.

Albumin is also vital to the function of aldosterone, which regulates fluid balance within the cells and the entire body. High levels of albumin prevent mutation, and low levels are an early predictor of morbidity and mortality. One of the many attributes of the nutritional supplement chlorella is its ability to increase the albumin level.

Platelet levels are also vitally important to the health of the person with cancer because cancer, by its very nature, forms tumors in order to grow. In order to have metastases, the platelets must aggregate and clump together. This means that if an individual's platelet count starts rising above the normal range, it is likely that the cancer is spreading. It also means, however, that by inhibiting platelet aggregation with enzymes like bromelain and herbs like turmeric, one can effectively inhibit one of the strategies that cancer uses to spread. Excessive platelet aggregation is also a cause of atherosclerosis.

Cholesterol is another important factor. I look at cholesterol levels because low cholesterol can indicate a suppressed immune system. The endocrine system utilizes cholesterol to make hormones, which are important to our vitality. Of course, cholesterol that is too high is a risk factor for heart disease.

Uric acid is still another consideration. Too low a level of uric acid can indicate overactive states, particularly in the lungs and liver. Too high a level indicates poor binding functions and may require folic acid, bromelain, quercetin, and other supplements to correct the condition.

EACH FORM OF CANCER IS UNIQUE

Just as each person is unique and must be treated in that way, so too is an individual's cancer. Two people who have the same type of cancer are likely to receive the same type of conventional treatment (particularly if they are in the same hospital), but the results of their treatment may be quite different. Why does one person's cancer spread to the bone, another's to the liver, and another's not spread at all?

Two people on the same chemotherapy protocol can react very differently and therefore need to be treated differently. For example, a common side effect of the chemotherapeutic drug Velban is neuropathy, which can be helped by taking lipoic acid, fat-soluble vitamin B_1, and a grape seed extract referred to as PCO. A common side effect of 5FU is mouth sores. This distressing and very uncomfortable symptom can be alleviated with simple herbs and an acidophilus mouth rinse. Not every patient taking the same drug will have the same reaction, but by treating each person individually, we can offer relief from side effects and greatly enhance the healing process that is so powerful and unique to each of us.

In my work, I strive to help people maintain their vital flow of energy; to keep their bodies healthy and well-nourished through the use of organic food, herbs, and nutritional supplements; to see a deeper meaning in life; to respect nature and honor the gifts it so humbly gives us; to understand the importance of spirituality and love, and to find peace within themselves. Healing encompasses all these factors to restore harmony and balance—a true state of total well-being.

2

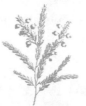

Cancer Defined

We do not see nature with our own eyes but with our
understanding and our hearts.

—William Hazlitt

Statistics about the war on cancer abound, but statistics can be very misleading. The truth is, cancer now strikes one in three and kills one in
four, up from an incidence of one in four and a mortality rate of one in
five in the 1950s. According to Dr. Samuel S. Epstein, a professor of
Occupational and Environmental Medicine at the University of Illinois
Medical Center and a frequent critic of the National Cancer Institute and
American Cancer Society, the key problem in the leadership of the cancer
establishment is a professional mindset fixated on diagnosis, treatment, and
research with relative indifference to cancer causes and prevention. While
focusing largely on smoking and dietary fat restrictions, organizations have
consistently discounted the role of avoidable exposure to industrial carcinogens
in air, food, water, and the workplace.[1] Studies of cancer mortality statistics

13

over the past twenty-five years have also shown that despite substantial advances in molecular oncology, progress has yet to impinge on mortality statistics. The focus upon cure of advanced disease rather than prevention of early disease is a major failure of the cancer establishment.[2]

Since there are now about eight million Americans living with cancer (breast, prostate, and colorectal cancers account for about half of these cases),[3] it is essential for those who take responsibility for their own health to understand the cancer process and how to stop it in its tracks. To the layperson, the material that follows may seem complicated and difficult to understand; however, this information is vital to understanding how the body functions.

WHAT IS CANCER?

On a physical level, cancer is a wild, uncontrolled growth of abnormal cells that can arise in any organ or tissue of the body. Whereas normal cells grow in an orderly, controlled pattern, abnormal cells reproduce themselves endlessly, causing a pileup of cells (a tumor). A benign (noncancerous) tumor has cells that closely resemble normal ones; its growth pattern is generally orderly and self-contained; it does not invade and destroy normal tissue; it does not metastasize (migrate via the lymph system or the bloodstream to attach itself to distant organs or lymph glands); it usually can be removed completely by surgery and is less likely to recur; and it normally does not endanger life unless it's growing in a tight space, such as the brain.

Normally, when old or sick cells die, the body produces just enough new ones to replace them. *Apoptosis*, or cell death, is a process by which sick cells are recognized and "allowed" to die off. Cancer cells are either not sick enough to die, or manage to protect themselves from the normal pattern of cell death. This gene malfunction allows an accumulation of cells to proliferate. When the collected defects finally free the cell from the body's normal restraints on cell growth, the cancer process begins. Tumors develop and often spread by invading other tissues in the body. This is called *metastasis*.

Knowledge of the early molecular events that must occur in order to create cancer has improved rapidly over the past two decades, particularly with the identification of two families of genes that are critical to cancer development—namely, *oncogenes* and *tumor-suppressor genes*. The development of cancer cells is dependent on the influences of these genes and on other regulators, such as hormones, growth factors, and cytokines.

Malignant (cancerous) cells look very different from normal cells. They are quite irregular in shape, have large, irregular nuclei, and are primitive in appearance because they generally fail to differentiate. These abnormal cells grow in an uncontrolled pattern; they never stop reproducing themselves; they grow at a faster rate than the normal tissue of origin; they do not properly perform the functions of the tissue of origin (or they don't perform the functions at all); and they often metastasize, invade, and destroy areas distant from the primary (original) site. They grow into tumors that interfere with the body's functioning by crowding organs and by invading and destroying surrounding healthy tissue and stripping the body of nutrients; and they can cause the body's muscle and fat to break down, thereby leading to *cachexia* (severe weight loss that can eventually kill the patient). Cancer cells also inhibit immune system functioning, causing some patients to contract deadly diseases, such as pneumonia.

A normal, or apparently normal, cell evolves slowly into a cancer cell by means of a sequential accumulation of alterations in the genetic material (DNA) that comprises *proto-oncogenes* and tumor-suppressor genes. Because it takes time for these alterations or mutations to occur, most cancers occur in older people. The accumulated damage to the gene is caused by *adducts*, chemicals that attach to the gene and disturb its function. When cancer occurs in infants and young children, it is usually because their apparently normal cells have one copy of a defective (or missing) oncogene, or, more often, a tumor-suppressor gene that was inherited from one of their parents.

Cancer, when left untreated or ineffectively treated, will prove fatal, sometimes within one to two years of diagnosis in the case of more aggressive forms of the disease. The majority of malignancies are fatal within five years. Even with aggressive conventional treatments, survival rates are sometimes limited because of recurrence of the tumor line, sometimes within five years of apparently successful therapy.

It is difficult for most people to choose a completely holistic approach to cancer treatment, even though this might be the best choice in some cases. For instance, certain cancers, such as early-stage breast cancer, prostate cancer, cervical cancer, and low-grade lymphomas, respond very well to herbal treatments, yet seem to be aggravated and sometimes worsened by surgical procedures or other conventional treatments. In other cases, a combination of both conventional and holistic therapies might prove to be the best approach. The more experience I have with cancer, the more I am able to recognize which approach will be best for a particular patient.

TYPES OF CANCER

Although there are more than a hundred varieties of cancer, when these varieties are classified according to the type of cell in which they arise, they fall into three general categories.

1. *Carcinomas*, the most common types of cancer, are tumors that arise in the epithelial tissues—the sheets of cells that cover all free surfaces of the body, such as the skin; the lining of glandular ducts (i.e., breast and prostate); and the lining of hollow organs such as the stomach and intestines. Some examples of carcinomas are:

- *Adenocarcinoma*, which originates in the epithelial tissues of glands, ducts, and mucous membranes in the breast, lungs, and colon.
- *Mucoid carcinoma*, consisting of cells that secrete mucin, found frequently in the stomach, colon, and rectum.
- *Squamous carcinoma*, arising from the thickened epithelium of the skin or the lining of the esophagus, tongue, and cervix.

2. *Sarcomas*, which are relatively rare, arise in supportive or connective tissue, such as cartilage, muscle, bone, fibrous connective tissue, and blood vessels. Sarcomas are very often malignant, increasing rapidly in size and invading neighboring tissues and the bloodstream. One example of a sarcoma is a *fibrosarcoma*, which is derived from the fibrous sheath of a large muscle; another is a *chrondrosarcoma*, which is derived from cartilage. Both carcinomas and sarcomas are solid tumors.

3. *Leukemias* and *lymphomas* arise from cells of the immune system such as leukocytes (white blood cells) and lymphocytes. They are usually composed of dispersed cells, although the lymphoma cells can occasionally form solid tumors. Leukemias are cancers of blood-forming cells that occur in bone marrow and other blood-forming organs. Lymphomas are malignant tumors that arise in the lymph system.

Other common forms of cancer include:

• *Melanoma*, a cancer of the cells that produce skin pigment. Melanoma is usually found on the skin, frequently in the form of a black mole, especially on the lower limbs, neck, or head. It is one of the most virulent forms of cancer for it can often spread rapidly through the bloodstream and lymphatic vessels to form metastases in many parts of the body.

• *Multiple myeloma, brain, and nerve tissue cancers.* These cancers affect either the spinal cord or the brain. Some common forms of these cancers include *astrocytoma, medullablastoma,* and *glioblastoma.*

• *Germ cell tumors* are cancers that affect those particular cells capable of developing into new cells of the same species, for example, ovum or spermatazoan cells. Examples of these cancers are *seminoma, embryonal carcinoma, testicular carcinoma,* and *yolk sac tumors.*

• *Childhood cancers,* such as leukemia, neuroblastoma, Wilms' tumor, some brain cancers, and retinoblastoma, are more frequently the result of genetic defects than are other cancers.

WHAT CAUSES CANCER?

The cell cycle is regulated by a series of signaling events that consist of positive and negative regulators. Their job is to control the process of cell reproduction, maintaining a balance between positive and negative regulators.

Two families of genes that play a role in the cell's signaling processes are oncogenes and tumor-suppressor genes. These genes are usually involved in the initiation of cancer. Damaged or misplaced genes, called *proto-oncogenes,* are simply genes with oncogenic potential.

Normal genes can be altered in a variety of ways, causing them to turn into oncogenes. To date, approximately seventy genes have been shown to be involved in carcinogenesis, some naturally occurring and others induced by a variety of endogenous causes.[4] All cancers are genetically determined to a certain extent, but it is the proto-oncogenes that are targets of a wide range of environmental assaults caused by such factors as chemicals and radiation. It usually takes more than genetic alterations to trigger a cell into cancer growth.

Normal cells become cancer cells by an alteration or mutation within the genetic material (DNA) of the cell. Genetic errors brought about by damage

---

CANCER GLOSSARY

Adjuvant therapy. Drugs or hormones given after surgery, chemotherapy, and/or radiation to help prevent recurrence or metastasis.

Angiogenesis. The formation and differentiation of blood vessels.

Apoptosis. Programmed cell death.

Differentiation. Occurs when cells mature and take on the specific forms and functions of the normal tissue from which they came.

Localized disease. Cancer confined to the area surrounding the original tumor.

Local therapy. Treatment aimed at eradicating the tumor and any cancer cells in the surrounding area.

Lymph nodes. Bean-shaped organs located along the lymphatic system which remove waste materials from the body. Cancer cells travel throughout the body through the lymphatic system. Lymph node dissection (removing and examining lymph nodes near the tumor) can help determine the extent of disease; thus this procedure is sometimes used to classify tumors by stage. However, since the lymphatic system is crucial in the ability to fight disease, we must find a better way to determine disease progression than by removing lymph nodes.

Metastasis. The spread of cancer from the original site to another part of the body. Regional metastasis indicates that cancer has spread to a nearby area, typically to the lymph nodes. With distant metastasis, the cancer has traveled farther away, typically to the liver, bones, lungs, or brain.

Mitosis. The proliferation of a cell. In cancer, mitosis occurs at an accelerated level.

Node-negative. The term indicating no cancer cells have been found in the lymph nodes.

Node-positive. The term indicating cancer cells have been found in the lymph nodes. This information is used to determine what course of therapy to follow.

Oncologist. A cancer specialist who determines what type of adjuvant therapy will be used to treat a cancer patient.

Palliative care. Therapy aimed at relieving symptoms, usually pain, rather than eradicating disease or prolonging life.

Recurrence. The reappearance of a cancer at the same site or the emergence of the same type of cancer at another site.

Remission. Shrinkage or disappearance of the tumor. Partial remission indicates that the tumor has shrunk, usually by 50 percent, but is still detectable. Complete remission indicates that the cancer has disappeared.

Stage. Tumors are classified according to the extent of disease. Tumor description, tumor size, lymph node involvement, and the presence of metastasis are all used to determine the disease stage. Stage I indicates the earliest cancers, typically small tumors confined to the original site. Stages II, III, and IV indicate more extensive disease. Letters may be used along with the numerals (Stage IIb, for example) to subclassify cancers based on specific tumor characteristics.

Survival. The length of time a person lives after treatment. Treatment success is often measured according to the percentage of people who survive five years. I do not agree with this measurement. With many cancers, including colon and breast, the conventional wisdom is that five-year survival indicates a cure, and that the cancer recurs within five years, it is not going to come back, but the truth is, cancer can come back at any time—sometimes up to fifteen or twenty years after an initial occurrence.

Tumor response. The term indicates the tumor has shrunk to some degree in response to therapy. Tumor response does not necessarily correlate with improved survival or better quality of life. As a matter of fact, many times it actually reduces the quality of life and shortens it. This is important to consider, particularly in late-stage cancers.

from outside the cell are referred to as growth-promoting proto-oncogenes, while tumor-suppressor genes function as growth-regulating genes. The activation of proto-oncogenes and/or inactivation of tumor-suppressor genes appear to cause a cell to become malignant.

Oncogenes

Oncogenes function as cellular messengers and come in a variety of forms. Some of them have been identified and are part of a large family referred to as *ras* oncogenes. These messengers attach to a cell's surface, initiating events through a series of receptors and intermediate compounds that control cellular function both within and outside of the cell. If a ras gene is mutated, it leads to an overexpression of a molecule called MAP (mitogen-activated kinase), which then causes uncontrolled cell growth. MAP is expressed five to twenty times more in cancers with the mutated ras gene. This mutated gene is found in 95 percent of all pancreatic cancers, one of the most difficult cancers to treat.

Proto-oncogenes

Proto-oncogenes are believed to be involved in normal growth and development. In general, they encode proteins, which are components of signaling pathways that regulate cell growth. These signaling pathways bind to specific membrane receptors and trigger a cascade of intracellular signals, and transcription of genes linked to proliferation follows.

There are three ways in which proto-oncogenes are transformed:

1. *Amplification* signifies the presence of multiple copies of the gene, which results in overproduction of the genetic product. It is interesting to note here that vitamin D's inhibiting effect on cancer is believed to be its ability to reduce such overamplification.

2. *Point mutations* occur as a result of a spontaneous or chemical carcinogenic reaction. They can then produce abnormal protein products leading to genetic damage.

3. *Translocation* occurs when a proto-oncogene moves from its usual location on a particular chromosome (where it may be benign) to a different chromosome where it can be activated by neighboring genes (which can act as promoters or enhancers of transformation) into a cancer cell.

Sometimes a compound is not carcinogenic on its own; when combined with other compounds, however, it will accelerate or stimulate a cancer-producing reaction. These compounds are referred to as *cocarcinogens*, substances that become cancerous only when combined with other substances. It is important to understand that many of the chemicals and hormones we ingest may cause little or no harm by themselves, but when combined with other chemicals they may react and initiate or promote cancer. For example, the action between hormone metabolites and DDT produces DDE, a very toxic by-product.

Estrogen is another chemical that can become quite toxic when combined with other chemicals present in the body. Most of these transforming activities take place in the liver.

Proto-oncogenes may be classified into four groups:

1. *Growth factors.* These factors occur outside the cell and encode homologous proteins. Although they appear normal, they are not. They stimulate cell signaling, such as platelet-derived growth factors.

2. *Growth-factor receptors.* These act as cell receptors receiving oncogenic information. Many growth-factor receptors contain protein tyrosine kinase activity, for example, erbB-2 protein, a newly identified proto-oncogene found in some forms of aggressive breast cancer.

3. *Signal transducers.* These are components of the intracellular signaling pathways. Signals are transmitted from cell-membrane receptors to the nucleus by second messengers. Cascades of protein kinases are involved in mediating these signals by way of proto-oncogenes. At this time, the most widely known and best understood is the ras gene. Cyclin-dependent kinases (CDKs) are a group of kinases involved in many cancers.

For example, CDK-1 plays an important role in the cell division of 40 percent of all cancers and an astounding 90 percent of all breast cancers. The expression of this protein facilitates the proliferation of vascular endothelial cells, which form the basis for creating blood vessels that feed new tumors, part of the process known as *angiogenesis*. CDK-4, another newly identified CDK, is involved with disturbing the control of one of the cell's phases of division. Suppression of CDK-1 and other CDKs is the target of many new cancer drug therapies. Currently, CDK-1 is also being used as a marker for assessing the aggressive nature of a cancer and as a risk factor for metastatic cancer growth.

4. *Nuclear transcription factors.* By binding to DNA in a sequence-specific manner, nuclear transcription factors activate gene expression within the nucleus of the cell. *Myc*, *fos*, and *jun* are three of the most well-known nuclear transcription factors.

Tumor-Suppressor Genes

Another class of cancer genes are the previously mentioned tumor-suppressor genes. Mutations that knock out tumor-suppressor genes are more threatening than the activation of oncogenes, previously thought to be the most important genetic cause of cancer. Mutations in tumor-suppressor genes should be viewed as markers for tumor susceptibility.

The most common genetic mutation that occurs in human cancers is in the tumor-suppressor gene p53. About 70 percent of all colon cancers, 30 to 50 percent of breast and ovarian cancers, 50 percent of all lung cancers, all small-cell lung cancers, and most prostate cancers are a result of a defect in the p53 gene. It is worth noting here that one of the many cancer-inhibiting effects of quercetin, a flavone found in onions and broccoli, is to prevent a defect in this gene.

An individual may inherit one defective copy of the tumor-suppressor protein gene p53 from a parent, giving that person a predisposition to develop cancer. Since p53 is a repair gene, when it malfunctions damaged DNA is able to escape, proliferate unchecked, and mutate into cancerous cells. As that person ages, she may then be more susceptible to external factors that can cause irregular cell proliferation. However, it sometimes takes an accumulation of ten or more mutations in critical genes before a cell becomes cancerous. Scientists have recently found that there is another gene, p34, that may be responsible for p53's ability to halt cell division. Approximately 90 percent of all breast cancers display abnormal p34 genes.

Another tumor-suppressor gene, the *Rb gene*, is implicated in a number of childhood cancers, such as Wilms' tumors and neuroblastoma.

Tumor-suppressor genes are regulators that control the expression of other genes. For example, normal cells contain dominant suppressor genes that down-regulate cancer genes. These dominant genes are lost, however, during any cell mutations. When this line of defense is lost, it is possible for tumor genes to be reexpressed rather than down-regulated—a situation that brings disastrous results.

Mutation

One well-known cause of cancer is a buildup of oxidative damage and mutations whereby the gene itself is altered and can then initiate the process of malignancy. The human body is composed of sixty-three trillion cells, plus or minus one hundred billion at any given time. Each day a cell undergoes around five thousand mutations, each of which could be capable of causing the initiation of cancer. Usually, mutations do not occur in both strands of the DNA helix and are therefore repairable.

A number of factors contribute to the ability of our cells to repair these mutations. Some of the ways the body is able to protect against the initiation of cancer are by:

- Inhibition of a mutation (by reducing the overall number of mutational changes).
- Repair of a mutation, once it has occurred.
- Inhibition of a mutation by "turning off" a damaged cell so that it cannot proliferate and do further harm.

The ability to inhibit an overproduction of mutational changes depends on dietary and lifestyle exposures to exogenous factors that can both cause and inhibit mutation. Many nutrients are protective against mutation initiation, promotion, and progression.[5] Chapters 3 and 4, in particular, will cite many epidemiological and biochemical studies supporting this fact. As substantiated throughout this book, food and herbs are truly the best medicine we have.

Indeed, some of the most significant benefits of all herbs and pure foods are their *antimutagenic* properties. Some of the most powerful antimutagenic foods are burdock, garlic, ginger, turmeric, and citrus peel. Studies have shown that in order to promote cancer growth, oncogenes, mutated suppressor genes (like p53), and carcinogens must all be present. Normally, oxidative stress and mutations within our cells are repaired by various enzymes found in herbs and whole foods. However, if mutations build up and our enzymes can't keep up with the task of repairing the damage, serious illnesses (like cancer) can result. The good news is that our dietary choices can and do effectively modulate genetic susceptibility to cancer.

Oncoviruses

One cause of mutational change, *insertional mutagenesis*, occurs when cells are infected by viral genes. This brings the cellular oncogenes under the influence of viral promoters or regulators that cause mutations by adding new DNA rather than altering existing DNA.

Some animal studies have indicated that viruses may be involved in carcinogenesis. Certain leukemialike diseases in chickens, cats, and inbred strains of mice can be induced in young animals by innoculating them with viruses isolated from leukemic animals. There is already some evidence linking the Epstein-Barr virus, perhaps one of the most common of all viruses, to two types of cancer, a carcinoma and a lymphoma. Another DNA virus group, the herpes virus, has been shown to have oncogenic potential, causing many types of cancers. The papilloma virus is the cause of cervical carcinoma. Among the RNA viruses and retroviruses, evidence is accumulating that links these viruses to breast cancer as well as leukemias, lipomas, fibrosarcomas, and osteosarcomas.

Two cancer theories propose the involvement of oncoviruses. One infers that exogenous viral infection occurs and that reverse transcriptase (reversing the genetic pathway code between RNA and DNA) is required to integrate the viral genome into the host genome. The other considers that oncogenes, some of which may represent proviruses, are inherited through endogenous genes that are acquired at birth and require only minimal mutation for expression.[6]

Factors That Can Induce and/or Promote Cancer

Cancer can be promoted by many factors, including toxic environment, devitalized processed and artificial food, high blood sugar, retroviruses, suppressed emotions, and stress. These conditions can also suppress the immune system, thereby inhibiting the action of immune cells responsible for attacking abnormally mutated cells. When a cell divides, the DNA of that cell is exposed to a reactive environment, and the possibility of genetic alterations is increased. Some of the more significant factors in the induction and promotion of cancer are:

Diet

A poor diet fails to provide proper nutrients for optimum cellular nourishment. It has been shown that up to 70 percent of all cancers are related to diets that are high in animal fat, low in fiber, and lacking in sufficient fruits and vegetables. Moreover, refined and processed foods have been stripped of the nutrients and enzymes that protect against cancer.

Environment

Toxic environmental chemicals such as pesticides and industrial by-products assault the body and overtax the immune system.

Heredity

Mutant genes can be passed from one generation to another. These genetic mishaps allow faulty messages to be transmitted, such as inactivation of tumor-suppressor genes at a time when they may be sorely needed to defend the body.

Proto-oncogene Activity

The threat of cancer rises when there is an increase in the number of genes that have oncogenic potential for mutation and overexpression. Viruses, particularly retroviruses that use reverse transcriptase, can cause genetic damage. Over a period of time, this cellular stress increases the potential for cancer development. What happens is that the retrovirus provides a pathway that is unavailable in a healthy cell. This path allows cancer cells to travel from a healthy cell's surface to its nucleus, where they transform the healthy cell into a cancerous one, and the cancer gains its foothold.

Free Radicals

Free radicals are by-products or waste material expelled by the cell, and they are normally not a threat to health and well-being. A problem arises, however, when too many free radicals overburden the body's means to eliminate them. This excess can circulate freely in the blood, damaging cells and eventually overtaxing the immune system. Free radicals can initiate irregular cellular behavior and DNA damage, causing some cancers to proliferate at a faster rate.

Radiation

Radiation creates cell damage in the form of hydroxal and hydrogen radicals. This may occur as the result of the sun's ultraviolet rays or the emission of radon gas by power lines, cell phones, or microwaves. Radiation therapy, when used for the treatment of cancer, can sometimes cause other cancers to form and/or cause cancer to spread more aggressively to other areas of the body.

CHEMICAL CAUSES OF CANCER

Chemical carcinogens can transform the cell through *somatic mutation* (nonreproductive cells or tissues) and alter existing DNA. Some of the most common of these carcinogens are:

• *Tobacco.* At the top of the list of substances that contain carcinogens, and perhaps the most publicized, is tobacco. Chemists have identified at least a dozen carcinogenic chemicals of the hydrocarbon type in the tars from tobacco. Tobacco smokers are at a greater risk than nonsmokers for cancers of the lung, throat, kidney, mouth, bladder, and pancreas. Scientists estimate that smoking accounts for about 30 percent of all cancers. Secondhand smoke is a major health hazard to nonsmokers as well.

• *Alcohol.* The association between excessive alcohol consumption and cancer of the mouth, larynx, throat, liver, breast, and esophagus has been well established.

• *Pharmaceutical estrogens.* Diethylstilbestrol (DES), a drug once given to pregnant women to prevent miscarriage, has been linked to cancer in their offspring. Estrogen replacement therapy prescribed for menopausal women increases the risk of uterine, breast, liver, and endometrial cancer.

Other carcinogens, perhaps not as well known but equally dangerous, are listed below:

• *Aflatoxins.* This carcinogen is a known cause of liver cancer. In some parts of Africa, where the level of aflatoxins in foods is high, cancer of the liver is quite common. Two foods at risk for aflatoxin contamination are corn and peanuts. However, there are reliable organic sources for these foods. The companies listed in Resources test for aflatoxins.

• *Alkylating agents.* This category includes such chemicals as mustard gas, which is associated with cancers of the lung and bone marrow. This is not a threat to most people, but in some areas of the world it is a concern.

• *Aromatic amines.* Aniline dye workers who are exposed to these chemicals have a higher than average risk of getting bladder cancer.

• *Arsenic.* This chemical element, used in metallurgy, can cause lung and skin cancer.

• *Asbestos.* An industrial chemical with over three thousand uses, asbestos is a danger to individuals in shipbuilding, mining, construction, and brakelining occupations. It may cause cancer of the lung and pleura.

• *Benzene.* Used in a variety of industrial processes and compounds, benzene can cause lymphoma and leukemia.

• *Chrome and nickel ores.* Mine workers who inhale these ores demonstrate increased risk of lung and nasal cancer.

• *Cycasin.* A product of the palm nut *Cycas circinalis* eaten by natives of the Pacific Islands, cycasin can cause kidney cancer.

• *Immunosuppressive drugs.* Immune-deficient individuals are more likely to develop cancer. Some of the drugs used to treat cancer, such as steroids, prednisone, interferon, and interleukin-2, as well as chemotherapy and radiation, can also *cause* cancer or other serious illnesses.

• *Polycyclic hydrocarbons.* Found in tobacco smoke, tar, soot, and fuel, these substances can cause cancers of the lung and skin.

• *Radiation.* Both natural and man-made radiation are known causes of a number of cancers including leukemia and cancer of the lung, breast, skin, and thyroid. Natural radiation is ultraviolet light and comes from the sun.[7]

More About Pharmaceutical Estrogens

Exogenous hormones are widely prescribed in the United States, primarily as oral contraceptives (OCs) during the menstrual cycle and hormone replacement therapy (HRT) after menstruation ceases. Each of these frequently used categories of drugs has a high potential to raise the risk of several common cancers, specifically breast and uterine cancers. The relationship of OCs and HRT to breast cancer risk is controversial, but several studies have shown a moderately increased risk after long-term use. Estrogen replacement therapy (ERT) is a major cause of endometrial cancer.

Numerous epidemiological studies have examined the relationship between oral contraceptives and the risk of breast cancer. Although there is still some controversy about this subject, most studies conclude that OC use at any age increases that risk.

The use of OCs also increases the risk of liver tumors. A case-controlled study of young women who died of cancer of the liver showed that the use of OCs was associated with a significantly elevated relative risk of hepatocellular carcinoma and that use for eight years or more was associated with significantly higher risk. Studies from Italy and the United States also provide evidence that OCs may cause liver cancer.[8]

The risks associated with the use of synthetic hormones should be carefully weighed by each woman. There are many herbs and nutrients that are extremely effective for relieving menopausal symptoms and protecting against heart disease and osteoporosis.

Depot-medroxyprogesterone acetate (DMPA), a progesterone, is a long-acting injectable contraceptive used in many areas of the world. One might assume that if estrogens alone can cause breast cancer, then DMPA should decrease breast cancer risk because the regimen prevents ovulation and does not include any exposure to exogenous estrogen. Unfortunately, this is not the case. In fact, the results of studies from Costa Rica and New Zealand suggest that progesterone may act like estrogen to stimulate breast cell growth.[9,10]

Based on the overall evidence from recent studies, long-term use of ERT may carry with it an increased risk of breast cancer. Whether or not adding a progesterone to ERT lowers breast cancer risk has not been well evaluated. In a Swedish study, women who received combined estrogen-progesterone treatment had a 4.4-fold greater risk of breast cancer with more than six years of use than women with no history of HRT use. The results of this study are compatible with results of the most recent studies of DMPA and breast cancer described above. Together these studies suggest that progesterone may enhance the carcinogenic effect of ERT on the breast. This phenomenon suggests that progesterone, in conjunction with the luteal-phase estradiol peak, could stimulate breast tissue mitotic activity and increase breast cancer risk.[11]

Case reports of endometrial cancer occurring in women after the use of estrogens have appeared in the medical literature for more than thirty years. Nearly all studies demonstrate a strong association between estrogen use and disease risk related to both dosage and duration of use.

More About Free Radicals and Cellular Damage

It is widely accepted among researchers that the switching on of cancerous growth is a multistage process. At any given time, most people probably carry one or more cells in some precancerous stage, and the process from stage to stage may be reversed or advanced by external factors. These external factors are carcinogens and anticarcinogens found in one's diet, environment, and personal habits.

Fortunately, foods, especially organically grown plant foods, contain many anticarcinogens. Most natural anticarcinogens act as scavengers of reactive oxidative waste in the body by blocking or reducing free radical damage and as enzyme inhibitors, selectively blocking cancer-cell metabolism.

Free radicals are unstable reactive molecules that contain unpaired electrons. The normal process of oxygen use promotes free radicals that cause molecular damage or *insults*. If the number of such insults exceeds what a human body can normally handle, free radicals can harm the cells. By altering genetic material, free radicals can disrupt a cell's cancer-prevention apparatus and impair its ability to do other chemical work.

The way free radicals do harm to the cells is simple. The cell is made up of many molecules that bond together, creating the cell structure. Free radicals cause chemical bonds to form between molecules that are usually independent. This process is called *cross-linking*. By not allowing the molecules in the cell to move independently, the flexibility of the cell is reduced. This process affects two areas of the cell: the inner nucleus, where the RNA/DNA is located, and the outer cell membrane.

The inner nucleus of the cell is the brain of the cell, the origin of the cell's orders. If there is damage to the RNA/DNA caused by free radical cross-linkage, it will be unable to give the cell correct information for performance and reproduction. A cell with abundant cross-linkage of its RNA/DNA will mutate, a condition that is apparent in any form of cancer.

The outer cell membrane consists of lipids (fatty acids) and protein. The lipid part of the cell membrane is very susceptible to free radical damage by a process referred to as *lipid peroxidation*. By turning the lipid portion of the cell membrane rancid, this process greatly reduces the membrane flexibility. This disrupts all of the metabolic traffic going in and out of the cell and impairs the cell's ability to get the nutrients it needs and remove its wastes. This is one reason why it is so harmful to ingest processed vegetable oil.

A variety of external factors can promote free radical formation in the human body:

- Pollutants
- Ultraviolet light
- Alcohol
- Margarine and other hydrogenated fats
- Cigarette smoke

- Radiation
- Hydrogen peroxide

If the genetic material is damaged by free radicals and isn't totally repaired, the damaged DNA is replicated in new cells. Fortunately, our cells have orderly systems for battling free radicals and repairing dangerous molecular by-products. These free radical fighters are sometimes referred to as *antioxidants*. I personally feel the term *antioxidant* (which means "against oxygen") is a misnomer. Some authorities say that the so-called antioxidant nutrients may even have negative effects in the body because they inhibit the mutation and removal of cancer and/or potential cancer cells. However, this can happen only if we try to manipulate nature by refining nutrients and by making them artificially. For instance, carrots and dark green leafy vegetables in their natural state are loaded with hundreds of different carotenoids and other phytonutrients that are protective against cell damage. Problems occur only when we try to outsmart nature. I call the specialized supplements that I recommend to my patients "cell-protective agents," not antioxidants.

Oxygen is obviously a requirement for human life, but it can also cause tissue damage, cellular damage, and even death, depending on its mixture and its reaction to other elements. The air we breathe is only 20 percent oxygen, most of the balance being nitrogen. If you were forced to breathe 100 percent oxygen for a prolonged period of time, it would cause enough lung damage to eventually kill you.

Why is oxygen dangerous? Because it is converted to hydrogen peroxide by tissues in the body. To back up a bit, let's look at the oxygen cycle that supplies the air we breathe. Plants take their energy source from the sun. As a by-product of this process, oxygen is released and becomes the air we breathe. After our cells have utilized oxygen, it is then converted into hydrogen peroxide, a free radical capable of causing extensive damage at the cellular level if it is not converted to water, the next step in this process. The trace mineral selenium is crucial at this juncture.

Understanding this process clearly illustrates the damage that free radicals can do; even more important, it demonstrates that cell-protective agents can be any agents that aid in the conversion of hydrogen peroxide to water, that inactivate free radicals, or that repair any damage caused by free radicals.

Some of the best cell-protective agents we have are certain phytonutrients found in the food and spices we eat, such as the carotenoids in carrots, saffron, squash, turnips, pink grapefruit, and all deep orange or dark green leafy vegetables. Turmeric, one of the most widely used spices in Asia, contains curcumin, another excellent cell-protective agent. The cells themselves also manufacture enzymes and compounds that offer excellent protection against free radical assaults.

The Importance of Glutathione

Glutathione is a primary molecule responsible for maintaining normal cellular metabolism, cell protection, and regulation. In its reduced form, glutathione is vitally involved in many cellular functions, such as antioxidation of reactive oxygen species and free radicals, detoxification of xenobiotics, and maintenance of the reduced biochemical state that characterizes healthy cells. In addition, it plays an essential role in DNA synthesis and repair, synthesis of protein, immune function, leukotriene and prostaglandin metabolism, and regulation of cellular proliferation.[12]

Glutathione is a sulfur-containing tripeptide composed of glutamic acid, cysteine, and glycine. In human cells, it is the most abundant nonprotein thiol. Glutathione exists in both a reduced state and an oxidized state (glutathione disulfide), but it is in the reduced state that just about all the vital functions of glutathione are carried out.

Studies have shown that without adequate levels of glutathione, many unwelcome conditions can occur, including premature aging, oxidative stress, exposure to toxins, and many chronic and degenerative disorders.

The dark brown spots that form on skin as we get older (sometimes referred to as liver spots) are believed to be related to low levels of glutathione, which can cause one to be prone to basal cell carcinoma, the most common and least dangerous form of skin cancer. The following supplements would protect those who are prone to this condition: Beta-Plex, lipoic acid, vitamins E and C, small amounts of zinc and selenium, grape seed extract, turmeric, and green tea.

In addition, a number of pathologic conditions, including peripheral neuropathies, cerebrospinal degeneration, Parkinson's disease, myopathies, macular degeneration, hemolytic anemia, AIDS, and several types of cancer, have been associated with decreased intracellular levels of reduced glutathione.

─────────── **WHAT ABOUT SUNSCREENS?** ───────────

I do not recommend using synthetic sunblocks because all they do is turn off the "alarm system" that gets people out of the sun when their skin starts turning red. When people use synthetic sunblocks, cellular damage takes place anyway, even though one doesn't feel the discomfort of reddening skin; moreover, without this warning signal, one is apt to stay in the sun for longer periods of time. The only commercial sun-protection product that I recommend is made by Aubrey (available in most health food stores). It doesn't oxidize when exposed to sunlight and contains shea butter and African nut butter. These provide natural protection by virtue of their high fatty acid content.

In healthy cells, glutathione disulfide is recycled back into the reduced state by glutathione reductase. This recycling of oxidized glutathione is aided by the ingestion of certain antioxidants that assist in maintaining adequate intracellular levels of reduced glutathione. It has been shown that certain anthocyans have the ability to regenerate reduced glutathione from oxidized glutathione even when faced with oxidizing agents, free radicals, and toxic exposure. These anthocyans are members of the bioflavonoid family and are found in certain fruits, vegetables, and plants such as berries, nuts, and grapes.[13]

In human studies, patients with varied conditions, such as cancer, lung disease, drug toxicities, kidney dysfunction, infertility, stroke, alcoholic liver disease, and radiation sickness, have shown functional improvements when taking oral reduced glutathione supplementation. In addition, many studies have shown the benefit of using reduced glutathione in combination with several chemotherapeutic agents to protect patients from the toxic side effects of chemotherapy while maintaining clinical efficacy. Reduced glutathione has also been shown to minimize the neurotoxic effects of cisplatin in the treatment of advanced ovarian, cervical, and gastric cancer.[14]

A recent study has demonstrated that by adding glutathione to the chemotherapeutic drug cisplatin, more cycles of cisplatin may be administered because the glutathione reduces the drug's level of toxicity. Patients undergoing this treatment show a statistically significant improvement in depression, nausea, hair loss, shortness of breath, and difficulty in concentrating; these are all negative side effects of cisplatin when taken without glutathione.[15]

Amazingly, oral administration of reduced glutathione has also been shown to increase its plasma levels. Studies have also demonstrated that reduced glutathione can not only be transported intact across the intestinal mucosa but also can be absorbed intact into isolated kidney cells via a sodium-dependent pathway.[16]

THE STAGES OF CANCER ADVANCEMENT

Once we understand how cancer progresses, the role of herbs, fruits, and vegetables in preventing and treating cancer becomes clear.

1. *Initiation.* In this stage, a series of genetic mutations transforms a normal cell into a latent cancer cell. The cell remains inactive and is not much different from a normal cell in its appearance or function, but it is vulnerable to change. This vulnerability makes it particularly susceptible to the ravages of free radical damage. This susceptibility can be inhibited by a diet of sulfur-rich foods, such as broccoli, cauliflower, and other cruciferous vegetables along with foods rich in carotenoids and chlorophyll (most fruits and vegetables) and flavonoids, such as green tea, grapes, berries, plums, and tangerines. Spices and herbs in this family include garlic, turmeric, and ginger.

2. *Promotion.* During this stage, the transformed cells are prompted by certain nutrients or metabolites to divide and multiply. As a result, minute precancerous masses are formed, but they are not yet malignant. This stage can be triggered by such agents as hormones (estrogens or xenoestrogens) and arachidonic acid (found in meat, processed oils, and all processed foods). Cervical dysplasia is an example of this stage. For this specific condition, I recommend a combination of folic acid, vitamin E, and carotenoids in order to inhibit promotion from dysplasia to cervical cancer. This protocol can actually reverse dysplasia as well. Other nutrients that help during this stage include turmeric, bromelain, quercetin, rosemary, and green tea.

3. *Progression.* During this stage, precancerous masses become cancerous and begin to divide rapidly. Here's where omega-3 fatty acids, fish and flax oils, lignans as found in pure seeds and nuts, and tangeretin found in tangerines would be helpful.

4. *Invasion and metastasis.* At this point, tumor cells cross tissue compartment boundaries and intermix with cells on the other side of the boundary. Tumor cells attach to basement membranes secreting enzymes that break down the membranes until the tumor cell is able to penetrate and migrate throughout the bloodstream. Helpful nutrients at this stage include modified citrus pectin, gotu kola, grape seed extract, omega-3 fatty acids, tangeretin (a flavone found in tangerines), and resveratrol, which is extracted from grape skins and leaves.

5. *Migration.* Cancer cells leave the tumor mass and migrate through the blood vessels or the lymph system and spread to distant areas. Even at this late stage, omega-3 fatty acids and good nutritional choices, including proteins like yogurt, tempeh, and steamed fish, can help, while quick-fix weight-gain, sugar-laced drinks and foods can actually make matters worse.

6. *Blood vessel formation (angiogenesis).* This is the point at which a cancerous mass forms blood vessels, allowing it to receive oxygen and nutrients. For a tumor to grow beyond a certain size, it must develop vasculature. Capillary blood vessels are needed for tumors to become larger than 2 centimeters. Vascular endothelial growth factor (VEGF) is one well-known angiogenesis inducer. It originates in the cell's own "intelligence." Cancer is an opportunistic disease whose mission is to take over. It seeks what it needs for survival. The strength of its course can be lessened by antiangiogenetic nutrients, such as flavonoids, particularly anthocyanins (found in foods with purple or blue pigments such as cherries, grapes, and plums). These nutrients, as well as most soy products, offer protection by strengthening vascular walls.

The Mechanisms of Metastasis

Cancer cells look different than normal cells or the benign tumor cells of the tissue in which they are found. Usually, the more abnormal the cell appears to be, the more malignant the cancer. The major difference between cancerous and benign tumor cells is that cancerous tumor cells have the ability to invade adjacent tissues and spread to distant sites. Cancer cells may eventually invade the bloodstream and establish colonies far from the original site. This is the process called metastasis.

Metastasis is one of the most devastating characteristics of a malignancy; indeed, most patients die as a result of metastases to distant organs (secondary tumor sites), not from damage done at the primary tumor site. Current evidence suggests that only a minority of the cells in a primary tumor express the constellation of phenotypic traits required to complete the many steps in the metastatic process.

In order for cancer to metastasize and develop into distant tumors, several steps must occur. It is here that many natural anticancer agents can play a life-saving role. These agents include tumor-cell adhesion inhibitors (such as modified citrus pectin), platelet aggregation reducers (such as turmeric and bromelain), angiogenesis inhibitors (such as genistein-rich soy products), and many more that are discussed in chapters 4 and 5.

Since metastases are a primary determinant of cancer morbidity and mortality, the use of nutritional and herbal interventions that may inhibit the metastatic process should be considered more seriously by oncologists for their patients with malignancies.

The first step of tumor invasion and metastasis occurs with detachment of the cancer cells from the primary tumor. The tumor cells then spread by piercing the protective membranes enclosing all tissue. Next, the cells make their way into the base membrane of a blood vessel and enter the bloodstream. There they secrete certain proteolytic enzymes, which digest the base membrane and enable the cells to slip between vascular endothelial cells and enter the vessel lumen. The cancer cell now lodges in the tiny capillaries and is free to travel to vital organs, such as the liver, brain, and/or lungs, or to remain in the lymph system. At this point, angiogenetic growth factors are secreted by the cancer cell to supply oxygen and blood to the secondary tumor. The tumor continues to grow until it takes over the host organ and starves that organ of its vital nutrients. Eventually, as the cancer proliferates, the organ becomes so infiltrated by the tumor that it can no longer perform its essential functions.

The bad news is that metastases are a primary determinant of cancer morbidity and mortality. The good news is that the use of certain nutritional and herbal interventions may inhibit the metastatic process by blocking vascularization. The process is called *antiangiogenesis.*

Cell Adhesion Molecules (CAMs)

Cancer cells communicate with each other and proliferate because of certain cell surface receptor molecules called *cell adhesion molecules (CAMs).*

CAMs are complex protein and carbohydrate molecules that occur on the plasma membranes of all cell surfaces. They control both intracellular and extracellular (cell-to-cell) communication. CAMs regulate organ architecture, cell migration, differentiation, apoptosis, mitosis, platelet aggregation, and the activity of the immune system.

There are three types of CAMs:

1. *Cadherins.* Cadherins inhibit both invasion and metastasis and reduce the expression of tumor cells. A well-known cadherin, E-cadherin, is strengthened by tangeretin, a flavone found in tangerines.

2. *Cell-surface lectins.* Lectins bind to the tumor cell and inhibit tumor cell-to-cell adhesion, thereby prohibiting completion of the metastatic process. A lectin called *galactose* is found abundantly in modified citrus pectin (MCP). MCP has been shown to inhibit tumor formation and growth in a number of cancers, including prostate cancer.[17]

3. *Proteoglycans (PGs) and glycosaminoglycans (GAGs).* PGs, proteins that form a major component of connective tissue, are attached to large carbohydrates called *GAGs.* GAGs are part of the extracellular matrix that forms such tissues as cartilage. Because they have a strong negative charge, GAGs are able to bind to many substances. Good sources of GAGs include glucosamine sulfate, cartilage (both bovine and shark), and hyaluronic acid. Hyaluronic acid offers major help in protecting the extracellular matrix (the "glue" that holds cells together), thereby acting as a defense against cancer's invasion.

Cancer-Cell Receptors

Cancer-cell receptors serve as a link between the extracellular environment and the cell nucleus. Signals are transmitted from the cell surface to the cell material (cytoplasm) and then to the nucleus. One such cell receptor is referred to as tyrosine kinase. The extracellular portions of the tyrosine kinase binds to specific ligands (sort of sticky-substance docking stations for intercellular messages). Ligand binding is followed by a process that leads to the activation of the receptor. A cascade of signaling events then takes place, causing cellular mutation, oncogene transformation, and tumor development.

What Influences Metastasis?

Tumor cells proliferate at a much faster rate than do normal cells. When a cell divides and the chromosomes are exposed to a reactive environment, the possibility of genetic alterations is increased.

In general, tumor cells have a higher sodium-to-potassium ratio than normal cells. Insulin, growth factors, and tumor promoters all increase the influx of sodium across the cell membrane, expel potassium, and stimulate anaerobic glycolysis (the breakdown of sugars into energy), which in turn increases the release of lactic acid.

Lactic acid production and its resulting increase in cellular glucose consumption enhances the ability of tumor cells to metastasize. Tumor cells consume three to five times more glucose than normal cells. *Avoiding all refined sugars and starches is an important dietary factor for inhibiting tumor cell proliferation. Cancer loves and feeds on sugar.*

Increasing the oxygen level in the blood, on the other hand, can inhibit tumor-cell proliferation since tumor cells favor a low-oxygen environment. Sometimes, however, if the body is toxic and nutritionally compromised, artificial oxygen therapies can encourage tumor-cell proliferation by increasing free radical damage to healthy cells. By using herbal nutrients, on the other hand, such as saffron extract (which is rich in aqueous carotenoids), one can enhance oxygen uptake of the cell and quench free radicals at the same time. This is another example of the wonder of nature and its healing properties.

Another factor in the inhibition of tumor-cell proliferation is temperature. Although it is possible to induce tumor death by raising the blood pH (this is the theory behind using cesium chloride), it is also possible to induce tumor-cell death by a drastic drop in pH through hyperthermia (heat therapy), which can decrease the extracellular pH. This is one of the many benefits of Epsom salt baths. High fevers have been reported to cause tumor regression—even, in a number of cases, complete spontaneous regression.[18,19] High fever induces systemic acidosis, which can cause such a significant drop in the intracellular pH that tumor cells can no longer live.

Tumor cells can suppress immune function, hide from our immune system, and spread in three ways:

1. By producing certain blocking factors that allow the tumor cell to go unrecognized by the immune system.

2. By producing immunosuppressing prostaglandins such as PGE-2. Cancer causes the failure of certain enzymes to transform healthy fatty acids into healthy tumor-suppressing prostaglandins. That failure marks a shift toward more unhealthy prostaglandins that actually assist in tumor growth.

3. By producing immunosuppressing cytokines or other angiogenic factors that lead to an increase in vascular permeability and eventually an increase in coagulation disorders. This is why we often see an increase in platelet count along with platelet aggregation, causing blood to clot in an abnormal fashion if cancer is progressing and spreading.

Many natural compounds can intercept tumor development by inhibiting some of these pathways. For instance, natural agents found in plants are commonly used to fight cancer by inhibiting fibrin production, platelet aggregation, and PAF. Specific natural agents and their functions will be discussed in chapters 4 and 5.

3

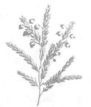

The Nutritional Challenge

And God said, Behold I have given you every herb bear-
ing seed, which is upon the face of all the Earth, and
every tree, in which is the fruit of a tree yielding seed;
to you it shall be for meat.

—*Genesis 1:29*

YOUR DIETARY CHOICES *DO* MAKE A DIFFERENCE

Heredity is often considered a major cause of cancer. This is partially true if
you make the same unhealthy dietary and lifestyle choices that your parents
did. For example, a diet rich in hydrogenated fats like margarine can influence
the initiation step in carcinogenesis, especially in relation to free radicals, and
a diet high in animal fats can influence the promotion stage of tumors by acting on initiated cells to elicit cancer growth. However, a healthy lifestyle and
diet may protect you. Diets rich in cruciferous vegetables and soy protein can
offer protection against genetically predisposed and lifestyle-induced cancers.
There is no substitute for a healthy diet of nutrient-rich whole foods.

Remember, nutritional supplements and herbs are not magic bullets and will not undo the harm done by a poor diet.

When supported with wholesome organic foods, the body is capable of restoring its internal balance even if confronted with illness or stress. This is due to "organ reserve": The functional capacity of human organs is four to ten times that required to sustain life. In truth, many of us are living unhealthy lifestyles by eating the wrong foods, breathing polluted air, drinking chlorinated water, depriving ourselves of adequate sleep, and exposing ourselves to many synthetic and toxic substances. Yet we marvel at the fact that we feel great, don't get sick very often, and have plenty of energy. However, we may not be aware that we are calling upon our organs to work at levels far beyond their normal operating capacity; by the time we become aware of a health problem, it is probably going to be a major one. To use a car as an analogy, we can drive our car hard with no maintenance at all for quite some time. However, when the engine overheats one day because there's no oil, we're going to have to deal with some major repairs—a situation that could have easily been prevented with a little routine maintenance.

A natural approach to healing cancer, as well as all chronic diseases, uses nutrition, diet, herbs, water, air, light, massage, touch, physical activity, scent, music, and most of all, love. It is a proactive way to live life—not waiting for "bad" genes to express themselves before developing a healthy lifestyle. Genetic expression is both a nutrient-dependent and a toxin-sensitive process. If there are imbalances of the essential macronutrients (protein, carbohydrates, fats), micronutrients (vitamins, minerals), and other phytochemicals in our dietary choices, the accurate transcription of genetic messages may not take place, disrupting the cells' adaptation capabilities.

Individuals whose adaptive capacity is thus reduced and whose environmental challenge is increased at the same time (perhaps by smoking or exposure to pollutants) can find their body systems unable to adapt to total environmental challenge, thereby putting themselves at risk for developing cancer or some other chronic disease.

Cancer cells favor an anaerobic metabolism. Like all other bacteria or viruses, cancer pathogens have a better chance to form in stagnation as opposed to an aerobic condition of oxygen exchange and movement. Assessing and correcting any and all nutritional deficiencies in order to promote a normal aerobic metabolism must be the first order of business to restore health and to either avoid cancer, bring it under control, or cure it.

HOW CANCER AFFECTS THE DIGESTIVE
AND ASSIMILATION PROCESSES

Cancer causes great stress on all metabolic processes, including assimilation, digestion, absorption of nutrients, and the elimination of waste products. Before selecting a specific diet for a cancer patient, it is necessary to strengthen the individual's vitality and digestive function.

Simply eating more food will not halt wasting in a person with advanced cancer nor will it extend or enhance the life of a person in the early stages of cancer. Frequently, in trying to pump high-calorie foods into a person with cancer, it's the cancer that gets fed, so any existing tumors grow faster.

The old saying "You are what you eat" should be "You are what you absorb." Poor assimilation leads to nutrient deficiencies. A person with cancer who is undergoing chemotherapy is in a difficult position because, with an accumulation of toxins, there is a need to detoxify. At the same time, however, the body is in a deficient state and needs help to build healthy tissue and become stronger. It is vital, therefore, that a proper nutritional balance be maintained so that both processes can take place.

After a patient has been through a series of conventional treatments, such as surgery, chemotherapy, or radiation, or when cancer is at an advanced state, the immune system becomes impaired, the body becomes malnourished, weight loss occurs, and anorexia (also called *wasting syndrome* or *cachexia*) follows. A loss of appetite due to chemotherapy, radiation, infection, depression, or the cancer itself frequently results in loss of vital muscle mass. There may also be metabolic disorders that cause changes in the way the body transforms food into energy. These may include:

1. Abnormalities in glucose metabolism (tumors cause an increase in the liver's production of glucose).

2. Abnormalities in protein metabolism, causing decreased levels of albumin in the blood (tumors fulfill their nitrogen needs at the expense of lean body mass). Albumin is the most abundant protein in the bloodstream. It is produced by a healthy liver and performs numerous functions that are vital to health. Maintaining optimal albumin levels is of the utmost importance in regard to the nutritional status of the person with cancer.

3. Abnormalities in lipid metabolism (tumors cause an increase in poor fatty acid utilization).

The goal of my nutrition program is to provide proper nutritional support for the cancer patient that will increase quality weight gain and improve blood count, immune function, digestion, and assimilation while at the same time inhibiting (or at least not feeding) the cancer.

The Importance of Good Digestion

The condition of the tongue is a reliable indicator of a person's health. A tongue that displays a white or yellow coating indicates poor digestion. A flabby tongue with bad breath signals a torpid liver. A clean, moist tongue is a sign of good digestion.

Nutrient absorption may be impaired because of a weakened gastrointestinal tract, and this results in poor digestion. Because of the many functions of the gastrointestinal tract, it is a vital component in maintaining good health and promoting healing. Its foremost function is to absorb nutrients, including vitamins and minerals that fuel the body by the process of digestion. It also contains a major part of the body's detoxification system as well as antibodies that act as the first line of defense against infection.

Everything we put into our bodies has an effect upon us. It can be good or bad, immediate or long-term, predictable or not, but one way or another there will be an effect. This is important to remember as you read the nutritional guidelines in this chapter because it will help you to understand the importance of proper nutrition, a fundamental aspect of good health that cannot be emphasized enough.

NUTRITIONAL GUIDELINES

Many of the diets recommended for treating cancer focus on the cancer and not on the individual. The variations in these diets are staggering and confusing—one says eat vegan with raw foods only; another suggests vegan with cooked foods; some eliminate fruits; most ban eggs, dairy, and meat. I recommend a diet that supports optimal personal health, a diet designed specifically for each individual's well-being and healing. Among my clients I have seen the need for very diverse dietary requirements. Although I believe that a vegetarian diet is morally, ethically, and generally a healthier diet, it is not appropriate for everyone. For example, when a person is extremely deficient and anemic (perhaps as a result of chemotherapy), I sometimes recommend a vegetable-beef soup made with organic beef. While not readily available in most supermarkets, hormone-free and naturally low-fat meats can be found in natural food stores. From a nutritional standpoint, they offer a bioavailability of certain nutrients (vitamin B_{12}, iron, zinc, protein) that is superior to vegetarian sources. On the other hand, I see people who have been eating animal protein and processed foods for most of their lives, and they benefit greatly from the cleansing offered by adhering to a vegetarian vegan diet. The bottom line for me is dietary flexibility: One's diet should be a source of strength to the body and a gift to the senses, not a fearful regime that offers no comfort.

First and foremost, it is essential to select foods of the highest quality. This means foods that are fresh, unprocessed, organically grown, nonirradiated, and free of chemical additives. Long before the health food revolution of the 1960s, Dr. Weston A. Price, a pioneering dentist, rightly placed the blame for the increase in dental cavities in America on the increased consumption of white sugar, white flour, processed oils, and canned foods. His book *Nutrition and Physical Degeneration* is a classic I recommend highly.

Eating refined carbohydrates, such as white sugar and white flour, can cause abnormally high levels of blood glucose, a common factor in cancer. The excess glucose feeds the fermentation process of cancer cells and suppresses the immune system. Elevated glucose levels are seen three to eight times more often in people with active cancer. Another sign that the metabolism is not properly oxidizing the products of sugar breakdown is high blood lactic acid levels. This is also frequently seen in people with active cancer. The liver converts excess lactic acid back to glucose, thereby feeding the cancer's growth. High lactic acid levels also contribute to the pain caused by cancer.

Why Organic Is Best

A balanced, healthy metabolism capable of inhibiting cancer requires a nutritionally adequate diet. Unfortunately, in today's society, where fast food makes up close to 40 percent of food intake, a diet devoid of fresh vegetables and fruits is not uncommon. Moreover, most of the produce available to us is picked before it is ripe and may retain traces of pesticides or other chemical additives.

Processing foods disrupts the natural makeup of nutrients and adds chemicals, such as artificial colors and flavors; environmental pollutants, including industrial chemicals and radiation, add toxicity to the finished product.

Recent findings have linked many cancers, including lymphoma, sarcoma, leukemia, colon, lung, nose, prostate, breast, and ovarian cancer to the pesticides and herbicides in our foods.[1] The increase in exposure to synthetic chemicals over the past forty years, along with the refinement of our food supply, may be responsible for the increase in cancer and other chronic illnesses.

Pesticides interfere with the enzyme systems of insects, many of which are similar to human enzyme systems. Measurements in human and animal tissues have shown that the enzyme systems are adversely affected by pesticides even at very low concentrations. There is no safe lower limit of dosage. Pesticide exposure eventually will result in illness. Preventive interventions must be taken now without waiting any longer for full scientific proof of the magnitude of the long-term effects.

Organic food is grown without exposure to chemical fertilizers or pesticides and without the use of growth hormones. Its nutritional quality is much higher than chemically processed food, particularly in trace elements, such as selenium and molybdenum, which are strong anticancer agents. It also nurtures the environment in which it is produced.

The healing power of fresh, organic food is more than the sum of its chemical nutrients. It contains many live enzymes released during the sprouting process when the plant is exposed to the sun's energy. We know, for instance, that eating broccoli supplies us with dithiolthiones that trigger the formation of glutathione S-transferase, which in turn prevents carcinogens from damaging a cell's DNA. By eating organic broccoli, we are assured that this process can take place unhampered by the chemical interference of pesticides or growth hormones. We derive vitality by eating foods that are vital themselves—it's as simple as that.

Findings from a recent study concur with this view and have demonstrated that commercial foods are likely to be inferior in nutritional content to organically grown foods. Analyses of the elemental content of both organic and nonorganic foods showed that many elements important for nutrition were present in greater amounts in the organic foods and that three potentially toxic elements (aluminum, lead, and mercury), though present, occurred in lesser amounts in the organic foods.[2]

Meanwhile, population surveys show that nutritional deficiencies continue to be prevalent among children, teenagers, the elderly, and the institutionalized, including those in hospitals. Food irradiation is a growing concern that needs to be addressed by government regulation. Irradiated foods can cause chromosomal damage, especially in small children. A number of grassroots groups are working against the irradiation of foods, and these groups deserve our full support. Commercially grown potatoes and many of the spices on our grocery store shelves are just two examples of foods that are commonly irradiated. The person with cancer, especially, should avoid irradiated foods. Microwave ovens, which change the molecular structure of food, should also be avoided.

Quality and Balance—Two Golden Rules

I have two golden rules when it comes to diet. The first is quality and the second is balance. To eat a balanced diet it is important to include a variety of foods. Eat many types of grains, fruits, and vegetables; don't get locked into a routine and eat the same foods daily.

Quality foods are fresh whole foods that are organically grown and then prepared and cooked so that the vitality that they freely give to us is not destroyed. We should honor and respect our food and give thanks every time we eat.

A proper diet should be balanced as follows:

- 40 to 60 percent complex carbohydrates
- 20 to 30 percent protein
- 20 to 30 percent healthy fats

These percentages should vary according to the season and the geographic location. There should also be a balance in the consumption of both raw and cooked foods. The advocates of raw food consumption claim that cooking destroys all enzymes and "kills" the food, but raw food is sometimes difficult to digest, particularly for cancer patients. One must always consider the individual's state of health as well as the time of year when making dietary recommendations. Generally, I suggest more raw foods and juices in the summer months and more cooked foods and soups in winter. Not only is this a healthy way to make food choices, since seasonal foods are fresher and give us specific nutrients particular to the season, but it also allows us to be in step with nature. In general, the colder the climate, the more fat one should consume. The balance of carbohydrates, proteins, and fats is very important to the modulation of eicosanoids/prostaglandins, a class of very active biological substances that regulate nearly every bodily function.

What About Fats?

Many health practitioners propose diets high in complex carbohydrates and low in either protein or fat—a low- or no-fat diet. Fats in general, and cholesterol in particular, have been completely misunderstood by the general public. Healthy fats, especially the essential fatty acids (EFAs) omega-3 and omega-6, are important for the proper regulation of prostaglandins (PGs), which are involved with many of the body's vital functions, including the immune system, reproduction, fuel storage, insulin control, and mental health. Even saturated fat (in moderation) is acceptable because it is stable and does not oxidize within or outside the body.

To be considered healthy and effective, all the double bonds of a fatty acid molecule must be in the *cis* configuration. Because cis double bonds are relatively unstable, they are often intentionally converted to the *trans* isomer in order to improve the shelf life, texture, and appearance of commercial oils and spreads. As a result, most fats in the typical American diet are denatured and devoid of any life-promoting essential components; rather, they are composed of life-destroying agents. Trans fats (listed as hydrogenated or partially hydrogenated on food labels) compete with normal EFAs at most structural sites and in many enzymatic reactions. A diet without healthful EFAs can cause a cascade of reactions that can lead to an acceleration of free radicals, an imbalance of prostaglandins, and many health problems.

Of the three varieties of prostaglandins, series 1 and series 3 are the good guys; they are capable of inhibiting carcinogenesis by suppressing the arachidonic acid (AA) cascade and inhibiting inflammation. Series 2 prostaglandins, on the other hand, are the bad guys; they encourage the development of arachidonic acid, which promotes tumor growth (see table 3.1). Overproduction of the series 2 eicosanoids/prostaglandins are found in every animal tumor, in every cancer cell system, and in every human tumor.

It is estimated that 80 percent of our population is lacking adequate EFAs, in particular the omega-3 fatty acids. There are many reasons for this. For one

Table 3.1 **Prostaglandins**

Prostaglandin	Role in Cancer Development	Type of Dietary Fat
Series 1	Inhibits carcinogenesis by suppressing arachidonic acid cascade	Essential fatty acids such as those found in evening primrose oil and borage oil
Series 2	Promotes carcinogenesis by encouraging development of arachidonic acid cascade	All hydrogenated or partially hydrogenated fats; margarine, animal fats, all saturated and refined fats
Series 3	Inhibits carcinogenesis by suppressing arachidonic acid cascade	Omega-3 fatty acids found in fish oils and flaxseed oil

thing, high-quality oils are difficult to find in most supermarkets. The commercially produced oils found on supermarket shelves are devoid of EFAs. By the time the refinement process is completed, they are also denatured, rancid, and toxic. In addition, hydrogenation, a process commonly used in nearly all processed foods, transforms EFAs into harmful trans fatty acids. Finally, our national mania with nonfat or low-fat eating has muddied the distinction between healthy and nonhealthy fats.

I have seen people avoid avocados, a powerhouse of EFA nutrition, and use fat-free salad dressings only to eat a bag of potato chips, loaded with harmful trans fatty acids, later in the day. We are either eating the wrong types of fats or no fat at all. The healthiest fats are found in seafood, olive oil, flaxseed oil, whole grains, nuts, seeds, and many green vegetables.

What About Dairy?

Many people blame dairy for many of our health problems. Although I do not advocate consuming large amounts of dairy, I wonder whether the problem is in the dairy product itself, or in what modern agriculture has done to the cow and the milk. We need to open our eyes and begin to ask questions about today's dairy industry. How are cows raised? What are they fed? Are they roaming freely and getting sunlight? Are they given antibiotics and growth hormones? Are they hand-milked or machine-milked? Is the milk then pasteurized and homogenized? Are preservatives or other additives such as synthetic vitamin D used?

I favor a moderate intake of organic milk products (unless one is allergic) in the form of yogurt and hard cheeses. However, organic goat products are even a better choice for most people, because goat dairy more closely resembles mother's milk and its enzyme configuration is easier to digest and assimilate. Also, goats are less likely than cows to be raised commercially, so the animals themselves are less contaminated by noxious chemicals.

THE IMPORTANCE OF PHYTOCHEMICALS

There are hundreds and hundreds of phytochemicals in plant foods that help prevent cancer. The chemicals that plants synthesize for self-protection against sunlight and insects and to help maintain their own growth enhance human health as well. Over the last twenty years, researchers have consistently found that those who eat the most vegetables and fruits have the lowest rates of cancer. Research has also shown that animals given vegetables and fruit before and after exposure to carcinogens are less likely to develop cancer.

In a recent study involving the intake of vegetables, fruits, and related nutrients in relation to the risk of premenopausal breast cancer, a strong inverse association was found between high intake of these nutrients and a low incidence of cancer. This study concluded that certain measured components found together in vegetables may have a synergistic effect on breast cancer risk.[3] However, other unmeasured factors in these foods may also influence risk. The implications of this data are profound. Ultimately, they could be used to design a diet that would not only provide increased protection against cancer, but also serve as an adjunct therapy for individuals with cancer.

Foods contain both major and minor constituents. The major ones, familiar to us all, are protein, fat, carbohydrates, and fiber. Of the many minor dietary constituents, some of the more familiar nutrients that research has found to be beneficial in cancer prevention include vitamins A, C, D, and K, folic acid, and selenium. In addition, there are a large number of substances, unfamiliar to most individuals, that inhibit carcinogenesis. Known as phytochemicals, they can protect against cancer in many diverse ways by:

- Scavenging oxygen radicals
- Preventing the formation of carcinogens
- Increasing the detoxification of carcinogens
- Inactivating mutagens and carcinogens
- Reducing damage to DNA and cellular membranes
- Slowing down the proliferation and promotion of the cancer process

Table 3.2 lists some of these phytochemicals, the foods in which they are naturally found, and the action they produce in the body. Many of these terms might be unfamiliar, but take the time to study the table. It's important to grasp the breadth of chemical protection offered to us by simple foods.

In order for phytochemicals to do their job, however, we need to eat enough plant foods, and far too few of us do. One review of over 200 studies that examined the relationship between fruit and vegetable intake and cancers of the lung, colon, breast, cervix, esophagus, oral cavity, stomach, bladder, pancreas, and ovary, showed a statistically significant protective effect of fruit and vegetable intake in 128 of 156 dietary studies. For most cancer sites, low fruit and vegetable intake produced about twice the risk of cancer. The review suggests that major public health benefits could be achieved by substantially increased consumption of these foods.[4] According to guidelines recommended by the National Cancer Institute, one must eat at least five half-cup servings of fruits and vegetables daily to lower cancer risk.

A 1991 study published in the *International Journal of Cancer* evaluated the relationship between cancer risk and the frequency of consumption of green vegetables and fruits in a series of case-controlled studies in northern Italy between 1983 and 1990. Though there were some uncertainties in biological interpretation, the data were consistent and strong for a pattern of reduced risk of seven common epithelial cancers with increased green vegetable intake; fruit intake was shown to be protective against cancers of the upper digestive tract and possibly the urinary tract.[5]

The Magic of Soy Foods

Soy foods are rich in isoflavones, phytochemicals that can cause cancer cells to differentiate and become more primitive, less specialized, and less deadly. The

Table 3.2 Phytochemicals in Food

Phytochemical	Food in Which Naturally Found	Action in Body
Limonene and nomilin	Citrus fruit	Stimulate detoxification enzymes that break down carcinogens.
Citrus pectin	Plant fiber of citrus fruit	Shown to inhibit metastasis in prostate cancer by competing with tumor cell surface galectins, which are essential for successful establishment of secondary tumor cell colonies.
Sulfur-containing compounds, sulforphane	Cruciferous vegetables (broccoli, cauliflower, kale, brussels sprouts, and other members of the cabbage family), onions	Protect against cancer.
Allyl sulfides	Garlic, onions, leeks, chives	Increase the production of glutathione S-transferase and other enzymes that enhance carcinogen excretion.
S-allylmercaptocysteine (SAMC)	Aged garlic	Detoxifies hormones and carcinogens.
Dithiolethiones	Broccoli	Trigger the formation of glutathione S-transferase, which may prevent carcinogens from damaging a cell's DNA.
Ellagic acid	Grapes, strawberries, raspberries, pomegranates	A polyphenol scavenger of carcinogens; prevents alteration in the DNA of cells. Also inhibits lung tumorigenesis induced by nicotine-derived nitrosamines.
Caffeic acid	Fruit	Enhances production of enzymes that make carcinogens more water-soluble.

Ferulic acid	Fruit	Binds to nitrates in stomach; prevents production of carcinogenic nitrosamines.
Phytic acid	Grains	Binds to iron and reduces free radical effects of too much iron.
Indoles	Cruciferous vegetables	Help detoxify estrogen.
Isothiocyanates	Cruciferous vegetables	Enhance glutathione S-transferase, which helps in carcinogen excretion.
Chlorophyll	Green vegetables	Antigenotoxin that inhibits the mutagenic activity of certain chemicals.

The following four classes of phytochemicals have demonstrated anticancer activity:

1. Protease inhibitors	Soybeans, chickpeas, other legumes	Reduce certain enzymes in cancer cells.
2. Phytosterols	Soybeans	Slow down the reproduction of cells in the large intestine, which may reduce risk of colon cancer.
3. Glycosides, saponins, and isoflavonoids	Soybeans	Interfere with the process by which the DNA of cells reproduce, which can prevent cancer from proliferating.
4. Genistein and daidzin (isoflavones)	Soybeans	Block the entry of estrogen into the cell, thereby causing cancer cells to lose their ability to function. Possibly help convert cancer cells back to normal cells.
Quercetin	Onions, broccoli, eucalyptus, blue-green algae, propolis	Inhibits the tumor-promoting PGE-2 series by blocking proflammatory reactions in the body.

mechanisms that enable them to do this involve estrogen-receptor-binding modulation of sex-hormone-binding globulin (SHBG), and inhibition of the enzymes protein tyrosine kinase (PTK) and 5-alpha reductase, a key enzyme involved in prostate cancer. Thus, soy foods have particularly beneficial effects on breast cancer, prostate cancer, and other hormone receptor-type cancers. Genistein and other soy isoflavones also have an antiangiogenesis effect on tumors. As noted in chapter 2, angiogenesis is the process that generates new capillary blood vessels, a critical step in the growth and proliferation of solid tumors. Genistein inhibits angiogenesis by neutralizing vascular endothelial growth factor (VEGF), a substance put out by tumors to encourage blood vessel nourishment.

Isoflavones also exert a mild estrogenic effect that may help relieve or eliminate the symptoms of menopause. The isoflavones present in soybeans are greatly enhanced and become more available during the fermentation process. Thus, one should be sure to eat fermented soybean foods such as tempeh, miso, shoyu (soy sauce), and natto along with the nonfermented soybean foods like tofu and soy milk. Studies of Japanese women have shown that those who consume miso soup daily have a significantly reduced risk for all types of cancer compared with those who consume little or none.

However, there are also findings that show miso consumption may be associated with a somewhat increased risk of digestive tract cancers, although some believe that faulty refrigeration is the culprit because it leads to bacterial growth in miso.

In addition, soy foods are a source of lignans, coumestans, saponins, plant sterols, phytates, and protease inhibitors, all of which contribute to the anticancer effects of soy.

It is important that dietary studies involving soy be carried out using whole soybeans rather than isolated compounds, since soybeans appear to contain several potential anticarcinogens. Unfortunately, studies continue to be carried out using genistein alone in cancer therapy.

FOODS THAT ARE GOOD FOR YOU

Vegetables

In 1996, the largest controlled study ever done to date on diet and breast cancer confirmed that high vegetable intake conferred a 30 to 50 percent protection against not only breast cancer but virtually all cancer sites and types.[6]

My number-one diet recommendation is to eat an abundant amount of fresh vegetables and fruits daily. Many homes today have replaced fresh fruits and vegetables with prepackaged foods that have been sitting in boxes, cans, cartons, or freezers for weeks. Tasting the difference between condensed frozen orange juice and freshly squeezed juice from organic oranges is proof positive of the superior value of fresh foods. Not only is the flavor sweeter and more delicious, but all the nutrients are at their freshest and most potent. This is true for all foods.

Botanically, there are nine vegetable families:

1. Cabbage/mustard (*Brassaceae*)
2. Lettuce/sunflower (*Asteraceae*)
3. Carrot/parsley (*Apiaceae*)
4. Beet/spinach (*Chenopodaceae*)
5. Cucumber/squash (*Cucurbetaceae*)
6. Mint/basil (*Lamiaceae*)
7. Tomato/pepper (*Solanaceae*)
8. Bean/pea (*Fabaceae*)
9. Onion/garlic (*Alliaceae*)

By including vegetables from each family, you receive the full spectrum of phytochemicals. It's a simple and natural way to provide a healthy diversity of vegetables in your diet.

Carotenoids

Eat at least one or two servings of carotene-rich vegetables, such as carrots, yams, squash, pumpkin, tomatoes, melons, and other deep orange or red-colored vegetables as well as dark leafy greens such as collard greens, kale, and dandelion every day; season your foods with paprika or cayenne pepper. If you carefully scrub organic carrots with a vegetable brush, you need not peel the layer where many nutrients reside. Low carotenoid consumption is correlated with the prevalence of many forms of cancers, including lung, bladder, stomach, prostate, and colon. Recent research shows that carotenoids other than beta-carotene (such as canthaxanthin, phytoene, lutein, xanthophylls, and lycopenes) offer better protection against cancer than beta-carotene itself. Xanthophylls are primarily found in edible yellow flowers, such as calendula, dandelion, and squash flowers, as well as in green leafy vegetables and egg yolks.

Carotenoids can protect phagocytes from auto-oxidative damage, enhance T- and B-lymphocyte proliferate responses, stimulate effector T-cell functions, enhancing their cytotoxic capabilities, and stimulate macrophage and natural killer-cell tumoricidal capacities, as well as increase the production of certain interleukins. Carotenoids protect the body, especially the lipids and organ walls in the cell, from oxidative damage. They also protect the skin from sun damage caused by sunlight reacting with fatty acids, which can result in oxidative damage to the body's DNA.

If you plan to add carotenoids to your diet in supplement form (see chapter 5), it is very important to take a full-spectrum natural carotenoid supplement, not simply synthetic beta-carotene. Carotenoids, whether in vegetables or in supplements, are best assimilated if taken with a fat such as flaxseed oil or olive oil.

Cruciferous Vegetables

Eat cruciferous vegetables daily, or eat at least five servings per week. Cabbage, broccoli, brussels sprouts, cauliflower, kale, collards, turnips, and radishes are among the most common. It is best not to eat them raw, because in their raw form they contain high amounts of goitrogens, thyroid suppressing agents that are removed during the cooking process. Since many people with cancer have slightly underactive thyroids, it's a good idea to avoid goitrogens when possible.

In addition to having special anticancer compounds called *indoles* and *isothiocyanates*, cruciferous vegetables are also high in vitamins A, C, and E; some contain anticancer minerals, and most are high in fiber. In experiments, indoles were added to the diets of mice before and during the administration of carcinogens (like those in cigarettes); the indoles stopped the growth of tumors developing in the stomach and lungs.[7] In some way not yet clear, indoles deactivate carcinogens or block them from damaging cells, acting at several different stages of carcinogenesis to stop both cancer promoters and initiators. It may be that indoles buttress the enzyme systems responsible for metabolizing carcinogens, and, in all probability, they increase the antioxidant

---
CRUCIFEROUS VEGETABLES ───

Broccoli	Chinese cabbage	Kohlrabi	Turnip
Brussels sprouts	Collards	Mustard greens	Watercress
Cabbage	Horseradish	Radish	
Cauliflower	Kale	Rutabaga	

---

action of glutathione compounds. However this works, cruciferous vegetables have proved to be terrific anticancer nutrients.

Another component in broccoli, called *sulforaphane*, also appears to block tumor formation in animals and presumably in humans as well. Organically grown broccoli produces a much greater amount of sulforaphane than the commercially grown variety. Sulforaphane is a potent inducer of phase II cellular enzyme activity, which is known to deactivate cancer-causing agents through detoxification.[8] Broccoli sprouts, which taste something like alfalfa sprouts, contain up to one hundred times more sulforaphane than does broccoli itself. Broccoli sprouts are available in some supermarkets and health food stores, or you can sprout your own. Sprouting seeds are very nutritious and cost-effective and provide a relatively easy way to acquire many vitamins, minerals, and important cancer-inhibiting phytonutrients. Besides mung bean sprouts, found in many Asian dishes, and the recently popular broccoli sprouts, other seeds and legumes that sprout well include red clover, buckwheat, chickpea, radish, chia, and sunflower.

Another compound found in broccoli and other cruciferous vegetables, called *indole-3-carbinol*, has been shown to increase the excretion of a form of estrogen called *2-hydroxyestrone*, which is linked to breast cancer. Clinical trials now in progress are testing indole-3-carbinol for treating some forms of cancer.[9]

Other Important Vegetables

Both red and white radishes and beets support the liver and have anticancer properties. They are best raw, either grated in a salad or as a fresh juice with carrots. One of the most remarkable and successful programs for treating cancerous tumors was begun in the late 1950s by Alexander Ferenczi, M.D., in a hospital in Csoma, Hungary, using nothing but raw red beets. According to Ferenczi, beetroot contains a tumor-inhibiting substance that he attributes to its natural red coloring agent, betaine.[10]

Celery contains abundant amounts of phthalides and polyacetanes, two phytochemicals that have been shown to inhibit cancer. They are able to detoxify many carcinogens and are of particular help in reversing some of the damage done by cigarette smoking. An excellent juice combination is two parts carrot, one part celery, and a half part beet.

Shiitake mushrooms should also be eaten on a regular basis since they foster many immune-enhancing activities, including stimulation of macrophages, increased cytotoxic activity of macrophages, increased production of interleukin-1 and -2, increased T-lymphocyte production, and enhanced CD-4 cell function.

Bitter melon (*Momordica charantia*) is a common vegetable eaten in Asia and the Carribbean Islands. It is available here in Asian food markets and some health food stores. The ripe fruit and leaves are a source of a guanylate cyclase inhibitor, which has been shown to inhibit prostate cancer, perhaps by regulating cyclic AMP and decreasing PGE-2 and the arachidonic acid cascade.

Asparagus is another vegetable with many anticancer properties. It has a cleansing effect on the lymphatic system and kidneys. It can be cooked or pureed and added to soups or drinks. It contains protein compounds called *histones*, which are believed to act as cell-growth normalizers on cancer-cell division. Asparagus therapy has been used to treat various forms of cancer, and reversal of the disease has been reported in a number of cases. As a form of therapy, asparagus should always be cooked, then put into the blender and liquefied at high speed to make a puree. It can then be stored in the refrigerator. The recommended dose is 4 tablespoons twice daily, which can be taken alone or mixed in any hot or cold beverage.

Potatoes, usually regarded only as a starchy filler, are actually a wonderful food. They are a rich source of alpha-lipoic acid, which is the most improtant intracellular and extracellular nutrient known today. Potatoes also contain a diverse amount of polyphenolic compounds and protease inhibitors and are a great source of vitamin C.

Avocados also have a very high nutritional value. They are perhaps the best overall source of essential fatty acids and glutathione and a very good source of protein. Avocados are easily digested, making them an ideal food for people recovering from surgery or for the very sick.

Other nutritious vegetables to eat include peas, string beans, zucchini, summer and winter squashes, eggplant, Swiss chard, and artichokes (both globe and rooted sunchoke). Artichokes are rich in nutrients that protect the liver. Eat all these vegetables raw or cooked, either whole, shredded, juiced, or in a soup broth. Soups or fresh juices are best for those in recovery.

Wild Greens and Flowers

Be sure to eat chlorophyll-rich dark leafy greens every day—both raw and cooked. Try to include wild greens like dandelion, chickweed, watercress, mustard greens, and my favorite green, nettles. Raw spinach and parsley are good sources of glutathione and chlorophyll. Parsley is also rich in poly-actylenes, which block the formation of tumor-promoting prostaglandins. Use romaine lettuce, arugula, escarole, chicory, and watercress in salad and forget about eating iceberg lettuce, which has no nutritional value at all. Eating watercress releases phenethyl isothiocyanate (PEITC), which can prevent nicotine-induced lung cancer. PEITC appears to partially block the metabolic activation of the tobacco-specific lung carcinogen NNK. In addition to watercress, other foods that contain similar compounds include Chinese cabbage (also called napa cabbage) and turnips.

Another wonderful wild green that can be added to your salad is purslane. This plant is rich in omega-3 fatty acids and antioxidants, such as vitamins E, C, and K, beta-carotene, glutathione, and psoralens. Psoralens are naturally occurring tricyclic furocoumarins that act as antioxidants and are found in other plants such as celery, parsley, parsnips, and figs.

Eat cooked greens such as kale, collard greens, mustard greens, and broccoli rabe. Learn to love the taste of bitter greens because they detoxify the liver. Of the wild greens, dandelion and nettles are both delicious sautéed with garlic. They are two of the most nutritious foods we can eat and they are both common weeds that grow everywhere. Another wild green, usually available only in the spring, is the young fiddlehead fern.

Dandelion root, which can be eaten as a food or used in tea, has shown antitumor effects in mammary carcinoma in mice, due to a cytolytic activation of macrophages. Both the root and the leaf have been used traditionally to treat various types of cancers.

Edible flowers also contain wonderful nutrients that can add color, flavor, and drama to many simple recipes. Flowers tend to be rich in many important phytonutrients, including large amounts of flavonoids and carotenoids, two of the most important nutrients for our health and well-being. Edible flowers can be added to many dishes or used as a garnish. Some of my favorites, which can be added to salads, vegetables, or soups, include viola, chive, rocket blossoms, coriander, nasturtium, rosemary, squash, bergamot, lavender, mint, sage, calendula, and borage. Even the dandelion flower can be eaten!

Garlic and Onions

Garlic possesses thiosulfinates such as allicin, found predominately in crushed raw garlic, and ajoene, a potent prostaglandin inhibitor found in steamed garlic. Along with onions, shallots, leeks, and chives, garlic should be eaten on a regular basis, as all these vegetables contain antitumor and immune-enhancing components.

Research completed at Pennsylvania State University has shown that garlic may keep normal cells in the breast from becoming cancerous. In this study, rats given aged garlic extract showed 66 percent less binding of a cancer-causing agent to normal cells than did rats that received no garlic when given the same cancer-causing agent. Even more impressive was the fact that the rats taking garlic plus selenium had a 99 percent reduction of the binding of the carcinogen.[11]

Results of another recent report on garlic support prior research showing that garlic effectively inhibits tumor formation in chemically induced cancers. Raw garlic powder and water extract of garlic both reduced chemically induced breast cancers by an average of 39.5 percent. A commercial deodorized garlic powder decreased adduct occurrences (chemical insults to the cells) by an average of 64 percent, and a commercial high-sulfur garlic powder reduced adducts by 56 percent.[12]

When working with a sulfur compound for use against prostate cancer, researchers at Memorial Sloan-Kettering Cancer Center in New York found that aged garlic, referred to as S-allylmercaptocysteine (SAMC), improved the breakdown of testosterone significantly. The SAMC aged garlic extract slowed the cancer cell's growth by as much as 70 percent compared to untreated cells. This compound in garlic also cut the production of two proteins in the blood, including the prostate-specific antigen or PSA. The PSA test is the most widely used blood test for prostate cancer screening.[13]

Fruit

Eat a variety of in-season fruit, preferably early in the morning or between meals. Look for nonhybridized fruit because it possesses a higher nutritional value and has less potential for allergens. Thus, choose pippin or Macoun apples rather than delicious or Macintosh, and eat a small amount of the core. Buy grapes with seeds and eat some of the seeds. They contain a group of flavonoids referred to as proanthocyanidin oligomers, PCOs for short. PCOs, also called OPCs, demonstrate a wide range of pharmacological activity, including antioxidant actions that are fifty times greater than vitamins C and E. Grapes, as well as many berries and some nuts, contain a phytoalexin component called *resveratrol* that has shown cancer chemopreventive activity. Resveratrol has been found to act as an antioxidant, antimutagen, and anti-inflammatory. It has also been shown to inhibit the development of breast cancer and induce antiprogression activity in human myelocytic leukemia. The highest levels of resveratrol (up to one hundred times more than grapes) are found in grape leaves.

Eat a variety of berries, figs, and other fruits. *Benzaldehyde* is the active anti-cancer principal ingredient found in figs and the bitter almond. Benzaldehyde has been shown experimentally to decrease drastically the uptake of thymodine and adenine, which leads to a decreased level of ATP (adesine triphosphate) within cancer cells, while having no effect on normal cells. It appears that benzaldehyde can arrest tumor progression and have a paralytic effect on tumor growth.[14]

Ellagic acid, a natural substance called a phenol, is found in many berries (pomegranates being the richest source) and nuts. It inhibits cancer formation and is believed to inhibit cancer mutation by latching onto DNA-masking sensitive sites on the genetic material that might otherwise be occupied by harmful chemicals.[15] Ellagic acid is particularly effective in the inhibition of lung cancer caused by tobacco.

Wild berries are a great source of many important nutrients, including a wide range of flavonoids and vitamin C. A few common wild berries include blackberry, black raspberry, thimbleberry, salmon berry, wild strawberry, huckleberry, cranberry, blueberry, and wild grape.

Cranberries are a good source of vitamin C, potassium, and many micronutrients as well as a number of organic acids, including benzoic acid, malic acid, quinic acid, and citric acid. Cranberry juice can prevent and treat urinary tract infections as well as inhibit the growth of several types of yeast. The anticancer effects of cranberries are similar to many other natural food phytonutrients; they work via the liver and its detoxifying enzyme systems. The most active anticancer constituent of cranberry is proanthocyanidin, which has an antioxidant capability ten times greater than that of vitamin E.[16] Never buy cranberry juice sweetened with sugar or corn syrup. It is very simple to make your own (see chapter 14). Get a guide book and learn about the areas of the country and seasons when various berries are available. In August, for instance, blackberries are everywhere in southern Oregon as well as in the Northeast. Go on a berry-picking hike—it's fun and a great way to begin to become more involved with nature. Berries are delicious and can be used in shakes, mixed with apple juice, or eaten as desserts—in pies, muffins, cobblers, or just plain with some yogurt.

Citrus fruits, including oranges, grapefruit, tangerines, and lemons, all contain abundant amounts of various flavonoids and terpenoids. These are potent activators of Phase I and Phase II detoxifying enzyme systems that occur primarily in the liver and act as important cancer inhibitors. The flavonoids found in grapefruit include naringin (the most abundant), naringenin, apigenin, hesperetin, and kaempferol. Naringenin slows the growth of human breast cancer cells. In addition, two important flavones found in citrus fruit are nobiletin and tangeretin. Tangeretin, found in tangerines, strengthens E-caderin, which inhibits cell-endothelial adhesion, a very important step in the metastatic process of cancer.

When eating citrus fruit, don't throw away the peel because it contains a remarkable anticancer substance called *D-limonene*, a monoterpene that has been used in a clinical trial in England as a monotherapy for people with pancreatic and colorectal cancers. Small bits of organic orange peel go well in salads or can be added to any tea. When adding citrus peels to tea, be sure to put a cover or a saucer on top of the cup while the tea steeps so that the aromatic oils don't escape into the air.

Rhubarb has also shown antitumor activity as a result of two of its compounds, rhein and emodin.

Whole Grains

Eliminate or reduce your intake of refined flours and replace them with whole-grain foods in the form of cereals, breads, or simply cooked in their whole form. Whole grains are filled with many important nutrients, including vitamin E, the B vitamins, minerals, protein, fiber, and many other important phytonutrients. Whole grains contain a substantial amount of insoluble fiber. Fruits and vegetables, on the other hand, contain soluble fiber. The combination of these two forms of fiber promotes bowel regularity and protects against colon cancer. It is estimated that colon cancer in the United States could be reduced by as much as one-third if people just consumed more whole grains, fruits, and vegetables and less refined "white" starches. Some of the best whole grains to eat are millet, quinoa, amaranth, buckwheat, brown rice, barley, oats, spelt, and whole-wheat berries. Choose a diversity of grains. Many of us eat too many wheat products, especially bread and pasta. We can all benefit by adding other grains to our diets. Amaranth, quinoa, and millet, for example, are delicious and actually have a much higher nutrient content than wheat.

Always use fresh whole-grain flour. Try to buy and eat grains in their whole form or consider buying a grain mill to grind flour fresh as you need it. The next best thing is to buy the whole-grain flour stored in the refrigerated section of your local health food store and keep it in the refrigerator or freezer at home. Much of the flour sold today has been sitting on the shelves for months. It is nutritionally inferior, has oxidized, and in many cases is rancid when you buy it. This is true even in natural food stores, when the flour is not refrigerated.

Recently, for the first time, a large study involving diet and breast cancer showed a relationship between an excess of starch intake, in the form of refined pasta and bread, and breast cancer.[17]

Protein

Dietary protein should be adequate, not excessive, to maintain nitrogen balance in a slightly positive state and to maintain lean body mass. Good digestion and assimilation of protein are also needed to build antibodies and a strong immune system. I believe that dietary protein intake should be in the range of 15 to 20 percent of total calories. Deficiencies in adequate protein digestion and assimilation are immunosuppressive. Studies have shown that protein calorie malnutrition is an important factor in the occurrence of pneumocystis carinii pneumonia in children being treated for cancer with chemotherapy.[18]

Protein foods should include fish, plenty of beans, lentils, and peas, plus a variety of whole grains, fresh nuts, and seeds, with an emphasis on almonds, sesame seeds, and Brazil nuts, the richest known source of selenium. As always with nuts and seeds, be sure you purchase them from a reliable source, as they are prone to rancidity. Other good protein sources are moderate amounts of fresh organic eggs and dairy products such as yogurt, goat cheese, and Parmesan cheese. As previously mentioned, goat's milk and goat cheeses are superior to cow's milk or regular cheeses, especially for the sick.

Organic Eggs

Organic eggs, because of their rich nutrient content and easy digestibility, are one of the best protein foods for people with cancer. One or two can be eaten one to three times per week; they are especially helpful when one is weak and needs to strengthen the digestive system. Eggs contain all eight essential amino acids and are rich in essential fatty acids. Although they are rich in cholesterol, they will not increase blood cholesterol to a dangerous level. In fact, when properly prepared, they are actually a good food for heart disease prevention because they contain eight times more lecithin than cholesterol. Besides protein, eggs are also rich in many vitamins and minerals, glutathione, sulfur, and phospholipids.

The best way to prepare eggs is to slow-cook them—soft-boiled or poached. They should never be cooked on high heat because heat reacts with fatty acids and forms dangerous trans fatty acids. Although eggs contain arachidonic acid (AA), which, as mentioned earlier, should generally be avoided, I feel that if the rest of the diet is high in omega-3 fatty acids and low in AA, moderate egg consumption will cause more good than harm.

Fish and Meat

Be sure to include fresh omega-3-rich fish like salmon and rainbow trout from clean waters in your diet two to four times each week. A recent study has shown that omega-3-rich fish oils impede angiogenesis and reduce tumor invasiveness.[19] Although a diet high in animal protein is not recommended, for some people moderate portions of animal protein once or twice a week can contribute to a well-rounded diet. I find that people who are anemic or have nutritional deficiencies sometimes need the type of nutritional profile that can be found only in meat. If meat is eaten, it should come from organically raised animals or wild game and always be hormone-free, especially for those whose cancer is of a hormone-receptor type, like breast cancer.

Nuts and Seeds

Nuts and seeds are another good protein source. Be sure to buy and eat nuts and seeds that are fresh, not rancid. Rancid nuts and seeds smell sour—not sweet and nutty as they should. Keep them in the refrigerator or freezer to preserve their freshness. They are rich in delicate essential fatty acids and protein as well as many vitamins and minerals. Organic nut butters, especially almond butter, are excellent nutritional sources. Flax, sunflower, pumpkin, and sesame seeds are all wonderful additions to a mixed salad. You can also grind flaxseeds and add them to salad dressings, cereals, or yogurt.

Yogurt

Lactic acid–rich foods, such as yogurt and fermented cabbage juice, can greatly enhance immune function and strengthen the intestines. Healthy bacteria in the intestines can resist many dangerous pathogens. Both the acidophilus and bulgaricus bacteria present in yogurt possess potent antitumor activity. Researchers have found that the dialyzate fraction of yogurt possesses the antitumor principals. Lactobacilli and bifidobacteria found in yogurt produce compounds within the colon that increase beta glucaronization and nitroreductase, which help the body to excrete carcinogens and hormones more efficiently. Researchers at the National Institute for the Study and Care of Cancers in Milan, Italy, found that the friendly bacteria found in yogurt inhibit not only gastrointestinal but also breast cancer.[20]

The gross protein value of yogurt is 9.5 percent greater than skim milk, from which it is made. Better protein availability leads to increased weight gain and higher food efficiency. Yogurt also contains higher levels of free-form amino acids than milk, mainly due to the proteolytic action of the lactobacilli. Studies have shown that the digestibility of the proteins in acidophilus milk, bifidus milk, yogurt, and buttermilk is improved because of the lactic acid produced by the fermentation process. *L. acidophilus* has also been shown to help prevent diarrhea in cancer patients who are receiving radiation therapy.

Soy Foods

Eat soybean products three to four times each week, particularly fermented soybean products such as miso, shoyu, tempeh, and natto. Their cancer-prevention properties exceed that of unfermented soybeans, soy milk, and tofu. During the fermentation process, innumerable valuable chemical reactions occur, resulting in the generation of many new substances. Fermented soy products are rich in isoflavones, including genistein, which has been shown to block the growth of a number of cancers, including prostate cancer. Soybeans are also an excellent source of protein.

I do not recommend eating commercially processed soy foods like soy grits, textured soy protein, and soy oil, which have been processed using hexane, a toxic chemical used frequently as an extraction agent by the food-processing industry.

General Guidelines for Protein Choices

Whenever possible, all foods should be organically grown. I realize that in today's world it is virtually impossible to eat 100 percent organic foods, but we need to strive for this and perhaps in so doing we will at least minimize the intake of contaminants. Also remember that not everyone will do well on the same diet. Individual constitutions and circumstances call for various dietary plans.

Fish: Two to four times a week. Salmon, halibut, trout, sole, cod. A diet that includes fish is, in general, the healthiest.

Soy foods: Three to four times a week. Tempeh, natto, tofu, miso, whole soybeans, soy milk, and tamari or shoyu (soy sauce).

Beans: Three to five times weekly. Lima beans, black beans, lentils, navy beans, kidney beans, white beans, aduki, chickpeas, and pinto beans, like soybeans, contain important isoflavones and protease inhibitors. Beans, because they do not contain all eight essential amino acids, are not considered a complete protein by themselves; however, by combining any dried bean with any whole grain, you will have a complete protein. This natural combination is found in many traditional diets throughout the world—tofu with rice in Asia, tempeh and rice in Indonesia, black beans and corn in South America, lentils and rice in India.

Seeds and nuts: Use sparingly throughout the week—make sure they are fresh and not rancid. Eat almonds, pecans, Brazil nuts, walnuts, sesame seeds, sunflower seeds, pumpkin seeds, flaxseeds, and milk thistle seeds in small snack-size portions of 1 to 2 ounces.

Eggs: One or two at a time—from one to three times a week. Eggs offer many of the ingredients needed to build and maintain health, including an abundance of high-quality protein and sulfur.

Yogurt: Eat only organic yogurt from reputable sources (see Shopping Guide, chapter 14) two to four times a week.

Cheese: Moderate intake of small portions (1 to 2 ounces) two to four times a week. Cottage cheese, some hard cheese, and Parmesan cheese. Goat cheese is preferable.

Meat: Because of its high-quality protein, meat in moderate amounts can fit into a healthy diet for those who enjoy it. I recommend eating organic meat in small portions (2 to 3 ounces) once or twice a week. Poultry, if eaten at all, should be organic without exception because of the growth hormones used in the feed of nonorganic chickens. Remember, each of us has different needs. Some require more animal protein, some less, and some need no animal protein at all. All of these high-protein foods should be organic or wild. Meat from wild animals or organically raised animals yields a much more nutrient-rich food and is far less toxic. Meat from wild animals contains higher amounts of protein and omega-3 fatty acids than commercially raised animals. Commercial meat is highly toxic because of the chemicals, growth hormones, antibiotics, and poor-quality food that is routinely fed to the animals. This is also true of nonorganic dairy foods.

Both meat and dairy do contain a potent anticancer fatty acid, conjugated linoleic acid (CLA), which has recently been shown to inhibit several cancer cell lines, including breast and colon cancer and melanoma. I personally have chosen not to eat meat, but I do eat plenty of fish, organic eggs, and organic dairy products.

Culinary Herbs

Herbs have antioxidant and antitumor activity. They also add wonderful flavor to food. Some common spices with antioxidant/antitumor agents include rosemary, sage, parsley, basil, oregano, marjoram, celery seed, caraway seed, orange and lemon peel, turmeric, nutmeg, clove, allspice, lavender, ginger, and burdock root. Common black pepper was historically used, as were many spices, to protect food (mostly meat) against rancidity and to cover up the taste if the food had already become semirancid. Black pepper exerts an antihepatotoxic effect by acting as a synergyst enabling other nutrients to perform their functions more effectively. It prolongs the life of antioxidants, allowing them to work for longer periods of time. For instance, taking black pepper with turmeric allows the turmeric more time to do its detoxification work in the liver.

Currently, a monoterpene extract found abundantly in the essential oil of lavender, referred to as *perillyl alcohol*, is showing great potential as an anticancer agent in clinical trials at the University of Wisconsin. Lemon grass and cumin contain farnesol, an isoprenoid that has been shown to inhibit tumor growth. Geranoil, one of the principal components of rose geranium oil, has slowed the growth of cancerous tumors in both human and animal cell cultures.[21] Milk thistle seeds, as well as turmeric, show great liver-protective effects against a number of toxins, including many chemotherapies. Milk thistle seeds can be bought at most natural food stores. Toast them lightly in a low-temperature oven for five minutes or put them in a dry pan and heat them on top of the stove, stirring with a wooden spoon until toasted. Sprinkle over salads or grain dishes—they are quite tasty.

Another common spice, used for several thousand years in the Far and Middle East, is black cumin. It is an annual herb with strong immunomodulating and interferonlike activity. Its active principal, nigellone, displays anticancer and immune-enhancing abilities. Studies have shown that 2 grams per day of this spice can significantly enhance cytotoxic T-cells and increase natural killer-cell activity. Black cumin in extract form inhibits cancer and endothelial cell progression and decreases the production of the angiogenic protein fibroblastic growth factor (FGF) produced by tumor cells. The fibroblastic growth factors contained in breast cancer, prostate cancer, and melanoma cells have all been shown to be suppressed by black cumin. The endothelial cells in these cancers reverted to a nonangiogenic state when exposed to the neutralizing influence of this common spice.[22]

It is amazing that so many common herbs and spices, used for centuries in traditional cooking, have such incredible promise for suppressing the initiation, progression, and invasion of cancer. (See table 3.3.)

Sea Vegetables

Learn to cook with various kinds of seaweed, or use them as condiments to sprinkle on your food. In some dishes, they can actually be used instead of salt. In fact, I suggest that seaweed be used in your daily diet as a salt substitute. You can use it in soups (miso soup with seaweed is a powerful cancer-fighting food), grain dishes, or salads or as a main vegetable. Dulse is delicious in salads.

Many species of seaweed, including wakame, kelp, and bladderwrack, have shown antitumor activity. Wakame has shown the strongest antitumor activity so far. Seaweed is nature's richest, most bioavailable source of organic iodine, a substance lacking in the average American diet and directly related to the high incidence of thyroid disorders. Many of my patients with ovarian or breast cancer are deficient in iodine and show signs of low thyroid function.

Seaweeds are also an excellent source of calcium and potassium and are rich in all minerals. They help in the removal of radioactive and toxic heavy minerals. I am thankful to herbalist Ryan Drum for teaching me the importance of this neglected food.

Table 3.3 Phytochemicals in Culinary Herbs

Phytochemical	Herb in Which Found	Action in Body
Phenolic diterpenes Carnosic acid Carnosol Rosmanol Ursolic acid	Rosemary Sage	Antioxidants, increase vitality and circulation; anticancer; cerebral antioxidant
Polyacetylenes	Parsley	Antioxidants
Thymol Carvacrol Rosmarinic acid	Basil Oregano	Antimicrobial agents
Phenol carboxylic acid Rosmarinic acid Acylated arbutin	Marjoram	Urinary tonics, antioxidants, anticancer
Phthalides	Celery seed	Moderate body's production of certain cancer-promoting substances
D-carvone	Caraway seed	Induces liver detoxifying enzymes; metabolizes and excretes carcinogens
Limonene Nomilin	Orange peel Lemon peel	Destroy cancer cells; increase metabolism of some cytotoxic drugs; antimutagenic
Curcuminoids	Milk thistle seed	Hepatoprotective effects against toxins, including many chemotherapies

Curcumin	Turmeric	Hepatoprotective; anticancer; anti-inflammatory; antioxidant
Eugenol	Nutmeg, clove, and allspice	Inhibits prostaglandin biosynthesis and suppression of thromboxane
Perillyl alcohol	Lavender	Antioxidants
Gingerol	Ginger	Antimutagenic
Lignans	Burdock root	Antitumor; antimutagenic
Acetic acid		
Piperine	Common black pepper	Antihepatotoxic synergist—makes other nutrients more bioavailable
Farnesol	Lemon grass	Inhibits tumor growth
	Cumin	
Geraniol	Rose geranium	Inhibits tumor growth

Super Green Foods

Chlorophyll, which gives plants their beautiful green color, is found in the chloroplast section of plant cells, where sunlight is converted to chemical energy in the process known as photosynthesis. Chlorophyll, like other plant pigments, is a powerful antioxidant and anticancer agent. In one study published in the journal *Mutation Research*,[23] chlorophyll proved to be a more effective antimutagen than all known anticancer vitamins, including vitamins A, C, and E. Chlorophyll works as an antioxidant and has an incredible ability to neutralize carcinogens such as aflatoxins.

Chlorophyll extracts have been shown to stimulate the growth of new skin tissue in wounds. Chlorophyll is especially active in wounds that refuse to heal using normal treatments. French scientists have shown that alfalfa can reduce damaged tissue caused by radiotherapy. Radiation burns have been repaired by other plants that contain significant amounts of chlorophyll, suggesting that this substance may be the common active constituent.

Chlorella

Chlorella is a one-cell blue-green alga that is highly nutritive as a food and also stimulates the immune system. It increases macrophage activity and has shown antitumor effects. Chorellan is a substance found in chlorella that stimulates interferon production. There are several papers on the prevention and/or inhibition of cancer using chlorella as well as documentation of its DNA repair mechanism.[24] One of the many benefits of chlorella is its ability to increase serum albumin levels. A drop in albumin level has many negative effects on the body. Of all the super green foods, chlorella is the one that impresses me the most.

Green Barley Grass

Young green barley leaves have potent pharmacological actions, including antioxidative activity, anti-inflammatory effects, and antiallergic activity. A flavonoid, 2-O-glycosyl isovitexin, was isolated and identified to be the major active component. Its antioxidant properties seem to be most active against lipid peroxidation, which means it can prevent fats in the body from oxidizing.

Fats and Oils

Lipids (fats and related substances) are essential components for proper cell communication and regulation. A major constituent of the cell membrane, lipids help give the membrane the permeability needed to maintain many cellular functions, including the fulfillment of the cell's nutritional needs, its metabolism, its genetic expression, and its capacity for intracellular, extracellular, and cell-to-cell communication. Unnatural and/or denatured fats, such as margarine or other hydrogenated oils, disrupt the metabolic process and interfere with the properties of the cell membrane. Oils must be fresh and not denatured in any way or they can become extremely volatile and dangerous, possibly causing and/or promoting cancer. These essential fatty acids can take on Jekyll and Hyde characteristics: They are vital and life-sustaining in their pure form, but dangerous and life-harming when processed.

In 1977, the World Health Organization issued a notice to all the nations of the world that the processed oils used in cooking and food preparation were of great danger to the health of all peoples. They even advocated legal action by governments against the production of such oils. Even though that warning was sounded more than twenty years ago, not one nation has taken any steps to outlaw the processing of oils or to formally warn people of their dangers.

Completely avoid all processed fats and oils or any foods containing processed oils, including hydrogenated or partially hydrogenated products. Just about all oils sold in supermarkets and any processed oils such as corn oil, safflower oil, or vegetable oil should be avoided completely. Cold-pressed olive oil is fine for all uses, but canola oil should be used only for baking because of the low temperatures involved. I do not recommend using canola oil in salads or for cooking at high temperatures because it is derived from a hard seed that requires technology for its processing—a fact that makes its purity suspect.

Flaxseed oil, rich in alpha-linolenic acid (ALA), and other related omega-3 fatty acids such as EPA-rich fish oil and evening primrose, borage, and black currant seed oils all contain gamma-linolenic acid (GLA), a substance found to kill a number of tumor-cell lines and cause a significant reduction in tumor growth in animal studies. Alpha-linolenic acid demonstrates significant anticancer properties, especially against breast cancer. Low levels of ALA were the first determinant of metastases and the most significant contributor to the spread of breast cancer in a recent study.[25]

Omega-3 fatty acids enhance the immune response in people with solid tumors by increasing T-lymphocyte production. Flaxseed oil, when taken with sulfur-rich proteins, such as yogurt or cottage cheese, forms a lipo-protein combination with a highly active electron system, which enables the free fatty acids in the flaxseed oil to penetrate the tumor-cell membrane and exert its cytotoxic activity. Meanwhile, the body's vital functions are also activated and enhanced by feeding healthy cells with these water-soluble electron-rich fatty acids.

Because of the delicate nature of ALA, flaxseed oil should only be used raw, never for cooking, and always kept refrigerated, away from heat or light. Flaxseed oil is always dated; check the label for date of pressing and date of freshness expiration. Recommended brands of flaxseed oil are Flora, Arrowhead Mills, Spectrum, and Barrens.

In addition to flaxseed oil, I also highly recommend using freshly ground flaxseeds (or flaxseeds that have been soaked in liquid overnight) and adding them to cereals or drinks. The lignans and/or their precursors, present in the whole seed, have demonstrated a broad spectrum of biological activities including antitumor, antimitotic, and antiviral activities. Some of the lignans found in flaxseeds that are being investigated as potential anticancer agents are gallic acid, ferulic acid, chlorogenic acid, and coumaric acid.

Choose unrefined nut or seed (such as sunflower and sesame) oils and extra virgin olive oil for your salads. An oil blend that I recommend as a salad oil (along with extra virgin olive oil) is called Udo's Choice, formulated by Udo Erasmus and made by Flora. It is available in most health food stores. Flaxseed oil and olive oil can also be combined in a basic salad dressing mix. (See chapter 14.)

In a double-blind, randomized, controlled trial, twelve healthy volunteers who were not at risk for colon cancer took either fish oil or corn oil supplements for four weeks. After a four-week rest, they switched to the opposite supplementation. There was a significant decrease in rectal cell proliferation after fish oil supplementation, compared to the corn oil supplementation. There was a reduction in the amount of tumor-promoting prostaglandin E2 released into the incubation medium from the biopsy specimens taken after fish oil supplementation, compared to those taken after corn oil supplementation. There was also a reduction in mucosal ornithine decarboxylase activity after fish oil supplementation. Ornithine decarboxylase is a tumor glycoprotein; increased levels of this enzyme have been seen in patients with familial colon polyps, who are at increased risk for colon cancer.[26]

I believe that the increased consumption of refined polyunsaturated fatty acids also plays a significant role in the rise of melanoma incidence in the United States. I discuss this further in chapter 8.

Juicing

Juicing is a wonderful and easy way to absorb a concentrated form of fresh fruits and vegetables. Many cancer clinics around the world use juice therapy as part of their treatment programs. The Gerson program was one of the first to emphasize freshly made juices for treating people with cancer. Juicing provides the most easily digestible and concentrated nutritional benefits of fruits and vegetables by eliminating much of the work of the body's digestive process.

Carrots, beets, apples, celery, and dark leafy greens are the most commonly used vegetables for juicing. Reliable brands of juicers are Acme and Olympic, which produce pulp-free juice, and Champion, which yields a pulpier juice.

Wheat grass, which is popular with many health food purists, can also be juiced but requires a special wheat grass juicer that can be purchased at most health food stores.

WATER

Drink spring water or filtered water. A good home filter system, such as Multi-Pure (see Resources), is a worthwhile investment. Fluoride, which is added to drinking water, has been banned in many countries and has been shown to be a risk factor in bladder cancer.[27]

It is important to drink water throughout the day—especially between meals. If you are drinking water with a meal, sip it between courses. While your food is being chewed, it should be mixed with saliva, not water or another beverage. This is essential for good digestion.

The amount of water needed by each individual can vary greatly. For instance, chemotherapy is a dehydrator and therefore calls for increased water consumption. On the other hand, someone who eats plenty of summer fruits, which usually contain high amounts of water, will not need to drink as much. The best advice is to learn to be aware of your body's needs. Drink before you become thirsty.

CHOOSE FOODS ACCORDING TO THE SEASON

Choose foods that are in season. Eat more raw foods and fresh fruits in the warmer months (during the spring, summer, and early fall) such as fresh salad greens, apricots, peaches, plums, cherries, and nectarines. During the colder months of fall and winter, eat more cooked foods, root vegetables, apples, and pears, as well as cooked greens like kale, brussels sprouts, and collard greens. After the first frost, these foods take on a whole new wonderful taste. Nature prepares certain foods to be ready at the exact time that we need them. It is no accident that citrus fruit ripens in the winter; that root vegetables drop their leaves, returning the energy into the roots at just the right time for them to be dug up for food; or that nuts that fall from the trees in autumn give us the important fatty acids that prepare us for the cold winter months.

Learn to optimize seasonal eating for healing too. For example, during the summer months, try a morning watermelon kidney flush. This is done by eating nothing but fresh watermelon for breakfast for three to seven days.

Other seasonal cleansing programs include fall programs, such as pears/apples/beets for the liver and gallbladder and grapes for blood detoxification, and winter programs, such as citrus cleanses, designed to detoxify the liver and gallbladder. Cleanses such as these should be supervised or guided by a nutritionist or health professional.

GOOD DIGESTION BEGINS IN THE MOUTH

Chew your food well and eat slowly. Food should not be swallowed until it is crushed and softened in the mouth. After being blended with saliva and swallowed, it enters the stomach prepared to mix with the many gastric juices that allow it to be broken down and assimilated as nourishment throughout the body. Antacids interfere with the digestive process. Those who lack the gastric juices needed for good digestion should take bitter herbs rather than antacids, which will only make matters worse. Dandelion, celandine, arugula, and watercress are helpful to digestion; they stimulate digestive juices and can be taken in a salad eaten before or after the main course. In the same way, lemon or vinegar mixed with oil (as in a salad dressing) helps to stimulate digestive juices that aid in breaking down fats.

Many people, particularly in America, consider mealtime a nonproductive time, which, therefore, should be finished as quickly as possible so one can go on to other, more important things. Another common bad habit is doing other things while eating—working, driving, reading, or watching television. It's not surprising that so many of us have digestive problems.

After you've shopped, prepared, and cooked your food with love and attention, there is still one more thing to do before taking the first bite. Remember to give thanks before you eat. May you enjoy all of your meals peacefully with relaxation and gratitude.

FOODS THAT ARE BAD FOR YOU

White Sugar, White Flour, White Salt

Avoid white sugar and white flour. Substitute Sucanat (pulverized whole sugar cane) for white sugar or use honey, rice syrup, and/or maple syrup as sweeteners. Substitute freshly ground whole grain flours for white flour. Substitute unrefined earth salt for refined salt and use sparingly. Sea salt has been refined and offers very little, if any, benefit over regular salt. Unrefined earth salt, such as Earth Salt by Herb Pharm (see Resources), which has a light pink color, contains many minerals other than sodium, and is acceptable when moderately used.

Over the past twenty-five years, intake of both artificial sweeteners and sugar has increased dramatically in America. Artificial sweetener consumption has jumped to about 25 pounds per year (up 5 pounds per person per year), and sugar intake has increased from 120 pounds to 140 pounds per person per year.

About 20 percent of calories in the typical American diet come from refined sugar. Thus, it is not surprising that so many manifest poor glucose tolerance curves, exacerbated by stress, low chromium and fiber intake, and sedentary lifestyles. Elevated blood glucose can cause hyperinsulinemia or insulin resistance, a condition that reduces the level of sex-hormone-binding globulin, and/or changes the regulation of insulinlike growth factor-1. Both of these are possible risk factors for hormone-dependent cancers. Insulin resistance can divert prostaglandin pathways toward tumor-promoting PGE-2, which is immune-suppressive, aggregatory, and vasoconstrictive and inhibits the biosynthetic pathways of estrogen binders. This, in turn, can cause an overproduction of estrogen, which has a negative effect on both breast cancer prevention and treatment. A diet designed to maintain low blood-glucose levels can selectively starve tumors, yielding a lower insulin output to help regulate prostaglandin synthesis. Insulin deprivation will inhibit tumor growth and cell division.[28] This can be achieved by removing all processed sugars and starches from your diet. However, don't overdo the Sucanat or honey either; unrefined sugars should also be minimized as you strive to keep quality and balance in your diet.

Processed and Canned Foods

Avoid colorings, flavorings, and preservatives in your food. Don't eat any refined or processed foods and limit your intake of commercially prepared foods as much as possible. Fast foods of any kind should be avoided completely. It is best to eat at home whenever possible.

Avoid nonfat or low-fat processed foods. Your diet should consist primarily of foods like vegetables, fruits, and whole grains, which are naturally low in fat. Avoid processed foods that have had the fat removed.

Avoid all foods that contain Olestra. Olestra, approved by the FDA in January 1996, became the first calorie-free fat substitute. For the mass market, this seemed like a dream come true. Procter & Gamble, the manufacturer of Olestra, uses it in salad dressings, ice cream, potato chips, and cheese as well as in other packaged snack-type products. Olestra looks, tastes, and acts like real fat, but because the digestive tract cannot break it down, it travels the length of the gut without being absorbed or contributing any calories to the day's total intake. Unfortunately, Olestra is not without side effects. The noticeable side effects can include diarrhea, intestinal cramping, and flatulence. The not-so-noticeable side effects are more serious. Olestra, when traveling through the body, takes with it the fat-soluble vitamins A, D, E, and K, and it also reduces circulating levels of carotenoids, including beta-carotene and lycopene. As little as six potato chips containing 3 grams of Olestra can reduce the absorption of carotenoids by 38 percent.

Avoid canned foods. They are inferior to fresh in every way, including taste. Canned foods lack many important nutrients, and a significant percentage of cans (as high as 85 percent) are lined with a plastic coating. This is done to avoid flavor-altering chemical reactions between the cans and their contents, but the unfortunate result is that small amounts of an estrogenlike pollutant, called bisphenal-A (BPA), leach from the plastic coating into the food. Although the amount of BPA found in canned food is extremely low in comparison with the body's own production of estrogen, the problem lies in the body's struggle to break down BPA and metabolize it efficiently.

Harmful Cooking Methods

Frying, barbecuing, or broiling meat, poultry, or fish, especially when using polyunsaturated fats such as safflower or corn oil, can produce potential carcinogens called heterocyclic amines (HCAs), which have been linked with many forms of cancer. If you do occasionally fry food, use sesame seed oil, olive oil, or butter and do not cook to a point where your food becomes burnt or blackened.

Fats and Oils

Don't use margarine or any hydrogenated fats. Use mostly olive oil and sesame seed oil. Although butter and clarified butter are saturated animal fats, they are slow to oxidize and contain butyric acid, an anticancer agent. Therefore, they are acceptable in moderation. In Ayurvedic teaching, ghee (clarified butter) is said to protect food from deteriorating, possessing a special capacity for picking up the medicinal benefits of the herbs and carrying them into the body. Olive oil, a monounsaturated fat, does not oxidize easily and is also a good source of squalene, the most potent inhibitor of angiogenesis (see chapter 5). Sesame oil, both unroasted and roasted, contains antioxidants that inhibit lipid peroxidation. Among the antioxidant constituents in sesame oil are the lignanphenols sesamol, sesamolinol, and sesaminol.

Buy only unrefined cold-pressed polyunsaturated vegetable oils, but do not use them in cooking. When exposed to air, heat, and light, these oils oxidize long before you can smell their rancidity. This oxidized form of polyunsaturated fat can cause increased levels of arachidonic acid and prostaglandin E2, which in turn can induce lipid peroxidation and abnormal cell growth. Eventually, this can lead to or promote cancer or other chronic diseases.

To explain further, oils that are polyunsaturated fatty acids naturally occur as healthful cis fatty acids in their double bonds. However, because of their delicate nature, they are subject to change through exposure to oxygen, light, and/or heat into harmful trans fatty acids. Trans fatty acids, which are not found in nature, incorporate themselves into the cell walls, altering the cell membranes and making them more permeable. This can lead to abnormal hormonal extracellular stimuli and the eventual promotion of breast cancer.

Women with a higher intake of trans fatty acids have more than three times the breast cancer risk than women with a low intake of these denatured polyunsaturated fats.[29] This cancer-causing artificial fat is contained in margarine, all commercial oils found in the supermarket, commercial cookies, crackers, snack foods, frozen foods, deli foods, mayonnaise, fried foods, and all foods labeled "partially hydrogenated." Read your labels carefully.

Beverages

Coffee

Cancer patients should avoid coffee. For those in good health, however, organic coffee is fine in moderation. Make sure that the beans are fresh and use drip-grind coffee rather than French-roast for less mutagenic potential (the French-roast method is stronger and uses higher heat). A good substitute for coffee is green tea or other herbal teas (e.g., nettles, dandelion, licorice, orange peel, red clover). Green tea infusion contains catechin polyphenols, which are nonspecific and broad-spectrum anticarcinogens. Black tea also contains some novel polyphenols called theaflavins, which occur through the oxidation process of green tea's catechins. Black tea's theaflavins and green tea's catechins are also strong inhibitors of HIV-reverse transcriptase.

Alcohol

Cancer patients should avoid alcohol. It depletes glutathione levels and stresses the liver. For healthy individuals, a glass of organic red wine with a meal is fine.

Wine is, after all, a rich source of two very important anticarcinogens—PCOs and resveratrol.

Smoking

Don't. Although smoking is not dietary, it often is associated with food and drink. The numerous deleterious effects of smoking and its links to cancer and heart disease do not need to be reemphasized here. Countless studies show significant increases in risk for cancers of the lung, bladder, esophagus, stomach, and pancreas in smokers as compared to nonsmokers. The relative risk factor of lung cancer for smokers versus nonsmokers is 13.6.[30] Among other harmful substances, cigarettes contain cadmium, a toxic metal present in tobacco smoke that accumulates in smokers. It is believed to be responsible for a significant amount of the harm caused by smoking. Other than as garden compost, there appears to be no safe way to use tobacco.

FASTING

One important aspect of improving health is increasing your body's ability to detoxify. Fasting can be one of the best and quickest ways to increase the elimination of wastes and enhance the healing process. It is very important that you

- Pick the right time to fast
- Fast for the right length of time
- Choose the right type of fast
- Support your body's detoxification and elimination processes with the appropriate nutritional and herbal program (most important of all)

Nutritional and herbal support is necessary during a fast because stored toxins, particularly in fat cells, are released into the blood and lymph system and brought to the liver for processing. These toxic substances, for example, the pesticide DDT, can reach toxic blood levels, cause toxemia to the blood and lymph system, and stress the nervous system. If you are going to fast, it is important that you be professionally guided by an experienced health care provider.

4

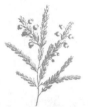

Herbal Medicine, Healing, and Cancer

Each tree, shrub, and herb, down even to the grasses
and mosses, agreed to furnish a remedy for some one of
the diseases named, and each said: I shall appear to help
man when he calls upon me in his need.

—*Cherokee prayer*

For hundreds, if not thousands of years, herbs have been esteemed for their healing value. Today, however, with the advent of modern medicine, herbs are considered inferior to drugs in many of the "developed" nations. In the United States, for example, most physicians consider herbs "unproven remedies," an ineffective relic of a primitive, unenlightened past.

I believe that herbs—growing in our gardens, around our homes, in fields, woods, and even in the cracks of city sidewalks—are God's wonderful gift to us. I often see burdock, red clover, dandelion, and plantain popping up in the most polluted places. They are manifesting in those places to heal the environment as well as each of us. In their simplicity, herbs offer us so much—food, comfort, and healing when we are sick. It is often the healing weeds—the ones we spend so much time, effort, and money attempting to eradicate from our lawns—that have the most to give. I keep these thoughts in mind as I prepare herbal compounds for my clients; I give God thanks, asking in my heart that those who take them be blessed and healed by them.

Charged with sunlight and alive with life, herbs have healing powers that synthetic drugs do not possess. In their humble way, they can contribute so much to the health and healing of those afflicted with cancer, stimulating the body's internal healing response and restoring equilibrium on all levels.

Herbs differ from drugs in that they work harmoniously with the body's innate capacity to heal, supporting the immune system rather than suppressing it as many drugs tend to do. When using herbs, however, certain cautions apply; for example, a few herbs can be toxic and should only be used with extreme care under the guidance of an experienced practitioner. Certain herbs should not be used during pregnancy, by those with high blood pressure, or when taking specific medications.

This being said, herbs given in proper dosage, as prescribed by a qualified professional, generally have fewer and less harmful side effects than many drugs, especially those drugs used in the treatment of cancer. When a drug company labels a particular herb toxic, it may only be partially true. The company's lab may have isolated one of the plant's components and found it to have harmful effects. However, what is not understood is the synergistic interplay among the plant's various components that tends to modify an isolated component's toxic effects and render the whole plant not only safe, but often healing. When reading information about herbs, it is important to be aware of the source. Some information can be misleading because it is written by people who do not have expertise in the medical use of plants.

Just as the healing potency of an herb depends on the interplay of its components, so too the potency of an herbal compound, consisting of various herbs, depends on the synergy among the herbs used. The purpose of prescribing a compound is to provide a protocol or formula that possesses entirely new capabilities beyond those of any individual herb the formula contains. Every protocol I prepare is unique to the individual client. It is also subject to change in strength and number of dosages over the course of treatment, depending on the client's health status.

This chapter presents the theory and practice of herbal healing, especially as it pertains to cancer. It covers classifications and descriptions of useful plants in the treatment of cancer, including mushrooms and sea herbs, and offers various healing formulas, plus general guidelines for some of my own.

THE EFFICACY OF HERBAL TREATMENT FOR CANCER

When I prescribe herbs and herbal tonics, I am often asked how they work and whether there are any scientific studies that validate their effects. The answer is that though there are not many studies of herbs in the modern medical literature, certain herbs and herbal remedies have historically been proven curative in certain diseases not just once or twice, or even in hundreds of cases, but in thousands—and not just for one or two years, or even hundreds of years, but for thousands of years.

Of course, for herbs to be truly effective, it is important for practitioners who work with them to study the action, dosage, and energetics of each herb in addition to knowing for which diseases it is curative. This requires careful study of the *materia medica*, but this alone is not enough. It is also essential to understand the client's symptoms as well as her constitution and lifestyle—all the factors that make that client a unique individual. Of course, experience also counts. Even after twenty years of experience, having worked with thousands of people, many of them cancer patients, my knowledge about herbs continues to expand.

Chinese Herbal Treatments

Today, most of the research on the use of natural herbal compounds is being done abroad. For example, the Chinese government has funded an intensive study of traditional Chinese herbal medicine. There are thousands of herbal formulas currently being used for cancer treatment in China, and over four hundred of them are described in three recently published books by M.Y. Chang, J.W. Yang, Y.Y. Hu, and M.S. Xuan. Most Chinese medicinal herbs and their combinations have been used for many hundreds of years, and I use many of them in my own practice. I am always astounded, therefore, when someone (sometimes a physician treating one of my patients) claims there is no evidence or proof that herbs are beneficial; that they may, in fact, be potentially dangerous; and are, in any case, a waste of money.

Fu-zheng

One Chinese herbal system, called *fu-zheng*, is widely used in Chinese hospitals as an adjunct to radiation and chemotherapy for cancer; in more progressive U.S. hospitals, it is beginning to be used in the same way. Fu-zheng successfully protects the immune system and increases survival rates by enhancing the effectiveness of radiation and chemotherapy without negative side effects. Interestingly, fu-zheng literally means to promote or enhance the natural host defense mechanism by strengthening one's resistance.

Studies show that a full 91.5 percent of patients in China who received both chemotherapy and fu-zheng therapy responded with tumor shrinkage, compared to 46.9 percent of patients who received chemotherapy alone. Doctors at Beijing Institute for Cancer Research also found significant differences in response rates as well as survival times between the two groups. It is important to note that in every study conducted, the group receiving fu-zheng herbs plus chemotherapy showed more improvement and longer survival time than the group that received chemotherapy alone. When fu-zheng herbal therapy was used as an adjuvant to radiation therapy to treat pharyngeal cancer, the five-year survival rate was more than twice as high (53 percent) as in a group not receiving the herbs (24 percent).[1]

The most common herbs used in fu-zheng are blood-vitalizing herbs, including astragalus, milletia, reishi, panax ginseng, schizandra, jujube, ligusticum, hoelen, salvia, ho shou wu, cordyceps, atractylodis, and codonopsis. Studies continue to demonstrate that these herbs have a dramatic impact on the enhancement of an immune system weakened by chemo and radiation therapies. They not only protect the immune and endocrine systems but also inhibit such diseases as influenza, upper respiratory infections, fungal infections, and chemically induced hepatitis. These diseases can cause serious complications for the person with cancer, requiring an interruption in treatment and a course of antibiotics that can lead to diarrhea and other debilitating problems.

THE QUESTION OF STANDARDIZATION

The belief that the medical effect of an herb—like that of a pharmaceutical drug—is due to a single active ingredient is a common misconception. This notion is responsible for a move to standardize commercially sold herbs to the so-called active ingredient, making them more like drugs. I regard this trend with apprehension. We need to respect and honor each herb as perfect in its own right; separating its constituents can create problems.

For example, many people today are using the herb St. John's wort (*Hypericum perforatum*) as a natural remedy for depression. Most over-the-counter varieties of this product are standardized to the hypericin content but, as recent information on this sacred plant indicates, hypericin is not the ingredient responsible for its antidepressant effects. St. John's wort has many constituents, including a number of flavonoids, that together with hypericin have a powerful healing effect. We should never overlook the possibility that when we standardize an herb for an active ingredient, we may remove the other beneficial ingredients—ones that may, in fact, enhance the effectiveness of the active ingredient or reduce the potential side effects of the active ingredient when taken alone.

While many pharmaceutical companies today are taking an interest in the healing power of herbs, some focus only on isolating their bioactive substances. By making molecular modifications to an herb's bioactive substance, they can produce synthetic products that can become proprietary or exclusive in terms of patenting.

These products have both benefits and drawbacks. On the plus side, some of the most effective cancer-fighting drugs have been developed from isolate components of herbs. For example, the vinca alkaloids, vinblastine and vincristine, two of the most widely used antineoplastic agents, come from the herb periwinkle (*Catharanthus roseus*). Vinblastine is used mostly for Hodgkin's disease, germ-cell cancers of the testis, and nonsmall-cell lung cancer. Vincristine is used for acute leukemia in children and adults, and has played an important role in combination therapies for Hodgkin's disease, non-Hodgkin's lymphoma, Ewing's sarcoma, neuroblastoma, multiple myeloma, and breast cancer.

Using plant-derived drugs such as the vinca alkaloids is the most aggressive way to treat a person with cancer, and the good news is that it can work well against fast-growing cancers. The bad news is that this is not always the best approach for less aggressive forms of cancer. In fact, many people who have the disease die from the cytotoxic agents used to treat them rather than from the cancer itself.

My hope is that someday cytotoxic, plant-derived drug agents will be combined with all the plant's constituents, thus making a full-spectrum medicine. Using this for cancer patients would spare the healthy cells without compromising the effectiveness of the drug on cancerous cells.

MY HERBAL PHILOSOPHY

As I've already mentioned, part of my protocol for each client I see is an individualized herbal compound that consists of a variety of herbs. Whatever condition the compound addresses, its primary purpose is to increase the client's vitality and restore immune function. I believe an appropriate herbal compound will:

1. Be more effective than a single herb because of the synergistic effect of many herbs when combined.
2. Address a number of symptoms as well as organ systems.
3. Mitigate any side effects that the principal components might have when taken as a single agent. (Some herbs can be very toxic when used alone but can be safely used when combined with other herbs that lessen their effects.)

Each compound I prescribe is dicatated by the patient's signs and symptoms. I strive to combine my understanding of individual typology with my knowledge of herbal energetics and the specific indications for an herb. This is more challenging than prescribing a specific herb to treat a certain ailment—say, for example, saw palmetto for prostate problems or ginkgo biloba for memory loss. However, it greatly enhances the accuracy and success of an herbal prescription because it takes into account factors other than the presenting ailment that may also affect the client's health.

For example, when I treat a woman with breast cancer, I choose an herbal combination that has many functions. It contains one or two antitumor agents that are effective against that particular cell line, some immune-enhancing plant agents together with detoxifying herbs that improve lymphatic and liver function, herbs that work on altering the cancer-promoting agents (in this case, hormones), herbs to enhance endocrine function (particularly thyroid function), plus herbs that will strengthen the woman's constitution. I do not have a "one-size-fits-all" formula for breast cancer. The compound for each breast cancer patient I see addresses the particular features of that woman's typology. I believe that this approach holds the best possibility of success in both treating cancer and preventing its recurrence. It is multifaceted and completely individual—just like each human being.

Especially when dealing with cancer, I believe it is important to consider the whole person rather than treating the condition with a disease-driven protocol. It is important to understand the client's constitutional patterns and biological individuality; to pay attention to diet, digestion, and sleep patterns; to get a sense of the client's mind, heart, and soul as well as body. This is the part of healing to which I am most drawn and in which I feel most gifted.

Often I am asked, "What is the pharmacological action of this herb?" or "What are the herb's active constituents?" Although these are concerns of mine and I strive to learn all the technical information I can, I believe it is also important to keep in mind that herbs have unique energetic qualities, and for each herb there are many applications. Although herbs can be used specifically for certain organ system imbalances, the true nature of herbs is constitutional. That's why, when I work with cancer patients, not only do I give each one an individualized formula, but I also pay attention to changing the formula as the individual's state of health progresses.

I believe that herbalism is both an art and a science. At its best, it is based on the following:

1. The latest scientific knowledge.

2. Historical knowledge (one must be proficient in the herbal *materia medica*).

3. The herbal medical system one is working within, such as TCM (Traditional Chinese Medicine) or American Eclectic medicine.

4. An innate intuitive ability (openness to listening inwardly for a sudden idea, a definite judgment, or a grasped meaning).

5. The virtue of patience—through patience so much is revealed.

6. A refined ability to improvise and be a "good cook." Knowing how to mix and match herbs for various effects, how to create formulas, how to prescribe supplements, and how to offer specific dietary guidelines are all necessary when formulating individual protocols.

7. Years and years of practice performed in humble goodwill to help people heal.

These seven factors are the basis of herbal wisdom, a state quite different from herbal knowledge. Practitioners who have developed such wisdom have a great deal of freedom to use their innate intuition and healing abilities in their practice. They know hundreds of applications for most herbs and understand their essential energetic qualities and how to use them constitutionally as well as for specific organ systems. This gives them many options when developing a protocol for a specific client.

Treating people individually, understanding each herb's energetic characteristics, and having the ability to relate them to the energetic characteristics of each client appear to be forgotten arts, even among holistic practitioners. Today, some are caught in the same "one-size-fits-all" approach as allopathic doctors, who tend to treat the disease and not the individual. I believe their clients would benefit greatly if these practitioners challenged themselves to delve deeper into the lives of their clients. By recognizing their clients' unique needs, they would be able to offer them the very best care from every perspective.

Three Stages of Cancer Therapy

In treating people with cancer, I have found that generally they need tonic therapy first to strengthen the vital force and the immune system. Second, they need liver and lymphatic detoxification, and third, cytotoxic therapy. As a rule, tonic therapy and liver detoxification are not available through conventional medicine, and its cytotoxic methods—radiation and chemotherapy—tend to suppress rather than enhance the patient's vital force.

In each stage of therapy I use two classifications of herbs:

Stage 1: Tonic Therapy
- Herbs that strengthen the individual's constitution and vitality
- Tonic herbs, adaptogens, and herbal immune enhancers

Stage 2: Liver and Lymph Detoxification
- Antioxidant, liver-detoxifying, anti-inflammatory, and antiangiogenic herbs
- Alternatives and lymphatics

Stage 3: Cytotoxic Therapy
- Gene-repairing, enzyme-inhibiting, and cytotoxic herbs
- Herbs that can alter the action of hormonal receptor-type cancers

See Herbal Classifications and Strategies beginning on page 96 for information about specific herbs that may be appropriate at each stage of therapy, depending on the individual being treated.

HERBAL MEDICINE AND THE IMMUNE RESPONSE

The Basics

This section explains some of the mechanisms by which herbs can be useful in the treatment and prevention of cancer.

Just twenty years ago, scientists had only fragments of information about how the many cells of the immune system interact to protect against disease. Through advances in cancer research, scientists now believe there are more than 100 million immune cells. There seems to be an immune cell specifically designed to hunt down and destroy every virus or bacterium. This relatively new understanding is leading to new ways of looking at defense mechanisms that can be used against diseases like cancer. With the use of advanced technologies, scientists are developing drugs and techniques that modify the body's immune responses. However, herbal researchers and traditional herbalists already know many herbs that work in harmony with the immune system in an equally remarkable way.

The immune system is the body's way of defending itself against invasion by foreign substances (pathogens). The immune response involves the coordinated efforts of several types of white blood cells. Invaders like viruses, bacteria, fungi, and protozoa all invoke and activate our immune system through a complex process to rid the body of pathogens. Once a pathogen causes the immune system to react, it is considered an antigen. Antigens are endogenous or exogenous substances that are alien to the body and induce an immune response that eventually leads to the formation of a specific antibody. Antibodies are soluble proteins produced by B-lymphocytes that bind to specific antigens.

The immune system is a complex array of organs, cells, and molecules distributed throughout the body. Each part of the system contributes to the growth, development, or activation of lymphocytes, the sophisticated white blood cells that originate in bone marrow and play a major role in the immune response. Some lymphocytes migrate to the thymus, where they develop into specialized types of immune cells. Some of these specialized cells gather in lymph nodes and other immune organs, including the spleen, tonsils, adenoids, appendix, and small intestine. Meanwhile, other white blood cells circulate throughout the blood and lymphatic vessels. Lymphatic vessels transport lymph, a colorless fluid that carries microorganisms and dead cells from distant infections into lymph nodes where they can be eliminated. Lymphatic vessels also transport white blood cells to infection sites throughout the body.

There are two general branches of the immune system that work together: humoral immunity and cell-mediated or cellular immunity. Humoral immunity relies on production of the antibodies produced from white blood cells, called *B-lymphocytes*. B-lymphocytes create a specific antibody for a specific antigen and form a memory that allows it to always remember that particular antigen and to be able to engulf and destroy it. With each exposure to an antigen, the immune system forms B- and T-"memory" cells. After recovery from chicken pox, for example, the immune system stores a few B- and T-memory cells for chicken pox. The next time the virus is contracted, memory cells multiply rapidly to stop the infection before it starts.

Vaccines work because of the immune system's ability to "remember." Memory cells can provide immunity for years, sometimes even for a lifetime. In the process of vaccination, dead or weakened live forms of an infectious organism stimulate the response of antibodies without causing the accompanying illness, but also without activating a cell-mediated immune response.

I believe that this weakens our overall immune system, fooling it into responding to a particular antibody response while perhaps causing confusion when the immune system is confronted with other unrecognized invaders or, even more disastrous, self-produced genetically damaged cells that are proliferating. In other words, it's possible that the immune system may fail to attack viral or cancerous cells because it is waiting for a vaccine to cause an antibody response rather than immediately issuing its own cell-mediated response (which, by the way, may cause an immune reaction without ever forming antibodies). More than a hundred years ago, Eli Jones considered vaccinations a significant cause of the rise in cancer, second only to the effects of fear and unrelenting stress to the nervous system.

Recently, there has been a significant increase in vaccine research. Scientists are trying to create specific vaccines for particular cancers and have already had some success in developing a vaccine to treat B-cell lymphoma. I'm sure research will continue in this area, although I am not very optimistic about major breakthroughs.

Cellular immunity, on the other hand, is the part of the immune system that is primarily responsible for the destruction of infected cells and tumor cells. Cellular immunity is made up of three broad categories of white blood cells: macrophages, natural killer (NK) cells, and T-cells. Many of the symptoms we feel when getting sick—like achiness and fever—are caused by activation of the immune system and not by the infection itself. This is why it is important to work with these symptoms and not suppress them. Cellular immunity relies on T-lymphocytes to activate the immune system. T-cells are made up of T-helper cells (also called CD-4 cells) and cytotoxic T-lymphocytes (also called T-suppressor cells and CD-8 cells). T-helper cells help and/or orchestrate the immune system. They help recognize the antigen and then bind it to the macrophage. They also make decisions about what type of immune response is appropriate.

The second group of T-cells, the CD-8 cells, destroy target cells and are responsible for down-regulating or suppressing an immune response. They turn off an activated immune system after it has finished its work in fighting an infection. Many people with AIDS who have a high level of CD-8 cells appear to live free of infections even when, overall, their T-cell count is low.

NK Cells, Granulocytes, and Cytokines

One form of white blood cells, natural killer (NK)-cells, are a class of trained assassins that bind to a target on a cell's surface and secrete cytotoxic substances that can destroy pathogens, such as viruses, as well as tumor cells. NK cells also help to form an antibody response by creating a cell-surface receptor. NK cells present the first line of defense against metastatic spread of tumors, so modulation of NK cells is crucial to cancer inhibition.

Another group of white blood cells, granulocytes, are made up of three particular cells called neutrophils, eosinophils, and basophils. Neutrophils are in charge of responding to a bacterial infection. Many people who are on chemotherapy develop neutropenia (low neutrophil count), which makes them susceptible to bacterial infections. Eosinophils are more involved in responding to parasitic infections or allergic responses. Basophils play a key role in allergic responses by forming mast cells that secrete inflammatory chemicals within the body, such as histamine, serotonin, and hesparin. Quercetin, found in many herbs and foods like onions, inhibits inflammation and allergic reactions through its ability to control mast cells.

The final important group of white blood cells, cytokines, are a diverse group of growth-regulating chemicals within the immune system that act as the local controllers of intracellular communication, playing major roles in cell immunity, growth, development, and apoptosis or cell death. Cytokines can affect cell growth both positively and negatively. For example, certain cytokines can stimulate cell growth in a manner that can block apoptosis while others can inhibit cell growth or initiate apoptosis. The cytokine families consist of interleukins, colony-stimulating factors, interferons, and growth factors. Because they are involved in cancer development and inhibition, modulation of cytokines is an important step in controlling cancer. What makes herbs so uniquely effective for this task is that they are modulators and understand the complexity of the body's innate healing capabilities. Their role is not to dictate to the immune system the way pharmaceutical drugs do, but instead to orchestrate, enhance, and direct the immune system to function optimally.

When activated, cytokines (which are then referred to as lymphokines) can activate other white blood cells, the monocytes and lymphocytes. Once monocytes and lymphocytes are activated, they become *macrophages*. Carbohydrate-proteins, called *mucopolysaccharides*, which are found in many herbs, such as echinacea and reishi mushrooms, not only activate macrophages but actually help them to bind to the antigen or tumor cell.

A healthly immune system can activate itself so efficiently that infected cells are destroyed and removed before they have a chance to develop into an illness. Herbs help the immune system in the fight against a serious illness like cancer; moreover, by keeping the immune system strong and vital, they can also help inhibit other pathogenic illnesses. Many people with cancer or AIDS die of secondary infections rather than the primary illness itself because their immune systems are compromised.

The stimulation of immune response is an important factor with regard to fighting cancer, but a serious problem arises when the cancer has multiplied and taken hold in the body. Because cancer seems able, to some degree, to hide itself from the immune system, it does not invoke as much immune response as it should. Helping this response along, therefore, is important. I sometimes recommend diaphoretic herbs, such as boneset, yarrow, and peppermint, along with hot Epsom salt baths, to activate a lymphatic-immune response. The immune system plays a critical role in preventing cancer by searching out and destroying newly transformed cells, a process referred to as immune surveillance.[2]

Summary of Basic Immune Cells and Their Functions

• B-cells and T-cells are white blood cells that bear the major responsibility for the immune response. They recognize and coordinate attacks against specific organisms.

• B-cells work by producing antibodies. Each B-cell is designed to make a specific antibody. Each antibody is designed to battle a specific microorganism. B-cells also develop into plasma cells that secrete thousands of identical antibodies.

• T-cells coordinate immune defenses and kill organisms in cells on contact. They also function by secreting potent chemicals called lymphokines, which direct the immune response. Lymphokines are particularly good at attacking cancerous cells or those infected by viruses.

• Phagocytes (from the Greek word meaning "eaters") are activated white blood cells whose main function is to gobble up everything that is unwanted by the body, from a speck of dust or pollen to a potent virus.

• Macrophages are a particular variety of phagocytes that play a versatile role. As scavengers, they rid the body of worn-out cells and other debris. They also play a vital role in initiating the immune response.

• Other white blood cells—neutrophils, eosinophils, and basophils—are also called cell-eaters. They release powerful chemicals that destroy microorganisms.

How Herbs Help Us Heal

Herbs, unlike man-made drugs, can assist the immune system throughout its entire response to an invader. One common way herbs intercede is by modulating, activating, and potentiating macrophages and T-cells to do a better and more efficient job in whatever area they are needed within this complex system. Drugs, or any man-made agents, can't do this. A plant, which is a living and breathing entity, has the ability to understand and work in synchrony with the body's internal needs, in harmony with the vital force within us, to heal and give life.

Immune activation is only one way that herbs, and many other foods as well, fight cancer. Cancer, because its inception and growth is a multistage process, provides many possible points of intervention where herbs can be used for their various anticarcinogenic activities. The following section gives some examples.

ANTICARCINOGENIC ACTIVITY OF PHYTOCHEMICALS IN HERBS AND FOODS

Many commonly used herbs, plants, fruits, and vegetables have been shown to possess cancer chemopreventive effects within their diverse pharmacological properties. Since cancer usually evolves over a long period of time, agents that inhibit or retard one or more of its stages could affect the overall course of the disease. Certain micronutrients (like the polyphenolic compounds found in tea) possess potent cancer-preventive abilities.

The blocking and suppressing agents found in specific herbs and foods (see table 4.1) are capable of the following anticancer activities:

- Inhibition of cancer formation by blocking or diverting carcinogenic material away from the cell, allowing it to be metabolized by the liver to a less toxic, more excretable substance.
- Prevention of cancerous substances reacting with the cell's DNA by meeting the carcinogen before it can do any damage and enhancing its excretion through metabolism.
- Repair of DNA that has been damaged by carcinogens.
- Retardation of cancer promotion by decreasing or turning off promotional factors that would otherwise be used for cancer promotion and proliferation.

One of the most important effects of the blocking agents found in herbs and foods is the inhibition of tumor formation by curbing the arachidonic acid cascade (see table 4.2). This effect is particularly evident in high-quality fats

Table 4.1 **Blocking Agents That Inhibit Carcinogenesis**

Blocking Agent	*Herb or Food Where Found*
Aromatic isothiocyanates	Broccoli
Curcuminoids	Turmeric
Coumarins	Red clover, dong quai
Conjugated dienolinoleic acid	Meat, dairy, whole milk yogurt (organic only and in small amounts)
Dithiolethiones	Brussels sprouts
Ellagic acid	Pomegranates, berries, nuts
Flavones	Licorice, ginkgo, onions
Glycyrrhetinic acid and related triterpenoids	Licorice
Glucarates	Yogurt
Indoles	Cabbage
Organosulfides	Garlic, broccoli, cabbage, brussels sprouts
Phenols (catechin)	Green tea
Tannins	Black tea, green tea
Terpenes	Aromatic oils, orange peel, lemon peel, rosemary

Table 4.2 **Blocking Agents Effective Against Tumor Promotion**

Blocking Agent	*Herb or Food Where Found*
Curcuminoids	Turmeric
Chalcones	Quercetin
Flavonoids	Grape seed extract, hawthorn
Glycyrrhetinic acid and related triterpenoids	Licorice
Inhibitors of arachidonic acid metabolism	Ginger, turmeric, boswellan, omega-3 fatty acids
Organosulfides	Garlic, onions
Phenols (catechin)	Green tea
Protease inhibitors	Soy, legumes
Tannins	Black tea, green tea

Table 4.3 **Suppressing Agents Effective Against Exposure to Carcinogens**

Suppressing Agent	Herb or Food Where Found
Aromatic isothiocyanates	Broccoli
Epigallocatechin gallate	Green tea
Inhibitors of arachidonic acid cascade	Turmeric
Inositol hexaphosphate	Legumes, grains
Protease inhibitors	Soy products
Terpenes	Orange peel

that include omega-3 fatty acids. Studies showing the ability of arachidonic acid inhibitors to prevent carcinogenesis have been more prevalent than studies of any other group of agents (with the possible exception of retinoids). Another important feature of blocking agents is their ability to prevent the attack of oxygen radicals. For example, the phenolic and polyphenolic compounds found in green tea are potent antioxidants. Their ability to inhibit cancer, however, is multifunctional and includes the capacity to activate certain detoxifying systems.

Suppressing Agents

Suppressing agents prevent the evolution of cancer in cells previously exposed to doses of carcinogenic agents (see table 4.3). They do this by:

- Preventing the endogenous formation of attacking molecules and/or inactivating those that might have already formed.
- Directly counteracting the consequences of genotoxic events.
- Producing differentiation.
- Selectively inhibiting cellular proliferation of potential cancer cells.

HERBAL CLASSIFICATIONS AND STRATEGIES

In this section, descriptions of some of the herbs commonly used to treat cancer are classified according to their primary actions. I generally prescribe herbs in the first two classifications—herbs that strengthen the individual's constitution and vitality and tonic herbs, adaptogens, and herbal immune enhancers—at the first stage of treatment, Tonic Therapy. Next, I prescribe herbs for the second stage, Liver and Lymph Detoxification. These are the herbs classified as antioxidant, liver-detoxifying, anti-inflammatory, antiangiogenic, alternative, and lymphatic. The third stage of treatment, Cytotoxic Therapy, includes herbs classified as gene-repairing, enzyme-inhibiting, and cytotoxic and, if needed, herbs that can alter the action of hormonal receptor-type cancers.

I have also included descriptions of herbs to treat specific symptoms of the cancer itself or the side effects of chemotherapy or radiation. It is important to keep in mind that while the herbs in this section are grouped according to their primary actions, individual herbs have many uses and, when combined, they have even more. There are as many combinations for unique formulas as there are herbs. This is why it is so important when taking herbs to work with a qualified herbalist or natural health care professional who is knowledgeable about herbs.

Herbs That Strengthen an Individual's Constitution and Vitality

Before prescribing herbs, it is important to assess the patient's vital state and nerve power. This evaluation takes many things into consideration:

- How is the patient's nervous system affected by stress?
- Where are the weaknesses of the endocrine system—adrenal glands, thyroid, reproductive organs?
- How does the patient's personality affect his or her overall health status?
- What hereditary patterns, if any, apply?
- What organ system weaknesses have manifested?
- Tongue diagnosis—for information about digestive function.
- Pulse diagnosis—for information about the vital state, including the strength or weakness of the individual.
- Eye diagnosis—for information about the health of the blood and vital organs.
- Urine evaluation—for information about the patient's constitutional health status.

When evaluating an individual, it is essential to be able to differentiate between conditions that impede function and those that reflect the positive eliminative or reconstructive action by the vital force. For example, in the case of an ulcerating tumor, do we stop it or assist in the body's elimination of necrotic tissue? Or in the case of a fever, at what point do we use antipyretics (to reduce the fever) as opposed to diaphoretics (to help it along)? It is sometimes difficult to know how to proceed, but one of the best indicators of the proper course to take is always the patient's condition. For instance, a person with high vitality and a good pulse can withstand a high fever while the fever kills cancer cells, but for someone who is weak, this may not be an option. The secret of good herbal and nutritional therapies is to recognize the vital resources inherent in the unique constitution of each individual. Descriptions of herbs to strengthen the constitution and vitality follow.

Pulsatilla *(Anemone pulsatilla)*

This herb, also called pasque flower, is often used as a remedy by homeopathic physicians but is seldom used by herbalists. The Eclectic physicians claimed it was very valuable, however, and found that the fresh plant extract was far more effective than any other preparation (perhaps because its life force was preserved). The Greek physician Pliny noted that the flower was named after the wind (*anemos*) because the flower, which is one of the first spring flowers to bloom, opened only when the wind blew. In many cultures, this plant represents the beginning of life.

I, too, have found pulsatilla to be a very beneficial remedy in the fresh extract form. Taken as a medicine to calm, soothe, and heal the nervous system, this herb is indicated when a person (either with or without cancer) is depressed and melancholy and is constantly anticipating death. There also tends to be much sadness and fear in such an individual, who usually weeps very easily. Usually the pulse of such a person is soft, open, and weak. It is indicated more frequently for women but may be used for men as well. I usually recommend a dose of 1 to 5 drops to be taken two or three times daily. It can be combined with other herbs. The nervous system must be healed before any other aspect of healing can take place; this is why pulsatilla is a friend (more like an angel) to many of the cancer patients I see.

St. John's Wort *(Hypericum perforatum)*

St. John's wort is a wonderful nervine, especially indicated for mild forms of depression with poor circulation and nerve injury. It can be used both internally and externally for nerve trauma. A specific for postoperative brain tumor surgery, it helps in three different ways:

1. It promotes healing from trauma and inflammation.
2. It helps with postoperative depression.
3. It acts as an inhibitor of neoplastic activity.

Hypericin, a constituent of *Hypericum*, possesses pronounced antiviral and antineoplastic activity. Many cancers involve a viral component in their initiation and promotion. Hypericin may be active against some of these cancers, including many forms of brain cancer. Hypericin will inhibit one form of leukemia that often occurs after radiation therapy.

Although hypericin can cause mild photosensitivity in high doses, its beneficial effects are light-dependent. It has been shown to inhibit protein kinase C and tyrosine kinase, both of which are important enzyme receptors involved in cancer-cell division.[3,4]

Besides the value of its components, hypericin and pseudohypericin, St. John's wort is also one of nature's richest sources of flavonoids, including quercetin.

Gotu Kola (*Centella asiatica*)

Gotu kola, native to India, is a popular medicinal plant in Ayurvedic medicine, the herbal tradition that has been practiced for centuries in India. Used for healing many skin afflictions, including leprosy, burns, eczema, psoriasis, and leg ulcers, gotu kola is also used to enhance mental concentration. It has a great ability to relax the brain, particularly when it is on overdrive and cannot focus efficiently. Many people, when told they have cancer, find it difficult to concentrate, in part because of the anxiety and fear associated with the disease, and also as a result of the many treatments and choices that are involved with having this illness.

Gotu kola is also used to treat mental retardation and many connective tissue diseases including lupus, scleroderma, cellulite, varicose veins, hemorrhoids, keloids, chronic urinary tract infections, as well as to aid in wound healing. The primary components in gotu kola are triterpenoids. Other constituents are various essential oils, fatty acids, sterols, and various polyactylene compounds. I believe this is one of the best herbs for people with cancer, and I now recommend its use more than ever before. Its benefits include:

• Promotion of healing in postoperative cancer surgery or postradiation therapy due to its ability to stimulate the rapid growth of the reticuloendothelial system. This increases healing, decreases inflammation, inhibits scar tissue formation, and inhibits the recurrence of cancer.

• Assists the nervous system with the stresses and fears associated with having cancer.

• Increases the formation of connective tissue components such as hyaluronan (also called hyaluronic acid), a natural substance produced by cells.

When large amounts of hyaluronan are produced, it can block the signals of ras, a cancer-causing gene, and stop the growth of tumor cells.

Dr. Eva Turley, of the University of Manitoba in Toronto, Canada, has found that a cell receptor called RHAMM can scramble the signals that allow ras to create mutated and cancerous cells. It can also stimulate the production of tissue plasminogen activator (TPA), which is associated with the ability to break down fibrin.[5] Fibrin formation, along with platelet aggregation, are important steps to tumor formation. It's amazing that a natural plant like gotu kola not only enhances wound healing but is also capable of distinguishing and inhibiting angiogenesis and tumor growth.

Scientists at the Amala Research Center in Kerala, India, have tested gotu kola against cultured tumor cells and found that gotu kola was effective in destroying 100 percent of the cultured tumor cells. The gotu kola used was a 5:1 concentrated extract. It was completely nontoxic to healthy cells, thereby displaying its selective toxicity to tumor cells only. In follow-up studies on animals, gotu kola extract more than doubled the life span of mice with tumors and displayed a remarkable lack of toxicity.[6]

Tonic Herbs, Adaptogens, and Immune Enhancers

Tonic herbs, adaptogens, and immune enhancers are herbs that enhance the immune system function, support and improve intestinal health, and can counter some of the damages of chemotherapy, radiation, and drug therapies. They contain a wide range of active constituents like polysaccharides and flavonoids that have been demonstrated to protect and strengthen immune response. They also maintain and strengthen the vital force within us and act as biological response modifiers in host defense mechanisms against cancer. These plants strengthen the immune system as well as protect the bone marrow, adrenal glands, liver, and other vital organs during chemotherapy and radiation.

Ginseng (*Panax*)

Ginseng has been used as a traditional medicine in Asian countries for more than five thousand years. More than five hundred scientific papers have been published on ginseng throughout the world. In China and Korea, ginseng is taken as both a medicine and a power food. Ginseng is most often classified as an adaptogen, which means that it enhances the ability to withstand a variety of stresses, including workload, pollution, physical and mental stresses, radiation, and exercise exhaustion. Ginseng is most noted for its antifatigue and antiaging effects. This has been attributed to a group of compounds in ginseng called ginsenosides. Saponins, yet another group of compounds found in ginseng, have been shown to inhibit proliferation of tumors induced by various chemicals and have demonstrated some antitumor activity.

Ginseng has been shown to enhance the overall activity of the immune system, including antibody response, natural killer-cell activity, interferon production, and the proliferate and phagocytic ability of the immune system. Red ginseng, which is produced from a steaming process, contains a ginsenoside (RH-2) and an acetylene alcohol, panaxytriol, that have proven to be the most active antitumor compounds found in ginseng. A large controlled study on ginseng done at one of the major cancer hospitals in Korea showed the potent preventive effect of ginseng against cancer. Those who took ginseng in extract form, as opposed to pills, powders, or teas, showed the lowest risk (0.14 percent) of getting cancer.[7]

I always recommend ginseng to those undergoing radiation therapy and feel it helps immensely to hasten the recovery and reduce the chance of scar tissue damage. In animal studies, panax ginseng has been shown to inhibit metastases to the lung and liver and to reduce elevated platelet and fibrinogen levels caused by the tumor cell lines. When panax ginseng extract was used with the chemotherapeutic agent mitomycin, it produced a much greater antitumor effect and also reduced the immune suppressing side effects that mitomycin had caused.[8]

Panax quinquefolium, better known as American ginseng, has been shown to revert cancerous liver cells to normal. Energetically speaking, American ginseng has more warming properties, is less stimulating, and is more soothing to the digestive and nervous systems. It enhances cerebral circulation, improves mental clarity, improves spleen and stomach function, and strengthens the nervous system. Panax red is the most stimulating and should be used only by those who are very deficient—for example, a person who has a weak pulse, very low vitality, anemia, and a very passive personality. In China, American ginseng is highly sought after. Wild American ginseng is an endangered species, therefore, I recommend buying it woods-grown rather than wild.

Uno de Gato (*Uncaria tomentosa*)

Uno de gato, commonly referred to as cat's claw, has recently become a popular herb in the United States. It grows as a woody vine in the highlands of the Peruvian Amazon and has many potent health benefits, including its overall boosting effect to the immune system. It is antimicrobial, antiviral, antihypertensive, and a digestive aid. An astringent, it balances the intestinal flora, inhibits dysbiosis, and helps to resist infection. Uno de gato also possesses mild antitumor activity.

In the 1970s, both the National Cancer Institute and National Institutes of Health tested uno de gato for its potenial use in cancer. But, as is frequently the case when dealing with herbs, they could not identify a single patentable agent, so the study was dropped. Uno de gato is made up of many complex constituents and is particularly rich in alkaloids (fourteen have been identified so far). Two groups of alkaloids, indole and quinoline, are believed to be its most active ingredients. Two specific alkaloids, isopteropodine (A1) and isorhynchyllin (A4), seem to be responsible for its immunostimulating effects.

Among the other biologically active compounds found in this plant are the phytosteroids beta sitosterol and campesterol, catechins (like those found in green tea), glycosides, and the flavones quercetin and rutin.[9]

Because this plant is very hard and woody, pills and capsules are of little value. I believe the best way to use this plant is in a high-quality extract, although a decoction, the traditional way of preparing this herb, is also of great benefit. To do this, boil 1 quart of water, add 1½ to 2 tablespoons of the herb, reduce heat, and simmer for two to three hours until the original amount of liquid has been reduced to about one-third. What's left (about 8 ounces) is the daily dose.

Virginia Snakeroot (*Aristolochia serpentaria*)

Virginia snakeroot is an herb that is seldom used today, although it possesses much value to those who are weak and have lost some of their vital essence. It promotes appetite and improves digestion. Aristolochic acid, under the trade name KC-2, has been shown to stimulate and strengthen the body's defense system. It specifically stimulates natural killer-cell activity. As an isolated compound, aristocholic acid has many side effects; as a whole plant extract, however, it is safe and well-tolerated.

Anti-inflammatory, Fibrinogenic, and Antiangiogenic Herbs

These herbs inhibit mutation and free radical damage while protecting, repairing, and detoxifying the liver. They also enhance Phase I (cytochrome P450) and Phase II (glutathione-S-transferase) enzyme systems, as well as other enzyme systems like N-acetyl transferase (NAT). The pro-oxidant/antioxidant shift (one of the main events that occur in cancers) is something herbs can address. When the balance of oxidative stress overpowers the body's means to regulate and detoxify, the antioxidant enzyme systems, Phase I and Phase II, create a friendly environment for neoplastic development and proliferation. Factors that cause this include genetic predisposition, exposure to estrogens and/or androgens, infectious agents, environmental and dietary factors, as well as normal aging.

One of the ways that liver-detoxifying herbs work is that they interact with energized molecules such as free radicals and, in so doing, they are able to spare glutathione (Phase II). Glutathione (GSH) is one of our body's most important antioxidant enzymes and is a significant anticarcinogen, especially in the liver, where the highest level of GSH is found. There, GSH combines with carcinogens to make the free radicals inert. GSH also plays a role in protecting the nervous system. The formation of oxidized DNA bases by active oxygen species is similar to damage caused by ionized radiation, which can act as a cancer initiator as well as a promoter. Another important action of antioxidants present in herbs is the ability to inhibit the arachidonic acid cascade.

The two main antioxidant-detoxifying enzyme-system pathways are:

Phase I. Xenobiotics (chemical compounds) that are insoluble in water are combined with compounds that make them water-soluble. While the resulting compounds may be less toxic than the original compounds, there is a chance they can become more toxic. Most compounds that undergo the Phase I system are primed for Phase II conjugation, although a few compounds may be directly eliminated through Phase I.

Phase II. Conjugation occurs during Phase II pathways, increasing water solubility and the ability to undergo significant ionization. The water-soluble compound created in Phase I is combined with substances such as glutathione that, except in rare instances, convert the intermediate to a harmless state that can be easily excreted with bile through the intestines or with urine through the kidneys. The major Phase II conjugation reactions are glucuronidation, glutathione amino acid conjugation, sulfation, acetylation, and methylation. Methylation is the pathway that processes and eliminates homocysteine. High levels of homocysteine are associated with many illnesses, including heart disease.

In addition, herbs that inhibit inflammatory pathways in turn possess fibrinogenic abilities (natural abilities to inhibit blood stickiness and clotting), leading to antiangiogenic activity. Their specific actions include:

- Inhibition of platelet aggregation
- Prevention of the formation of fibrin
- Acceleration of the degradation of fibrin or fibrinogen
- Inhibition of the fibrin-stabilizing factor
- Possible activation of the plasminogen-plasmin system
- Inhibition of cyclooxygenase-2 (COX-2)

This fibrinogenic action of some herbs can enhance the cytotoxic effects and make them more target-specific in both radiation therapy and some chemotherapy, while at the same time inhibiting the toxic side effects of these therapies, including scar tissue formation resulting from radiation or postoperative healing and excess nerve damage. Cancer itself, in general, usually causes an acceleration of fibrin, thrombic obstructions, and blood clotting.

Research into the enzyme system that underlies some of the inflammatory processes of arthritis, heart disease, allergies, and cancer is causing pharmaceutical companies to seek anti-inflammatory drugs that can modulate prostaglandins and fatty acids, actions already available to us in many herbs and natural enzymes.

Two types of enzymes, cyclooxygenase enzymes 1 and 2 (COX-1 and COX-2), are involved in the functions of cartilage cells and joint-lining cells. COX-1 is necessary for a healthy gastrointestinal tract and good kidney function, while COX-2 is induced by tissue injury and leads to inflammation and pain. It is found in tumor tissue and its overexpression increases cancer invasiveness and resistance to cell death. Many drug companies are trying to develop COX-2 inhibitors as a new line of cancer-fighting drugs, particularly for colon cancer. Bromelain and quercetin, along with herbs like turmeric, horse chestnut, and licorice, act as powerful nontoxic anti-inflammatory agents, especially when taken together.[10]

Turmeric (*Curcumin*)

Curcumin as well as other curcuminoids present in turmeric have been extensively researched recently and are thought to be responsible for this plant's liver-protective and antioxidant properties. Turmeric, the main spice in curry blends, works against environmental mutagens and inhibits the mutagenicity of cigarette smoke. Turmeric has been shown to be a much stronger cell-protective agent (antioxidant) than vitamin C, and has protected against DNA damage induced by lipid peroxidation by 85 percent, compared to beta-carotene at 50 percent and vitamin E at 57 percent.

The antitumor effect of curcumin results from a combination of mechanisms. Curcumin reduces the induction of ornithine decarboxylase activity, reduces polyamine synthesis, and blocks oxygen free radicals. Turmeric also inhibits cyclooxygenase, lipoxygenase, and the production of arachidonic acid, which are all proflammatory, tumor-promoting, and have inhibitory effects on the immune system. Curcumin also enhances the production of several important cancer-fighting cells.

Turmeric has a long history of use in the treatment of cancer. In recent studies, turmeric extract has been demonstrated to be cytotoxic to both human chronic myeloid leukemia cells and Dalton's lymphoma cells. Curcumol and curdione isolated from the volatile oil of turmeric have shown an inhibitory effect on sarcoma 180 in mice. Turmeric is used in China to treat early-stage cervical cancer.[11] An ethanol extract of turmeric, applied externally for the treatment of skin cancer (where all other treatments failed), has relieved pain, reduced itching, and promoted healing. Turmeric has been shown to be extremely effective at inhibiting recurring melanoma in people at high risk and has demonstrated antihepatotoxic effects against a variety of chemical toxins, such as carbon tetrachloride. It has also been shown to inhibit both azomethane-induced colon cancer and DMBA-induced breast cancer.[12]

A new study on turmeric administered in the diet or applied topically has shown a significant chemoprotective effect on oral precancerous lesions.[13] In addition, another study involving the chemopreventive effects of curcumin derived from turmeric along with epigallocatechin-3-gallate (EGCG) from green tea has shown that the combination of these naturally occurring botanical constituents demonstrates synergistic interaction in inhibiting growth of squamous cell carcinoma.[14]

A recent study demonstrated the potent free-radical scavenging effects of curcuminoids present in turmeric in a study involving nitric oxide. Curcumin reduced the amount of nitric oxide generated from sodium nitroprusside. Because this compound is implicated in inflammation and cancer, the therapeutic properties of curcumin against these conditions might be at least partly explained by its free-radical scavenging properties, including those directed at nitric oxide.[15]

Another recent study has demonstrated a connection between nitric oxide production and tumor angiogenesis. It seems that elevated levels of nitric acid correlate with tumor growth. Nitric oxide appears to be critical for vascular endothelial growth factor (VEGF), which is an angiogenesis activator.[16]

Very often, part of my protocol for inhibiting cancer will consist of combining bromelain with turmeric extract tablets containing 95 percent curcumin, and one or more medicinal mushroom extract capsules (reishi, maitake, shiitake). I believe that turmeric, which possesses anticancer, antioxidant, anti-inflammatory, fibrinolytic, and liver-protective properties, has a synergistic effect with the enzyme therapy of bromelain.

Bupleurum (*Bupleurum chinense*)

One of the most widely used herbs in Traditional Chinese Medicine, bupleurum is useful for conditions associated with constrained liver *chi* (stagnation).

Stagnation refers to poor blood and energy flow that usually involves dampness and/or cold. It may also be useful in treating premenstrual symptoms, such as emotional instability, abdominal bloating, dizziness, and/or other menstrual problems. It is cooling and is therefore useful in conditions of heat with manifestations that include bitter taste in the mouth, dry throat, dizziness, and a feeling of constriction and fullness in the chest and flanks.

Bupleurum is also used as a predominate herb in formulas for the liver, such as hepatitis. One such formula that I use is called Minor Bupleurum (Xiao Chai Hu Tang). This formula has been found extremely effective at inhibiting cancer by enhancing the immune system, inducing apoptosis, and inhibiting angiogenesis. It has also been shown to increase the effectiveness of the standard chemotherapeutic drug 5-fluorouracil (5-FU). It is most useful in breast and liver cancers, but can also be used to treat colon cancer. Bupleurum saponins exhibit anti-inflammatory activity similar to prednisone.[17,18]

Schizandra (*Fructus schizandrae*)

The dried berry of schizandra, like astragalus, bupleurum, ginseng, and ligusticum, is commonly used in traditional Chinese medicine for its adaptogenic properties and as a restorative remedy for immune enhancement. Schizandra is referred to as the five-flavored seed because its taste includes the five tastes of sour, bitter, sweet, acrid, and salty. In Shen Nong's *Herbal Classic* (written about two thousand years ago) and in the *Compendium of Materia Medica* (written by L.I. Shizhen in 1596), schizandra was referred to as a valuable tonic—an adaptogen with a diversity of indications for its use. It has a stimulatory effect on the central nervous system without being excitatory and enhances both mental and physical capabilities.

Classically, schizandra is used for lung and kidney deficiency. It is considered astringent in nature, and is widely used for the treatment of stress-induced nervous system exhaustion and fatigue, insomnia, weakness, depression, forgetfulness, liver disease, diarrhea, and chemical toxicity. It is also used for regulating gastric secretions to balance pH levels and for a variety of liver ailments. Schizandra is especially effective at lowering serum transaminase levels. Recent studies from China have found schizandra and its active components to be effective against viral and chemically induced hepatitis. It was found to lower SGPT levels in patients with chronic hepatitis C virus while increasing liver protein and glycogen synthesis.[19] An elevated level of this particular liver enzyme is a clear indication for the use of schizandra in the individual's protocol. It is, without a doubt, one of my favorite herbs, and I use it as a general tonic herb as well as a detoxifier to help rid the body of chemical toxicities, including chemotherapy and radiation therapy.

Schizandra is also an antioxidant that has demonstrated its superiority to vitamin antioxidants against oxygen free radicals. In addition, various ethanol-soluble lignans found in schizandra have powerful liver-protective properties against a variety of chemical toxins. Besides hepatitis and other liver ailments, schizandra is also helpful in certain types of intestinal infections, including chronic gastritis.

Soviet studies indicate that schizandra improves vision, particularly in adjusting to darkness. To review schizandra's effects, this herb offers:

- Antitoxic and antioxidant activity against many chemical toxicities.
- Protection of DNA from damage, most notably by carbon tetrachloride, which is activated within the body to a deadly liver toxin.
- Assistance in the liver's detoxifying enzymes by stimulating the biosynthesis of protein and liver glycogen.

One lignan component, gomisin A, inhibited the development of chemically induced preneoplastic lesions in rats. The results of this study indicate that gomisin A, one of the main lipid-soluble lignans found in schizandra, appears to be an antipromoter agent in hepatic carcinogenesis.

Schizandra is also considered adaptogenic and a tonic, according to a review of its traditional use as well as a review of the scientific studies that demonstrate its ability to increase work capacity, exercise capacity, mental capacity, and adaptability to darkness and other environmental stresses in both animal and human studies.[20,21]

Green Tea

Green tea provides broad protection against four major categories of carcinogens:

1. Indirect chemical carcinogens (such as benzopyrene in diesel fuel)
2. Direct chemical carcinogens (such as nitrates in processed meats)

3. Physical carcinogens (such as ultraviolet light)
4. Tumor promoters (such as the pesticide DDT)

Green tea inhibits tumor initiation by preventing the formation of carcinogens, helping the liver to detoxify, and protecting DNA by producing enzymes that speed carcinogen removal and enhance DNA repair activity. It also inhibits tumor promotion by blocking abnormal cell growth, slowing the production of hydrogen peroxide and other reactive free radicals, and enhancing the immune system.

Green tea does contain caffeine, and caffeine, to the surprise of many, possesses anticancer activity. Caffeine is able to induce apoptosis within cancer cells and it also enhances the cytotoxicity of radiation therapy and alkalating chemotherapeutic drugs, including carboplatin, cytoxin, busulfan, and valalbine, all commonly used in cancer therapies.

The polyphenolic compounds present in green tea demonstrate chemo-preventive activity in animal tumor models. Epidemiologic studies have also shown that green tea consumption might be effective in the prevention of certain human cancers. The National Cancer Institute recently investigated the effect of green tea polyphenols on the induction of apoptosis and the regulation of the cell cycle in human and mouse carcinoma cells. The study concluded that green tea offers protection against a wide variety of human and mouse tumor-cell lines by causing cell cycle arrest and inducing apoptosis.[22]

Another recent study has demonstrated growth inhibition of human lung cancer-cell line PC-9 by green tea polyphenols, specifically epigallocatechin gallate, one of its main constituents. Green tea appears to intercept cell division during the mitotic stage of cell growth.[23–25] Still another recent study involving green tea has shown a strong inhibitory effect on stomach cancer growth in humans. Findings from this study recommend drinking green tea to protect against stomach cancer.[26]

Alteratives and Lymphatics: Herbs That Detoxify

These are the herbs that increase the body's elimination of waste material and improve nutrition. Detoxification, an area of extreme importance to our health that is largely overlooked by conventional medicine, takes place at three levels.

1. *Intracellular,* the interplay of electrolyte functions and the diffusion of chemical ions across the cell membrane (such as lymph glands). Each cell goes through a process of utilizing what it needs for energy and what it needs to detoxify. Cells detoxify into the lymph and blood systems. Herbs referred to as lymphatics and blood purifiers fall into this category. Thuja and red root are examples.

2. *Organismic,* intermediate metabolism (such as liver detoxification). Some examples of herbs that assist the liver (as well as the kidneys and spleen) in detoxification include the popular hepatic bitter herbs, dandelion and celandine, both of which have tumor-fighting ability. Dandelion is an amazing plant that heals and provides nutrition. While it is sad that so many chemical toxins are directed at ridding our lawns of this wonderful herb, the good news is that, with all of our efforts to destroy this plant, it triumphs and remains with us, offering its healing properties.

3. *Organs of excretion,* the elimination of unusable end products and chemical wastes from the kidneys, bowels, skin, and lungs. Some examples are nettles and horsetail, which support the kidneys; butternut, pectin, and a trio of plants used in Ayurvedic medicine, called *triphala;* and diaphoretic plants including elder, yarrow, and boneset, which enhance elimination through the skin.

Each step of metabolism involves an understanding of the nervous system. What is the balance between the parasympathetic (anabolic) and the sympathetic (catabolic) nervous systems, and how does this relate to the breakdown and excretion of waste materials? Eliminative functions are often thought of in terms of the kidneys and large bowel but, in fact, problems of detoxification and the body's ability to eliminate waste is more complex. Some of the indications that help determine the most appropriate herbs for an individual's protocol include:

1. *The average level of body temperature.* Many cancer patients have a subnormal temperature that contributes to their illness and inability to get well. A basal metabolic temperature reading taken before getting out of bed in the morning provides important information.

2. *The degree of tissue hydration.* A parasympathetic individual will urinate frequently during the day, more than once during the night, and will usually also experience low blood pressure, dry skin, and low levels of aldosterone, cortisol, and perhaps DHEA.

3. *Functional organ state.* If the patient shows over-relaxation or overcontraction, this indicates the need to use herbal stimulants or relaxants. For

example, boneset is a relaxing diaphoretic, while dry ginger or prickly ash are stimulating diaphoretics. Constipation can be caused by lack of tone (over-relaxation), which would call for a liver/bowel stimulant, such as butterbur, or it can be the result of tension (vasoconstriction), which would call for a bowel relaxant, such as fringe tree or magnesium.

4. *Acid/alkaline base.* Is an excess of systemic catarrh (mucus) produced by the body? It is important to review the patient's diet, taking note of the balance between acid and alkaline foods. A high uric acid level calls for reduction or elimination of meats, shellfish, and alcohol and the addition of berries, folic acid, bromelain, and quercetin. Herbs that help with uric acid reduction include celery seed, nettles, fringe tree, and pipsissewa. Diuretic herbs are classified as those that increase the excretion of water and promote the elimination of waste.

Turkey Corn (*Corydalis formosa*)

Corydalis is a classic alterative with analgesic properties. It is most useful in advanced stages of cancer when the patient has swollen lymph glands, dry and scaly skin, and a toxic system. Corydalis is used extensively by practitioners of Chinese herbal medicine for pain, especially abdominal pain. Corydalis is one of the primary ingredients in both the Eli Jones compound, called Scrophularia, and a Chinese herbal formula I often prescribe called SPES. Along with butterbur, corydalis is one of the best nontoxic analgesics for people suffering from the pain caused by cancer.

Thuja (*Thuja occidentalis*)

Thuja is an herb that I use in many of my herbal tonics. It has a wide range of uses in addition to cancer. Its indications are cancers of viral origin, colon/rectal cancer, uterine cancer, and breast and lung cancer. It is also effective in precancerous conditions like polyps and warts. Recently, West German researchers have reported results demonstrating that thuja enhances the immune system by stimulating T-lymphocytes and increasing interleukin-2 production. Thuja also possesses antiviral and immune-modulating abilities that may allow for greater tolerance of chemotherapy and radiation therapy.[27]

Poke (*Phytolacca americana*)

Eli Jones considered this plant the most valuable of all plants in the treatment of cancer. He believed the anticancer effects of poke were most useful against cancers of the breast, throat, and uterus. Poke is indicated for cancer of the breast when the breast is hard, painful, and purple in color. I often combine poke with other lymphatic herbs that may include thuja, echinacea, baptisia, figwort, red root, tiger lily, ocotillo, and corydalis. Poke is helpful in fibroid tumors that are not cancerous. Its internal and external use is indicated for sore nipples and sensitivity or inflammation of the breast. For acute mastitis, poke is used both externally and internally. It is the main ingredient in my lavender and poke oil compound. Poke is one of the best lymph remedies we have and a well-known alterative that needs to be used with care, because an overdose could be toxic. Use only with the guidance of a health care professional.

Poke's specific indications include glandular enlargement and hardness, especially of the lymph nodes in all areas of the body. For tonsillitis and/or sore throat, I combine it with red root, echinacea, propolis, thuja, goldenseal, and baptisa, add a small amount of glycerin and/or aloe, and use it as a throat spray. In chronic skin conditions, such as boils, ulcerations, psoriasis, or eczema, it is used locally as well as internally for its alterative properies, particularly its effects on the lymphatic glands.[28–30]

Modern research has reported that pokeweed contains a potent viral inhibitor that is capable of reducing the infectivity of the tobacco mosaic virus. Since then, three proteinaceous substances have been purified and shown to have antiviral activity: pokeweed antiviral protein (PAP), PAP II, and PAP-S, also referred to as phytolaccins. The PAPs are not only inhibitory to plant viruses, but are also effective against animal viruses, such as influenza A2, polio type-I, herpes simplex type-I, and herpes simplex type-II. Poke increases white blood-cell production and increases mitosis in lymphocytes.

Burdock (*Arctium lappa*)

Burdock contains antitumor activity and a substance capable of reducing mutation called the B-factor, for burdock factor. Benzaldehyde, a constituent of burdock, has been shown to have antitumor activity. Burdock is traditionally classified as an alterative and is an ingredient in the Hoxsey/trifolium compound. The highest levels of lignans are found in the seeds, the part of the plant I use most frequently. Methanol extracts of burdock seed have induced differentiation of myeloid leukemia cells and demonstrated potent anticancer action against lymphocytic leukemia.[31,32]

Gene Repairing, Enzyme Inhibitors, and Cytotoxic Herbs

These herbs have more direct anticancer and/or antitumor effects. They are capable of inducing cell death by selectively removing cells in which DNA has been damaged.

These are herbs that either increase the innate immunity and cytotoxicity of one's immune system, or have direct antitumor/antineoplastic activity. The most common antitumor active principals found in plants are terpenes and alkaloids.

Gene repairing is a mechanism in which some plant compounds genetically alter cancerous cells to revert back to normal cells, possibly by inhibiting cell division through means of a DNA repair mechanism or by extinguishing the malignant information that can eventually kill the cancerous cell. One known mechanism by which plants can genetically affect cell proliferation of preneoplastic cells is by inhibiting certain enzymes that promote cancer growth. Two such enzymes are tyrosine kinase, which is a crucial enzyme involved in the promotion of many cancers, including melanoma, and ornithine decarboxylase (ODC). ODC as well as other cancer-promoting enzymes trigger mitogen-activated protein (MAP) kinase activity, which in turn implies a proportional increase in tumor invasiveness.

Genes involved in the invasive and metastatic phenotype of cancer cells are potential candidates to serve as markers of tumor aggressiveness. The interaction between cancer cells and laminin, a major basement membrane glycoprotein, is considered a determining event in tumor progression. Among the several cell-surface proteins that are able to interact with laminin, the 67-kd laminin receptor (67LR) is involved in the chemotactic migration of malignant cells toward laminin. Compared to a normal tissue counterpart, 67LR expression is increased in a variety of human cancers, including breast, prostate, colon, gastric, ovarian, endometrial, lung, thyroid, and hepatocellular carcinoma; furthermore, this increase in 67LR is also associated with the biologic aggressiveness of the cancer cells.[33] Laminin accumulates between invading cells and host tissue. It aids cancer-cell growth by promoting adhesion.

Catechin, a flavonoid found in many plants, including green tea and the Chinese herb fo ti (*Polygonum multiflorum*), inhibits the invasion of a variety of tumor-cell lines. At least one of the mechanisms by which catechin inhibits tumor-cell growth is its ability to bind tissue-type plasminogen activator (t-PA) to laminin, which leads to partial inactivation of t-PA and cancer-cell growth. Tissue-type plasminogen activator is an enzyme that facilitates tumor invasion.

Herbs contain agents that can also inhibit the malfunction of tumor-suppressor genes by stopping or inhibiting them from mutating and causing DNA to become jumbled. Quercetin, a flavone found in many plants and foods, including eucalyptus, ginkgo biloba, and onions, can inhibit the tumor-suppressor protein gene p53, a critical suppressor gene involved in at least half of all cancers, including breast and prostate cancers. This keeps cell growth in check and prevents cancer transformation.

Enzyme inhibitors found in plants can block certain enzyme pathways that cancer uses to proliferate. One common cancer enzyme pathway, called lactate dehydrogenase, works by blocking anaerobic glycolysis. During this conversion, pyruvic acid is converted to lactic acid without the body being under any physical exertion. This creates a healthy acid blood environment for cancer that is referred to as *lactic acidosis*. Some plant agents that inhibit lactate dehydrogenase include oxalic acid found in rhubarb, sorrel, and spinach; allicin, found in garlic; and gossypol, from cottonroot.

Herbs that contain antitumor alkaloids can directly inhibit cancer growth because of their inhibitory activity against reverse transcriptase of RNA tumor viruses. The mechanism of action occurs within the cell cycle process. There it interacts with adenine-thymine (A:T) template primers, stopping DNA synthesis at the initiation of the polymerization processes.[34] Many cancers, particularly leukemias, lymphomas, and brain tumors, are believed to be initiated by tumor viruses such as the Epstein-Barr virus (EBV), and use reverse transcriptase to promote infiltration. The HIV virus also uses reverse transcriptase to promote its growth.

A more direct antitumor mechanism of plant compounds has to do with inhibiting tubulin polymerization. This is the way that most chemotherapies work. These antitumor compounds are called antimitotic agents. Taxol, a nat-

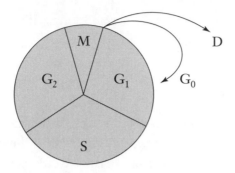

G_0 = Resting
G_1 = Synthesis of purines and pyrimidines
S = Synthesis of DNA
G_2 = Synthesis of components for mitosis
M = Mitosis
D = Differentiation

Figure 4.1 **Cell Life Cycle**

ural product derived from the yew tree (*Taxus brevifolia*), which has become a popular chemotherapuetic agent for the treatment of ovarian and lung cancers, has a unique mechanism of action. Rather than inhibiting microtubulin formation at the M-phase (the mitotic phase of the cell, during which time the cell is dividing) the way other plant alkaloids do, taxol inhibits cell division by decreasing the concentration of tubulin required for assembly, thereby keeping it in the Gap-I phase longer than it should and not allowing the cell to get to the mitotic phase for division (see figure 4.1).

Sundew (*Drosera rotundifolia*)

Sundew contains the same active components as the Venus's-flytrap plant. I have been using sundew for several years and feel it is most valuable. It repairs genetic malfunction, is cytotoxic, is antiviral, lowers cholesterol, and enhances the action of antibiotics. Its action as an effective nontoxic treatment for many types of cancer is similar in many ways to that of Venus's-flytrap, although sundew has been used much more frequently in traditional medicine. Sundew was traditionally used for irritated mucous membranes, particularly of the gastrointestinal tract and lungs. It's great for coughs, both bronchial and dry.

Mistletoe (*Viscum album*)

Popular throughout Europe, mistletoe is one of the most widely used plants for hypertension and in the treatment of cancer. It is the main therapy used to treat cancer by anthroposophical physicians. Iscador, a fermented extract of *Viscum album*, reduces the leukocytopenia produced by radiation and chemotherapy. Mistletoe is tumor-inhibiting and cytotoxic to a number of different tumor types. It also increases natural killer-cells. *Viscum's* cytotoxic components include viscumin and viscotoxins. Viscumin is a lectin component that causes agglutination of tumor cells. Mistletoe also contains polysaccharides, which stimulate nonspecific immune function, and polypeptides, which have a cytotoxic action on tumor cells only.

Periwinkle (*Catharanthus roseus*)

Vincas, a group of natural alkaloids that possess antineoplastic activity against many cancers, are present in minute quantities in the periwinkle plant. It takes about 500 kilograms of the plant to make a single gram of the alkaloid. The vinca alkaloids include the anticancer agents vincristine and vinblastine. They exert their cytotoxic effects by binding to a specific site on tubulin and preventing polymerization of tubulin dimers, disrupting the formation of microtubules, which eventually disappear with continued use. The primary cytotoxic effect of vinca alkaloids is their ability to stop cellular division. The cytotoxic mechanism of the vinca alkaloids is the same as many other plant alkaloids such as colchicine, podophyllotoxin, and taxol. Periwinkle was used traditionally for treatment of diabetes and high blood pressure as well as cancerous tumors.

Isatis (*Radix isatidis*)

Isatis is a commonly used herb in Traditional Chinese Medicine. It is classified as bitter and cooling and is used primarily to remove infections that produce excess heat. This includes viral, bacterial, and fungal type infections. It is very effective against acute mononucleosis and hepatitis, mumps, herpes infections, and streptococccus infections. Its most noted compounds are indoxyl-B-glucoside, B-sitosterol, isatin, and indirubin. Indirubin possesses strong anticancer activity; it is particularly effective against CML (chronic myelocytic leukemia). In a clinical trial of 314 patients with CML, 82 achieved complete remission, 38 partial remission, and 87 had beneficial effects. The total effective rate was 87.3 percent. There were no reported serious side effects, and no inhibitory effects on the bone marrow were seen. Indirubin was also found to inhibit breast and lung cancer.[35]

Camptotheca acuminatea

The alkaloid camptothecin is extracted from the wood, bark, and fruit of the *Camptotheca acuminatea*, a tree native to China where it is called the "tree of joy." It is one of the newer cytotoxic drugs. The chemotherapeutic drug CPT-11 is camptocetheca. The drug Topotecan, recently approved for ovarian cancer, is a synthetic spin-off of camptothecin. Camptothecin possesses noteworthy broad-spectrum antineoplastic activity against several lines of leukemia as well as many solid tumor cells in animals.[36]

I have never used this plant and do not intend to because, like taxol, it is one of the recent naturally derived cytotoxic agents. By the time it has been isolated and synthesized in a lab (as these agents are), it can no longer be considered herbal medicine, as I practice it. I list *Camptotheca* here only because it is the herbal version of some of today's most commonly used cancer drugs. It's important for us to be aware of this trend toward the use of herbs for their traditional healing properties, although conventional medicine still insists on tracking down the toxic constituents rather than realizing the healing benefits of the whole plant.

Herbs That Can Alter the Action of Hormonal Receptor-Type Cancers

These are the herbs that adhere to hormonal receptor binding sites, thereby competing with hormones (e.g., estrogen), causing a decreased hormonal effect. By occupying the receptor sites without activating them (or at least not overactivating them), these herbs prevent estradiol molecules in the circulating blood from occupying those sites, which then leads to a net decrease in estrogen response. These plant compounds, sometimes referred to as phyto-estrogens, can also inhibit the aromatase enzyme, which can decrease the conversion of androgens to estrogens. Both saw palmetto and nettle root extracts have been shown to inhibit aromatase. Inhibition of aromatase is very important in the prevention and treatment of both breast and prostate cancers. When aromatase is inhibited, it leads to the deactivation of cancer-driving hormones (such as sex-hormone-binding globulin, a hormone that increases as we age), which would otherwise bind to receptor sites.[37]

In some breast cancers, for example, the aromatase enzyme is responsible for causing androgens to convert to estrogen. Flavones, such as those found in Chinese skullcap, and isoflavones, like those found in red clover and soy products, interrupt that process and actually redirect androgens for ultimate elimination rather than conversion into estrogen.

In prostate cancer, the importance of androgens to fuel the cancer is significant; at least 75 percent of all tumors in men with metastatic prostate cancer are androgen-dependent at initial diagnosis. Also, the enzyme 5-alpha-reductase is at least in part responsible for converting testosterone into its more active cancer-promoting form, dihydrotestosterone (DHT). That is why certain herbs such as nettle root and saw palmetto, for instance, which inhibit the enzyme 5-alpha-reductase from testosterone, can be effective at both preventing and treating prostate cancer when combined with other herbs.

Androgens in prostate cancer, as well as estrogens in breast cancer, also alter intracellular glutathione levels and the activity of certain detoxification enzymes. Physiologic levels of these hormones are capable of increasing oxidative stress, perhaps due to increased mitochondrial activity.[38] Because of this, it is important to include herbs that can enhance the detoxification and excretion of cancer-promoting hormone metabolites. Another example of this in breast cancer is to enhance detoxification and reduce the levels of the estrogens estradiol-17B and 16-alpha-hydroxylase. The liver plays a key role in the metabolism of hormones and carcinogens, and it can use all the help it can get.

One interesting note on the subject of breast and prostate cancers is that they can both manipulate hormones, causing estrogens to fuel prostate cancer and androgens to fuel breast cancer. This means that the drug tamoxifen used in treating breast cancer and flutamine used in treating prostate cancer start out inhibiting cancer, but over time their effects can actually be reversed and they can promote cancer.

A major advantage of implementing natural healing by the use of herbs and diet is that nature has an innate intelligence that is not merely directed at removing superficial symptoms but in restoring balance as well. Only nature in the form of herbs can bring us into balance, lift our spirits by elevating our mood, bind to cancer-promoting hormones, detoxify the liver, strengthen the endocrine system, enhance the immune system, assist in regulating body temperature, remove obstructions and accumulated toxins—and all in collaboration with our own innate healing vital force.

Red Clover (*Trifolium pratense*)

Red clover blossoms are an excellent alterative, and one of the main herbs in the trifolium compound and the Hoxsey Formula, a classic combination of alteratives, tonics, and eliminative herbs used to treat many glandular disorders, skin afflictions, coughs, and various cancers. Traditionally, red clover was used as a blood purifier as well as for irritable conditions of the larynx and air passages, especially if accompanied by a spasmodic cough.

On an emotional level, red clover can have a healing effect on the heart. Recent investigation of this plant has shown it to be rich in isoflavones, such as biochanin A and genistein, which exert powerful antiestrogen, anticancer, and antiangiogenic effects. Red clover seems to be most active against prostate, breast, and colon cancers and melanoma.

Coumarin, which is another main active ingredient in red clover, as well as the popular Chinese herb dong quai, has been shown to stimulate macrophages and reduce the recurrence of metastatic melanoma. Twenty-seven patients who had recently undergone surgical excision of malignant melanomas received either 50 mg a day of coumarin or a placebo in a randomized, double-blind trial. During a follow-up period of two-and-a-half to three years, there were two recurrences of melanoma in the thirteen patients treated with coumarin, compared to ten recurrences in the fourteen patients given placebo.[39]

Licorice (*Glycyrrhiza glabra*)

Licorice is an antiviral, anti-inflammatory, antitumor, and antiulcer herb and it increases the production of interferon and natural killer-cell activity. Licorice inhibits Epstein-Barr virus expression, which is associated with development of certain cancers. It also possesses liver-protective and antiallergenic activity. Triterpenes, mainly glycyrrhizin, possess blocking ability against tumor-promoting agents. A recent study done in Japan demonstrated that glycyrrhizin can inhibit liver cancer caused by hepatitis.[40] The flavonoids and isoflavonoids in licorice possess hormonal regulating ability, and the polysaccharide fraction has immunostimulating activity.

Licorice affects adrenal function by increasing the production of cortisol, DHEA, and aldosterone. Low levels of DHEA are found in many women with breast cancer. Licorice, by increasing cortisol, produces anti-inflammatory actions and may inhibit the growth of leukemia and lymphoma cells by affecting glucocorticoid receptor sites on their plasma membranes.

Chinese Skullcap (*Scutellaria baicalensis*)

Chinese skullcap (huang qin) differs from American skullcap. It inhibits many viruses including tumor viruses and the HIV virus by inhibiting reverse transcriptase; it is anti-inflammatory and induces cell death in a number of cancer cell lines including two sarcomas and cervical cancer. It also inhibits human hepatoma cell growth by 50 percent. Chinese skullcap has a particularly high flavonoid content, over 35 percent. Its flavonoid content is believed to be responsible for most of its anti-inflammatory, antiviral, antiretroviral, antitumor, and antimicrobial effects. It also stimulates the immune system. In addition, *baicalein*, a saponin, inhibits cancer-cell multiplication and induces cell death *in vitro*. A number of Chinese formulas used to treat cancer feature this herb. It is used traditionally to cleanse heat, dry excess moisture, and remove toxins.[41,42]

Herbs to Treat Specific Symptoms

These are herbs that can alleviate the symptoms of cancer itself or the side effects of conventional cancer treatments like chemotherapy and radiation.

Red Root (*Ceanothus americanus*)

Red root is one of my favorite herbs, and is excellent for spleen and lymph disorders. It strengthens the lymph system and helps remove wastes from the body. It is also a stimulant to the digestive apparatus, the portal circulation, the liver, and especially the spleen. I have found it to be a specific for increasing platelet counts that may have dropped as a result of cytotoxic drug use. It is also good for enlarged spleen, liver, and/or lymph nodes, as well as excessive bleeding.

Red root will work well with echinacea, baptisia, licorice, thuja, usnea, propolis, and poke for sore throats, inflamed tonsils, and many respiratory tract infections.

Red root raises the activity of T-cells and is a good herb to include in a compound to treat low-grade infections such as Epstein-Barr virus. Red root also improves digestion and assimilation, especially when loose stools occur. In Chinese medicine, red root would be classified as a true spleen remedy.

My own personal constitutional tonic always contains red root. It is particularly helpful for those who have had their tonsils taken out at a young age.

Wild Geranium (*Geranium maculatum*)

Wild geranium is a powerful astringent, and is used specifically with the cancers that cause excessive bleeding. I have used geranium for this purpose many times and have been very impressed by its ability to assuage this serious problem that plagues so many cancer patients. I usually combine geranium with others herbs such as yarrow or red root, and if I feel the mucous membranes need soothing, I add comfrey.

Horse Chestnut (*Aesculus hippocastanum*)

Horse chestnut is traditionally used for diseases of the venous system, including varicose veins, thrombophlebitis, bruises, painful leg cramps that occur at night, brain trauma, edema of the ankles, postoperative edema, and the fluid accumulation caused by cancer. It reduces capillary permeability by acting on the connective tissue barrier between blood vessels and tissue. By increasing the capacity of the inner walls to accept moisture, it enhances the ability of tissues to drain. Horse chestnut, because of its ability to inhibit both increased vascular permeability and collagenase activity, may also act as an angiogenesis inhibitor.

The two most active principals found in horse chestnut are aesculin, a coumarin derivative, and aescin, a saponin. It also contains many more constituents, and its medicinal effects are due to the synergy of all these constituents rather than to any single one.

Slippery Elm (*Ulmus rubra*)

This herb contains an abundant amount of plant mucilage which gives it a "slippery" texture. An effective remedy for irritated states of the mucous membranes of the chest, lungs, stomach, and intestines, it is an excellent herb for convalescence and debilitated states, especially when digestion is weak and overly sensitive. Slippery elm is a safe herb that can even be given to infants. It brings relief to acid conditions of the stomach and should be included in any herbal protocol for ulcers, diverticulitis, inflammation of any internal tissues, hemorrhoids, irritable bowel syndrome, constipation, or diarrhea, and for lung conditions such as bronchitis, pleurisy, and tuberculosis. It can also be used externally for the treatment of tumors, cysts, or ulcers because its action is to soften, soothe, and draw. To use externally, mix 1 teaspoon of slippery elm powder, 1 teaspoon of fenugreek seed powder (optional), and 30 to 60 drops of echinacea and/or calendula extract. Apply to the boil as a warm paste. Leave on for twenty to thirty minutes. After the boil has been drawn out, apply a healing herbal salve such as calendula to the area.

Slippery elm is indicated for people who are undergoing radiation to the respiratory or digestive area. It is amazing how a tea of this common herb can bring so much relief to the pain and suffering caused by this form of treatment. A cold water infusion is also a good way to use this herb. Soak 1 tablespoon of cut slippery elm bark in 12 to 16 ounces of water for several hours or overnight. Heat gently being careful not to boil; strain and drink. The powder can also be mixed into food such as oatmeal by using 1 to 3 teaspoons per bowl.

HOW TO USE HERBS

After an herbalist or doctor determines which herbs are appropriate for a particular condition, the next steps are to determine:

- Which form to use (fluid extract, decoction, infusion, extract, pills, etc.)
- How to administer the herbs (by mouth, bath, inhalation, enema, transdermal)
- The amounts to give, the frequency, and the time of day for doses to be given
- How to combine the herbs into appropriate formulas

Good overall health must be achieved before improvement can be expected. This means that before one can aggressively attack the cancer or try a radical detoxifying diet, one must increase vitality and strength by:

- Improving digestion and assimilation
- Regulating the body temperature
- Normalizing circulation

Other Useful Herbs in Cancer Treatment

This section contains an alphabetized list of other herbs commonly used in cancer treatment.

Agrimony (*Agrimonia eupatoria*)

Agrimony is used in both Western and Eastern herbal traditions to treat a wide range of urinary problems, including incontinence, cystitis, and kidney stones. It

---

————— HERBAL GLOSSARY —————

Actions of Herbs

Alterative. Stimulates changes of a defensive or healing nature in metabolism or tissue function when there is chronic or acute disease.

Analgesic. Relieves pain.

Anesthetic. Decreases nerve sensitivity to pain.

Antifungal. Kills or inhibits fungi.

Antigen. Induces the formation of defending antibodies.

Antimicrobial. Kills or inhibits microorganisms.

Antioxidant. Prevents oxidation by slowing down the formation of lipid peroxides and other free-radical oxygen forms.

Antispasmodic. Relieves or prevents spasms.

Antiviral. Inhibits the proliferation and viability of infectious viruses.

Aromatic. Alters mood through scents via a plant compound that forms gases that can be smelled when brought into contact with air.

Astringent. Causes the constriction of tissues; usually applied topically to stop bleeding, secretions, and surface inflammation and distention.

Demulcent. Soothes internal membranes.

Diaphoretic. Increases perspiration.

Diuretic. Increases the flow of urine.

Expectorant. Stimulates the outflow of mucus from the lungs and bronchial mucosa.

Herbal Preparations

Compress. Soak a cloth in a hot decoction of herb, squeeze out most of the liquid, and apply the hot cloth to the affected area. Once it has cooled, repeat the process.

Decoction. The method of choice for making tea out of bark and seeds. Use 1 to 2 teaspoons of herb per cup of cold water. Bring mixture gently to a boil. Keep covered and simmer for about ten minutes. Prepare no more than twenty-four hours in advance of use.

Fluid extract. An extract of an herb that is made according to official pharmaceutical practice, with a strength of 1:1 (each ounce of extract has the solutes found in an ounce of the dried herb).

Fomentation. This is a hot, wet poultice used on painful and inflamed areas; it is usually made by dipping a towel in tea, applying it hot or warm to the swollen tissue, and changing it when cool.

Infusion. The method of choice for making tea out of leaves or flowers. Add 1 to 2 teaspoons of dried herb (or 2 to 4 teaspoons of fresh herb) to a cup of boiling water. Infuse for ten minutes before straining. May be taken hot or cold, but do not prepare more than twenty-four hours in advance of use.

Plaster. Mix enough ground herbs or powdered seeds with boiling water to make a paste. Apply paste to a specific area, such as a boil, cover, and leave on for several minutes to several hours, as directed by the herbalist. Heat is sometimes applied over the plaster.

Poultice. Mix chopped herb or powdered seeds with boiling water to make a pulp. Place the pulp in a piece of cloth and apply to the affected area while hot. Replace when cool.

Tincture. An herbal extract made by steeping the herb for about six weeks in a mixture of water and alcohol. The strength should be listed, usually as a ratio (1:5).

Table 4.4 **Dosage Guidelines**

100–120 drops (depending on viscosity) = 1 teaspoon

5 ml = 1 teaspoon

25–30 drops = 1 ml

1 dropperful = 1 ml

50–60 drops = ½ teaspoon

30 ml = 1 ounce

15 ml = 1 tablespoon

is also useful for sore throats and diarrhea. It is astringent and anti-inflammatory and contains tannins, coumarins, flavonoids, volatile oils, and polysaccharides.

Aloe Vera

Several biologically active substances are found in the leaf juice of the aloe plant. These include polysaccharides such as emodin, which has shown anti-leukemic activity, and acemanna, which has shown antiviral and immune-boosting activity. Aloe has anti-inflammatory, antitumor, and antiangiogenetic activity and inhibits platelet aggregation. Lupeol and salacin account for aloe's pain-relieving effects. Aloe has also been shown to provide a protective effect against injury from radiation treatment. When making an herbal tonic, I often use an aloe leaf extract as a base for the herbal extracts.

In clinical trials, one highly concentrated, specially grown and processed aloe product called T-UP has demonstrated the ability to increase T-lymphocytes, which in turn produce cytokines that destroy microbes and cancer cells. T-UP is, to my knowledge, the most potent form of aloe made. It has been shown to effectively inhibit many cancer-cell lines, particularly cancers of viral origin.[43]

Amla (*Emblica officinalis*)

Amla is a small fruit that grows in India. In Ayurvedic medicine, amla is classified as a rejuvenative and restorative tonic. Amla is known to be nature's richest source of vitamin C, about twenty times higher than an orange. In a popular Indian daily rejuvenizer amla is called *chyvanprash*, combined with a blend of delightful aromatic herbs to create a sweet, jamlike herbal concoction. It is esteemed for its power to enhance health and reverse the aging process. Amla is a rich source of other antioxidants, including bioflavonoids, vitamin E, polyphenols, the vitamin B complex, and carotenoids. Studies have shown that amla can elevate levels of the important antioxidant enzyme, superoxide dismutase (SOD). Beyond its curative powers, its reputation as a powerful enhancer of health is being demonstrated in clinical research. Clinical effects include accelerated repair and regeneration of connective tissue, enhanced interferon and corticosteroid secretion, and increased lean body mass.[44]

Andrographis (*Andrographis paniculata*)

Andrographis was traditionally used to treat a host of illnesses in China, Thailand, and India. It was used to fight both bacterial and viral infections, reduce fever, control diarrhea, reduce inflammation, lower blood pressure, relieve pain, treat ulcers, induce abortions, protect vital organs such as the liver, and lower blood sugar. It contains a group of unique active principals called *andrographolides*. Andrographolides have important immune-activating and cancer-inhibiting abilities, making this an important medicinal herb in cancer therapies. Andrographis extract (as opposed to pure andrographolide isolate) has been shown to inhibit the proliferation of cancer by causing differentiation-inducing activity upon dividing cells. Some of the tumor-cell lines that have been inhibited by andrographis include stomach cancer, breast cancer, prostate cancer, lymphocytic leukemia, melanoma, and non-Hodgkin's lymphomas. Many studies have confirmed andrographis extract as a potent nontoxic plant extract having cytotoxic effects against a number of cancers.

A study reported in the *Journal of Chinese Medicine* in 1977 found andrographis inhibited skin cancer even after it became metastatic. It also demonstrated antiprostate tumor effects by lowering PSA counts and by inhibiting *in vitro* tumor growth. Another study, involving breast cancer, demonstrated andrographis's tumor-inhibiting ability to be equal to that of tamoxifen. Andrographis is safe and free of side effects; however, it is contraindicated for pregnant women. Besides being cytotoxic, it provides liver and kidney protection; acts as an effective antidiarrhetic; helps to regulate immune functions against second-line pathogenic infections that could otherwise be life-threatening to a person with cancer; and strengthens the nervous system, which enhances vitality.[45]

Ashwagandha (*Withania somnifera*)

Ashwaganda is one of the most revered plants in Ayurvedic medicine. It has recently been shown to have antitumor, immunomodulatory, and radiosensitizing effects in experimental tumors *in vivo*, without any systemic toxicity. I recommend it during and after radiation therapy.[46,47] Ashwagandha significantly increases white blood-cell count, reducing leucopenia caused by radiation and immune suppressive drugs. It also has a normalizing effect on red blood-cell count, hemoglobin, and platelet count.

Astragalus (Huang chi root)

In Chinese medicine, astragalus is known to strengthen the body's natural defenses that involve the immune system. It is one of the main herbs used in fu-zheng therapy to enhance the immune system during chemo and radiation therapy. It seems to increase not only interferon levels but also natural killer-cell and T-cell activity. It also makes the T-cells more aggressive. Astragalus has been shown to have liver-protective activity against a number of toxic substances, including carbon tetrachloride.

In Traditional Chinese Medicine, astragalus is prescribed for spleen deficiency characterized by chronic weakness, low vitality, fatigue, diarrhea, spontaneous sweating, and lack of appetite. It's a true blood builder.

Astragalus also possesses antitumor activity and inhibits platelet aggregation. It has been shown to increase tenfold lymphokine-activated killer-cells (tumor-fighters). It protects the heart, liver, and kidney from the toxicity of chemotherapy and has been shown to potentiate and reduce the overall toxicity of interleukin-2 against two specific forms of cancer—renal-cell carcinoma and melanoma.

She-Quan-Da-Bu-Tang, a Chinese formula that includes astragalus and ligusticum, has proved most effective in enhancing cellular immunity, specifically interleukin production by the body, in addition to potentiating the activity of chemotherapeutic agents, inhibiting recurrences, prolonging survival time, and reducing the adverse toxicities of antineoplastic agents.

Astragalan, an extract of the whole plant, has demonstrated immune-enhancing abilities, but the active constitutents of astragalus are believed to be the result of a combination of ingredients rather than one single agent.[48]

Atractylodes (*Atractylodes macrocephala*)

Atractylodes contains three cancer-inhibiting components: atractylin, atractylon, and butenolide B, which have demonstrated the strongest activity against esophageal cancer. Atractylodes improves defective IL-2 production and restores immunity in people with cancer who have had immune-suppressing therapies like chemotherapy. In Chinese medicine, atractylodes is classified as a spleen remedy for excess dampness. It is used for loose bowels, edema, and decreased urination.[49,50]

Bee Pollen

Bee pollen is one of the most nutrient-dense rejuvenative healing foods we can include in our diets. It contains all known nutrients and many unknown healing agents. Add 1 to 2 tablespoons per day to any food or drink. One should be careful not to cook it or expose it to high temperatures because many of its important enzymes will be destroyed. Bee pollen has been shown to contain an unidentified anticarcinogenic substance that slows the growth of breast cancer.[51]

Bitter Melon (*Momordica*)

Constituents of the ripe fruit and leaves of bitter melon inhibit guanylate cyclase, which is elevated in many cancer cells. The aqueous extract of bitter melon is found to block the growth of prostatic cancer in rats. The crude extract is preferentially cytotoxic for leukemic cells versus normal cells.[52] It has also demonstrated antioxidant activity against free radicals and lipid peroxidation.[53]

Black Cohosh (*Cimicifuga racemosa*)

Through its influence on the vasomotor centers and on the nerve ganglia, black cohosh has a beneficial influence on the heart. It is an antispasmodic and is very effective at relieving certain types of pain, particularly muscular rheumatism. Specific indications for this herb are flulike deep muscular body aches that are worsened by cold. Traditionally used as a woman's remedy, black cohosh is indicated in ovarian neuralgia, dysmenorrhea, nervous excitement, dull headaches, and depression. In general, it is also used as a stomach remedy that improves digestion by relieving excess stress. Because of its nervine qualities, it is also advised for the treatment of nervous coughs.[54] Pharmacological studies have demonstrated that *Cimicifuga* contains substances with endocrine activity that cause a selective reduction of the serum concentration of pituitary luteinizing hormone (LH) and are able to bind to estrogen receptors, thus affecting the reproductive and central and peripheral nervous systems.

Black cohosh is a good example of an herb with many diverse and helpful actions. It has a wonderful balancing effect on hormones, relieving many of the symptoms of menopause without the risks associated with HRT use. It is one of the many plants that I recommend for women who have had breast cancer to safely help them through menopause.

Bloodroot (*Sanguinaria*)

Bloodroot possesses antitumor, antiviral, and antimicrobial actions. Both the isoguinoline alkaloids sanguinarine and chelerythrine (also found in celandine) have been shown to uncouple oxidative phosphorylation and inhibit reverse transcriptase enzyme which is required for the replication of an RNA virus. These and other alkaloids in bloodroot have been shown to exert a therapeutic effect against Ehrlich carcinoma (in mice) and a significant necrotizing effect on sarcoma 37 (also in mice). Bloodroot was traditionally used as part of a paste to treat forms of skin cancer. Eli Jones believed bloodroot to be most useful in cancer of the rectum.[55]

Boldo (*Peumus boldo*)

One of the most widely used herbs in South America, boldo is an excellent general tonic. It has been used traditionally to treat liver and bowel dysfunctions. It aids in digestion by stimulating the secretion of bile.

Boswellan (*Boswellia serrata*)

Boswellan, also known as Indian frankincense, contains gumlike resinous constituents referred to as boswellic acids. These exhibit potent anti-inflammatory, analgesic, ulcer-protective, lipid-lowering, and anticancer activities. Traditionally used in Ayurvedic medicine to treat a variety of disorders, including osteoarthritis and rheumatoid arthritis, *Boswellia serrata* has been found, in recent studies, to contain a group of triterpene acids that demonstrate potent antitumor activity. These acids were found to inhibit the synthesis of DNA, RHA, and protein in human leukemia cells. They have also been shown to inhibit topoisomerase I and II (enzymes that catalyze the passage of individual DNA strands through one another) by interacting with binding sites on the DNA molecule.[56]

Boswellan is one of the herbs in Super-Tonic (see Resources), and is a great natural anti-inflammatory agent that inhibits cancer by working synergistically with other natural botanical agents, including turmeric, licorice, green tea, bromelain, and quercetin. Studies have shown its positive effects on cell-mediated and humoral components of the immune system and its ability to increase body weight, total leukocyte count, and humoral antibodies.[57]

Buckthorn (*Rhamnus cathartica*)

Buckthorn contains antitumor activity from two different components, emodin and dihydroxyanthroquinone. It is listed as a safe laxative and diuretic that is helpful when there is bowel or renal obstruction.

Bugleweed (*Lycopus virginicus*)

Bugleweed is specifically indicated for an overactive thyroid gland, usually with the heart palpitations that often accompany this condition. It is an astringent, has mild sedative properties, and is also useful for loose coughs. It works somewhat like digitalis in controlling excessive vascular excitement. It improves the appetite, reestablishes normal secretions, and improves blood production, thereby making it a useful plant medicine for debility.[58]

Bugleweed's astringent properties make it useful for conditions of excess bleeding. It is particularly helpful in cases of lung cancer when the patient is coughing up blood, is having difficulty breathing, and has a racing heartbeat. It contains phenolic, caffeic, chlorogenic, and ellagic acids.

Butterbur (*Petasites officinalis*)

Butterbur has neurosedative and spasmolytic properties and is useful for both gastrointestinal and respiratory spasmodic complaints. It is a good remedy for painful coughs, such as whooping cough. It is a tumor analgesic, therefore very useful for the pain caused by tumors. It has also shown anticancer properties.[59,60]

Celandine (*Chelidonium majus*)

An anticarcinogenic, celandine is indicated when there is an enlargement of the liver, constipation, indigestion, and a strong urinous odor. It is particularly well-suited for cancers of viral origin. Celandine has been shown to possess anticancer and antimicrobial activity. Animal experiments have shown its tumor-inhibition activity in cases of sarcoma 180 and Ehrlich carcinoma. Celandine is effective in conditions where liver and digestive function is impaired.[61,62]

Chaga (*Inonotus obliquus*)

A fungus that grows on birch trees, chaga (as well as the birch tree bark itself) is rich in betulinic acid, which has been shown to inhibit the growth of human melanoma by inducing apoptosis. Betulinic acid is converted from betulin in birch bark. Animal studies have shown betulinic acid is more effective and less toxic than any other cytotoxic therapy presently being used to treat melanoma. It is believed to down-regulate the mutant p53 suppressor gene responsible for allowing proliferation of oncogenes.[63] Using 1 ounce of chaga to 12 to 16 ounces of water, simmer for fifteen to thirty minutes. Then allow it to steep for one to four hours. Strain and drink 2 to 4 cups a day. Chaga makes a pleasant-tasting tea.

Chaparral (*Larrea tridentata*)

Also known as *creosote bush*, chaparral as been used by Native Americans to treat a variety of illnesses, including cancer. Chaparral contains an ingredient called *nor-dihihydroguairetic* (NDGA), a potent antitumor agent. NDGA inhibits aerobic and anaerobic glycolysis (the energy-producing ability) of cancer cells. The flavonoids present in chaparral have strong antiviral and antifungal properties.

Chaste Tree Berry (*Vitex agnus-castus*)

Chaste tree berry is native to the Mediterranean but has spread to central Asia. It is the fruit of this herb, containing volatile oils with a peppermintlike scent, that is used medicinally. *Vitex* has unique effects on the reproductive system. It appears to have a *corpus luteum* effect, causing an increase in luteinizing hormone production, while inhibiting the release of follicle-stimulating hormone (FSH). *Vitex* is therefore a specific for corpus luteum insufficiency. It allows for a better shift to occur during and after ovulation, giving a better ratio of estrogens to progesterone. By assisting in a better output of progesterone, it can also inhibit excess androgen output.

I have recommended *Vitex* with great success for a number of imbalances and health conditions, including premenstrual syndrome symptoms, such as bloating, breast swelling, water retention, emotional stress, and menstrual cramps. I have also recommended it for menopause and cystic ovaries, and to increase the production of breast milk, to help with acne, and, in general, to treat all conditions that may be caused by overproduction of FSH, which can produce excess estrogen and/or androgen hormones and low progesterone.

Vitex, because of its hormone-balancing effects, should be considered for use in the prevention and treatment of breast, endometrial, ovarian, and prostate cancers. It can be combined with isoflavone-phytosterol-rich plants, as well as lymphatic and liver detoxifiers, for a comprehensive herbal compound.[64]

Chrysanthemum Flowers (*Dendranthema morifolium*)

Chrysanthemum is used primarily to treat fevers and headaches. It has antibiotic effects against streptococcus, staphylococcus, and shigella. It is used to treat the common cold, flu, and other upper respiratory infections. It is also used to treat hypertension.

Cleavers (*Galium aparine*)

Cleavers is used as a diuretic for inflammatory states that are accompanied by renal burning and irritation. The herbalist John Scudder recommended that it be used for nodulated growths or deposits in skin or mucous membranes.

Eli Jones used it for cancer of the tongue when there is a nodular feeling and the lump is tender to the touch.

Codonopsis (*Codonopsis pilosula*)

Codonopsis is referred to as "poor man's ginseng" in China. It is classified as a "sweet *chi* tonic" and used for disorders of the spleen and lungs. It stimulates the growth of red blood cells, enhances T-cell transformation, and stimulates phagocytosis.

Colchicum (*Colchicum autumnale*)

Colchicum, as well as colchicine (the active principle in colchicum) are both used predominately as a gout remedy because of their ability to reduce uric acid levels. Colchicum is also an antimitotic, and is being explored as an antileukemic drug for acute lymphoblastic leukemia in children, chronic myloid leukemia, and some skin cancers.

In vitro studies using colchicine have shown anticancer activity against various cell lines.[65] In its pure form, colchicine is too toxic for human use as an antitumor drug, but colchicum, as a whole plant extract that includes colchicine along with other components, may be effective and have substantially fewer side effects. Colchicum, because of its ability to reduce uric acid, should also be considered for people who are undergoing cytotoxic therapies that interfere with uric acid excretion. Hydrourea, which is used to treat chronic myloid leukemia, is known to cause this problem, for example.

Coleus (*Coleus forskohlii*)

Coleus is used in Ayurvedic medicine for a wide range of ailments, including cardiovascular disease, hypertension, eczema, asthma, convulsions, painful urination, colic, and insomnia. To date, its main active compound, forskolin, is found in no other plant. Forskolin has unique effects within the cell process and is most effective when the entire plant is used, rather than when it is isolated out and used by itself as a drug. The unique biological activity of forskolin includes the activation of an enzyme, adenylate cyclase, which increases cyclic adenosine monophosphate (cAMP) in the cells. Forskolin has also been shown to inhibit a number of membrane and channel proteins. Forskolin is a smooth-muscle relaxer and inhibits the platelet-activating factor (PAF), which plays a major role in the inflammatory and allergic processes.

Besides forskolin's ability to lower blood pressure and inhibit asthma and other allergic conditions, it is of great value in psoriasis. The very property that allows it to control psoriasis also allows it to play a unique role in suppressing cancer growth. What do cancer and psoriasis have in common? Uncontrolled cell division in both conditions, as well as increased levels of another cell regulator, cyclic guanine monophosphate (cGMP), which overrides and dominates cAMP. Forskolin can help normalize the balance between cAMP and cGMP, thus normalizing cell division. By way of inhibiting PAF, forskolin also inhibits inflammatory processes that allow cancer metastases to occur. It has also been shown to activate white blood cells, making it an immune activator. Other beneficial effects of forskolin include improved nutrient absorption, critical for people with cancer; increased thyroid function (low thyroid is a condition commonly found in women with breast and ovarian cancer); increased salivation; and strengthening of the heart muscle and increased blood flow, specifically cerebral blood flow. I usually use a fluid extract of forskolin in an individual's tonic or a tablet extract containing 18 percent forskolin. The dose would be 50 to 100 mg two to three times per day.[66]

Condurango (*Marsdenia cundurango*)

Used especially for gastric and breast cancer, indications for condurango are ulcers in the corner of the mouth or cramping pains in the stomach. It has repeatedly been found to be beneficial in cancer treatment, increasing the appetite, reducing pain, and restoring weight. Antitumor glycosides have been isolated from condurango.[67]

Cotton Root (*Gossypium*)

Cotton root contains a number of constituents, including the polyphenol *gossypol*, which has been shown to possess antiviral, anticancer, and antibacterial activity. It also inhibits arachidonic acid and the proflammatory prostaglandins. New research on cotton root is showing possible applications for prostate, breast, and adrenal cancer by decreasing the hormone metabolites that may be promoting tumor activity.[68,69]

Dandelion (*Taraxacum officinale*)

Dandelion is a rich source of nutrients, including chlorophyll and carotenoids. In addition to being a great food, it is also a great medicine. Dandelion is one of the best liver remedies because it enhances the flow of bile, and it is therefore used to treat a variety of liver ailments. In China, dandelion has been used to treat breast cancer. The leaf of the dandelion is an excellent diuretic, comparable to Lasix; yet, dandelion replenishes potassium and other minerals that are normally depleted by diuretics.

Dong Quai (*Angelica sinensis*)

Dong quai, also known as tang kwei, is rich in two groups of constituents that have demonstrated immune-enhancing, antiallergenic, antibacterial, and anticancer activity. They are coumarins (such as othole, angelicin, osthenol, umbelliferone, archangelicine, bergapten, and ostruthol) and flavonoids (such as archangelenone and caffeic acid). The coumarins activate white blood cells, making them capable of destroying tumor cells. Angelica is widely known for its healing and tonic effects on female health. It is useful in menopause for relieving hot flashes. A smooth-muscle relaxer, it is also very helpful in relieving cramps and promoting menstruation. In Chinese medicine, it is used to regulate the menstrual cycle of those with deficient blood. The symptoms include pale face, tinnitus, blurred vision, heart palpitations, and pain from stagnant blood. Angelica also contains vitamin B_{12} and is therefore useful in the treatment of anemia caused by chemotherapy.[70]

Echinacea (*Angustifolia* and *Purpurea*)

Echinacea is perhaps the best-known herb for the enhancement of immune function. It promotes T-cell activation, interferon production, natural killer-cell activity, antibody binding, lymphatic function, and macrophage phagocytosis. Echinacea increases the reticulo-endothelial layer to boost production of alpha, beta, and gamma globulin, which increases antibodies. Echinacea inhibits hyaluronidase, thereby assisting wound healing and indirectly inhibiting cancer growth. This occurs through the activation of hyaluronic acid. Echinacea has been shown to possess antitumor activity in several studies and it also enhances the effectiveness of antibiotics.

Echinacea was traditionally used by American Indians of the western plains, and was the herb most widely used by Eclectic physicians. It was used primarily as a blood purifier to treat various conditions such as abscesses, boils, gangrenous wounds, poison ivy, spider and snake bites, scarlet fever, and influenza.

Recently there has been much confusion about echinacea's active compounds and the correct length of time to continue its use. The Eclectics and all other clinicians who have used echinacea over the years suggest that it can be used for long periods of time for chronic health conditions, with no side effects or contraindications. Echinacea works best as a preventive and should be referred to as an immunomodulator.

I recommend echinacea both as a tonic herb and an herb for acute infections, often combining it with other herbs. The two most common herbs the Eclectics combined with echinacea were baptisia and thuja. These three herbs have a synergistic effect and work well together for treating many acute and chronic infections.

I believe echinacea is one of the most valuable herbs in use today and it is often the main ingredient in the personal and specific tonics I recommend to patients. These tonics may be taken for a month or more.

Many people have the mistaken belief that echinacea should be used only for a short period of time (seven to ten days) and then stopped for the same amount of time before resuming its use. I do not believe this is true. I do believe, however, that echinacea, or any immune booster, when used to fight off an acute infection, should be taken frequently and in fairly high doses (½ teaspoon five to six times a day). Using echinacea in this way activates the immune system by stimulating cell-mediated immune function in order to ward off any invaders that are trying to take over. If echinacea is being used as a tonic herb, the dose is much less; perhaps 20 drops two to three times a day. Echinacea is then acting as an immune modulator, a blood purifier, and a tonic.

Through immune modulation, echinacea is a very valuable herb in cancer treatment and prevention. It activates specific antitumor immune-fighting cells, makes macrophages cytotoxic, and has some direct tumor-destructive constituents, namely the essential oils.[71-73]

Eclipta (*Eclipta alba*)

Eclipta encourages liver regeneration and has been shown to inactivate hepatitis B surface antigens. Its hepatic-protective properties help to guard against liver cancer and enhance the liver processes that aid in detoxification of carcinogens and hepatotoxic chemotherapies.[74]

Eucalyptus (*Eucalyptus solium*)

Eucalyptus is rich in the essential oil camphor and is useful for nausea and vomiting when there is a sour taste in the mouth. The Canadian cancer-fighting drug referred to as 714X is a camphor-based formula used in many cancer clinics around the world.

False Bittersweet (*Celastrus*)

False bittersweet was one of the principal ingredients of Compound Scrophularia Syrup, a well-known formula that was used in the treatment of cancer by the Eclectic physicians. *Celastrus* is an alterative and improves the elimination of waste from the body. It contains tannins, volatile oil, and a unique bitter principal called celastine.[75]

Figwort (*Scrophularia marylandica*)

Figwort, another main ingredient of the Compound Scrophularia Syrup, is especially useful when cancer has invaded the lymph system and there is marked evidence of cachexia, toxic blood, and puffiness in the face with full, pallid lips.[76]

Foxglove (*Digitalis*)

Foxglove contains cardiac glycosides, most notably digoxin, which was used to treat a variety of heart conditions in the past. Today, digoxin is seldom used because lenoxin, its synthetic version, is generally used instead. As a whole herb, however, digitalis (which happens to have beautiful bell-like flowers) contains many other constituents, including other glycosides. One of these, digitoxin, appears to possess strong cancer-inhibiting effects. Studies with both human and animal models have shown it to inhibit certain tumor cell lines, including both ER-positive and ER-negative breast cancer. One possible mechanism for this might be the interaction between cardiac glycosides and the estrogen-receptor target site Na/K ATPase. This, by the way, is the target site for tamoxifen, a currently popular breast cancer drug. Digitoxin inhibits cancer growth in a dose-dependent manner, but the therapeutic dose is far below a potentially toxic dose. Only skilled herbalists or doctors trained in the use of this plant and the constitutional uses of cardiac glycosides should use digitalis because it can be toxic.[77]

Fringe Tree (*Chionanthus virginicus*)

This herb, seldom used today, has much value for the liver and other digestive organs. It has no cancer-inhibiting effects that we are aware of, but it has a specific use in cancer therapies. It is indicated when the patient is suffering from jaundice, acute dyspepsia, acute or chronic inflammation of the liver, or irritable liver. It is very helpful for people with cancer, particularly those with obstructions in the digestive tract, bile ducts, or tumors of the liver.

Ginkgo (*Ginkgo biloba*)

Many people would not think of using this popular herb for any kind of cancer protocol. Ginkgo is recognized primarily for restoring brain health by dilating peripheral blood vessels, increasing cerebral vascular circulation, and oxygen utilization. But ginkgo is also a free-radical scavenger that stimulates the immune system, is anti-inflammatory, inhibits histamine release, and is fibrinolytic. Ginkgo extract enhances the cytotoxic effects of radiation while reducing the overall toxic effects.[78]

Goldenseal (*Hydrastis*)

Indications for use of goldenseal are a broad, indented, and lightly coated tongue and evidence of dyspepsia, constipation, flatulence, and distress in the bowels. Goldenseal is also used to treat breast and stomach cancers.

Berberine, a main compenent of goldenseal, has potent antitumor activity, particularly against malignant brain tumors.[79]

Gromwell (*Lithospermum*)

Traditionally used by Native Americans as a natural birth-control agent, a daily infusion of gromwell can inhibit ovulation. It contains antigonadotropic properties, and its active compound is lithospermun acid (phenylcarboxylic acid). Both bugleweed and motherwort contain similar compounds.[80] Traditionally, gromwell was also used as a diuretic for chronic and acute cystitis. This plant may be thought of as the herbal version of lupron, a drug often used in prostate (and sometimes breast) cancers because it shuts down reproductive output throughout the endocrine system, particularly the adrenal glands. In women, it can stop ovulation.

Guaiacum

Guaiacum is a powerfully stimulating diaphoretic. It is often combined with other herbs, particuarly sarsaparilla, for the treatment of arthritis, lymphatic swelling, and many skin conditions.[81]

Ho Shou Wu (*Polygonum multiflorum*)

Ho shou wu is widely known for its antiaging, youth-preserving ability. It can sometimes prevent the graying of hair. Specific indications include deficient blood with signs of dizziness, blurred vision, weakness in the knees and lower back, and all signs of premature aging associated with liver and kidney deficiency. It contains emodin and rhein, two laxative agents that also possess anticancer activity, as well as lecithin. It is useful in cases of constipation and in the treatment of chronic debility with intermittent fevers and chills. Ho shou wu is also excellent for lowering cholesterol levels.

Jaborandi (*Pilocarpine jaborandi*)

I use jaborandi primarily for xerostomia, the dry mouth often induced by radiation that can cause much discomfort. I usually combine jaborandi with echinacea, prickly ash, and kava; dilute the mixture with aloe; and recommend its use as a mouth spray several times a day. Jaborandi is also very good for certain types of fevers, specifically when the skin is tight and the person is not sweating.

Jujube (*Ziziphus jujuba*)

Jujube, a sweet red date, is a delicious fruit and an effective herbal remedy that has been used in China for over twenty-five hundred years. It is a mild sedative and aids in increasing muscle strength and weight gain, improves stamina, is antiallergenic, increases immune system resistance, and augments natural killer-cell activity.[82]

Combined with kava kava, passionflower, and gotu kola, it is very helpful in reducing anxiety and balancing mental activity. Jujube also possesses analgesic and anticonvulsive properties and can significantly increase sleep time and quality. This herb contains betulin, betulinic acid, and the glycosides jujuboside A and B and is a good source of many vitamins and minerals. Several alkaloids have been found in the seed and fruit.[83]

Juniper Berries (*Juniperus communis*)

Juniper berries are a strong diuretic and kidney stimulant and should be used only in small amounts. When I use juniper in a compound, it normally comprises no more than 5 percent of the herbal mixture. It is excellent for helping the body to excrete excess uric acid and other waste materials. Many patients who are receiving chemotherapy experience negative effects on their kidneys and can suffer from gout, a painful arthritic condition brought about by the buildup of uric acid.

Lapacho (*Tabebuia avellanedae*)

Lapacho, also referred to as *pau d'Arco*, contains anticancer compounds, the main one being lapachol, which suppresses tumor formation and reduces tumor viability. Lapacho has proven to be particularly effective against leukemia. In South America, lapacho is often combined with yerba maté as a tonic. The major components found in lapacho are flavones, such as quercetin and quinones. American research has shown that lapacho inhibits some solid tumors, such as Walker carcinosarcoma 256, Ehrlich solid carcinomas, and Ehrlich ascites cell tumors. Lapacho is also a mild analgesic for cancer patients and is completely safe as a whole herb.

Lapacho has also demonstrated properties as an antioxidant, antibacterial, antiparasitic, and antifungal, which is why it is commonly used to combat yeast infections.

The best way to take this herb is in a decoction, drinking up to 1 quart of tea daily.[84,85]

Ligustrum (*Ligustrum lucidum*)

Ligustrum is one of the main herbs used in China to offset the toxicity of chemotherapy and radiation therapy. It is used in fu-zheng therapy, along with schizandra, reishi, ginseng, and astragalus. As a single agent, ligustrum is used for toning the kidneys and liver and, in cases of deficient yin, to treat such symptoms as dizziness, tinnitus, blurred vision, and low back pain. Ligustrum protects the liver during chemotherapy.

When combined with astragalus, ligustrum has shown notable immunopotentiating actions, far beyond the effects of either herb alone. This synergy has also been demonstrated when ligustrum is combined with echinacea, baptisia, and thuja.[86] Ligustrum's active ingredients include an alkaloid, tetramethylpyrazine, ferulic acid, chrysophanol, sedanoic acid, and 1 to 2 percent of essential oils.

Lotus Seed (*Nelumbinis nuciferae*)

Lotus seed is traditionally used in Chinese herbal medicine as a spleen tonic. It is excellent at stopping diarrhea, both chronic and acute. It strengthens the spleen and lymph systems and improves the appetite. I sometimes combine it with red root and codonopsis for a weak spleen.[87]

Mayapple (*Podophyllum*)

Traditionally, mayapple was used by Native Americans for treating cancer. It contains a group of resinous components, referred to as *podophyllotoxins*, that possess antitumor activity. One of the podophyllotoxins, podophyllin, is used externally to treat venereal warts and herpes. Podophyllotoxins taken alone are too toxic for internal consumption, but when used properly, in balance with the other constituents of mayapple, they are not toxic. However, too much mayapple (even as a whole plant extract) has a cathartic effect. The plant needs to dry and be aged before its medicinal constituents can be extracted.

Milk Thistle (*Silybum marianum*)

Milk thistle is a liver protector that stabilizes and strengthens the structure of the cell membrane. It is a great free-radical scavenger and it protects the liver against damage caused by drugs and heavy metals, including chemotherapy. Silymarin, a flavonoid in milk thistle, has been shown to provide substantial protection against different stages of UBV-induced carcinogenesis. The antioxidant properties in silymarin are believed to be the protective factors.[89]

The anticancer drug cisplatin is known to be toxic to the kidneys. Silymarin protects kidneys and liver from this toxicity.[90] Silymarin has also demonstrated a synergistic effect when combined with cisplatin and doxorubicin in the treatment of ovarian cancer.[91]

A recent study has shown silymarin's exceptional anticarcinogenic effects through an apparent down-regulatory effect on certain breast cancer-promoting enzymes, namely cyclin-dependent kinases.[92]

I always supplement the diet of people who are undergoing chemotherapy or radiation therapy with silymarin. It is best to take it before bedtime.

Milletia (*Jixueteng*)

Milletia (both the root and vine) is an important herb in the treatment of anemia, a frequent condition in postsurgery cancer patients undergoing chemotherapy or radiation. It increases white blood cell counts and treats systemic weakness and irregularities in the menstrual cycle. Its unique active compound is milletol, one of the main herbs in a formula called Marrow Plus (see Resources).[88]

Nettles (*Urtica dioica* and *Urens*)

I consider nettles equal or superior to all of the super green foods on the market today. Nettles are very high in chlorophyll, protein, and minerals. There are many benefits from eating nettles regularly. Especially good for anemia, upper respiratory diseases, allergies, and poor lymphatic function, nettles is a weed that grows freely and abundantly once planted. It can be cooked and eaten like spinach or dried and mixed in salad dressings, soups, and smoothies, or as a tea, alone or with other herbs. Be sure to wear gloves if picking nettles because they are prickly; the prickles disappear when the leaves are cooked or dried.

I utilize the root and seed, in extract form, for prostate cancer. The root extract reduces the androgen-binding capacity of the sex-hormone-binding globulin. The phytosterols, B-sitosterol and sitosterol B-glucoside, are found in the root, and lignans are found in the seed. The phytosterols found in the root are potent immune-activators and possess anti-inflammatory activity as well.

Nux Vomica (*Strychnos nux vomica*)

In cancer treatment, nux vomica is one of the most important plants for those whose vitality, digestive system, and nervous system are underactive and weak. It contains the alkaloid strychnine, as well as other alkaloids, and is therefore a very toxic plant that needs to be diluted and used with utmost care. I usually combine it with other herbs in a dose of 1 to 5 drops two to four times daily before meals. It provides a powerful stimulant to the nervous and digestive systems, which is so often needed by those who have cancer, particularly those who have been battling it for some time and are tired and losing strength.

Orange Peel (*Citrus aurantium*)

Orange peel is a bitter with a pleasant aromatic flavor. A terpene compound (*D-limonene*), found abundantly in the oil of orange peel as well as in other citrus fruits, has been shown to destroy cancer cells and to increase the metabolism of some cytotoxic drugs. I recommend a commercial product called Citrus Power, an orange peel oil capsule.

Small amounts of the extract or the dried or fresh peels make a delicious tea. Try a tea of lemon balm, chamomile, ginger, fennel, fenugreek, and orange peel. This is a tasty after-dinner tea—both a digestive aid and a mild sedative.

Orange peel can also lower cholesterol and dissolve gallstones. Interestingly, one side effect of many cholesterol-lowering medications is an increased risk for developing gallstones.[93,94]

Peony Root (*Paeona lactiflora*)

Traditionally, peony has been used to treat anemia because of its ability to nourish and build blood. It has also been shown to inhibit many allergic and inflammatory reactions. Peony contains glycosides, which have an immunomodulating effect and are able to exert a down-regulating effect on B-lymphocyte proliferation and interleukin-1 production of macrophages. This herb has also been shown to inhibit the overexpression of certain aspects of the immune system in diseases such as rheumatic arthritis. Peony's unique immunomodulating effects are believed to be mediated through the pineal gland.[95]

Phyllanthus (*Phyllanthus amarus* and *niruri*)

Phyllanthus has been shown to be effective against hepatitis B and other liver disorders. An aqueous extract of the plant not only inhibited viral DNA polymerase *in vitro* but was also shown to possess *in vivo* antiviral activity against the hepatitis virus. It is useful as a preventive against liver carcinoma.[96]

Pipsissewa (*Chimaphila*)

Pipsissewa is a good lymph and urinary tonic. Eli Jones considered it specifically useful for breast cancer in large-breasted women when the cancer also involved the lymph system. It was also used for prostate and bladder cancers. Pipsissewa contains arbutin, an effective urinary antiseptic that works against alkaline bacterial infections. It also contains the flavones quercetin and kaempferol.

Prickly Ash (*Zanthoxylum*)

A diaphoretic and alterative, prickly ash is used for xerostomia (dry mouth). It contains many complex alkaloids, coumarins, amides, and volatile oils. Chelerythrine, one of its many alkaloids, has displayed antimicrobial and antiviral activities. Fagaramide, another alkaloid contained in prickly ash, is a potent prostaglandin inhibitor.

Propolis

Propolis is a gluelike resin made by bees and used by them as a building material and antiseptic agent within their hives. Propolis is one of the best infection fighters and healing agents available. A concentrated extract of propolis can be used externally for healing wounds. It should be applied to the wound, allowed to dry so that it can form a hard shell-like coating, and then reapplied once a day until the wound has healed. Internally, propolis is excellent for bacterial, viral, and fungal infections, sore throats, and mouth ulcers. Studies have shown it to be particularly helpful for those who are undergoing radiation therapy.[97]

I usually recommend taking 10 to 20 drops three to six times a day, using a 50 percent extract. Propolis, like all bee-produced products, contains a vast number of constituents, many of which have demonstrated cancer-inhibiting properties. Two phenolic compounds found in propolis are caffeic acid phenethyl ester (CAPE) and apigenin (which is also found in chamomile). Apigenin inhibits the enzyme *hyaluronidase*, which in turn inhibits the breakdown of hyaluronic acid, a component of the extracellular matrix, the glue that holds cells together. In order for tumor invasion to take place, there must be a breakdown in the extracellular matrix.[98]

Queen's Root (*Stillingia sylvatica*)

John Scudder claimed that queen's root, a top-rated alterative used by Eclectic physicians for treating cancer and syphilis, increased the excretion of waste. *Stillingia* is one of the key ingredients of the Hoxsey/trifolium formula. It is indicated for irritated mucous membranes, specifically those of the airways. It is a good general lymphatic remedy that was primarily used to treat scrofula (a tubercular infection of the lymph glands in the neck), various skin conditions, and sore throats accompanied by a dry cough.

Rabdosia (*Rabdosia rubescens hora*)

This herb has been used traditionally to treat many forms of cancer, particularly breast and esophageal cancers. It contains several terpines that have demonstrated anticancer activity. Among its active constituents are rubescensine B, oridonin (a diterpene), cyclopentanone, and ponicidine. In addition, it contains essential oils and tannic acid, both of which possess anti-cancer activity.

Rabdosia is widely used in the province of Hunan, China, to treat esophageal cancer. One study reported the treatment of moderate and advanced esophageal carcinomas with this single herb between 1974 and 1987. Of the 650 patients in this study, 40 survived over five years, 30 over six years, and 23 over ten years. A total of 20 patients were still alive after twenty years.[99] Other studies have shown that DNA synthesis in Ehrlich ascites cells was inhibited by 74 percent after treatment with oridonin. Alcoholic extracts of this herb are highly toxic to HeLa cells, and oral administration of rabdosia extract has demonstrated remarkable inhibition of mice-bearing Ehrlich ascites cells and S-180 sarcoma cells.[100]

Rabdosia has also been shown to work synergistically with and potentiate the cytotoxic drug cisplatin.[101] Its cytotoxic effects against esophageal cancer are stronger than two popular chemotherapeutic drugs, bleomycon A5 and 5FU, and since it is a whole herbal extract, it is nontoxic.

This herb also possesses antispasmodic, smooth-muscle-relaxing, anti-inflammatory, and analgesic effects. Its essential oil has antibacterial activity and it has been traditionally used to treat sore throats.

Rehmannia

Rehmannia is an herb found in many traditional Chinese herbal formulas. Its specific indications include dry conditions with heat, low-grade fevers, muscle wasting, constipation, and dry mouth with throat pain. Its main active ingredients are beta-sitosterol, mannitol, stigmasterol, capesterol, arginine, and rehmannin. Rehmannia has liver-protective effects against a range of toxins, including carbon tetrachloride. It is an anti-inflammatory and a diuretic and has the capacity to lower blood pressure.

Rosemary (*Rosemarinus officinalis*)

Rosemary is a powerful antioxidant that increases overall vitality and improves circulation and mental outlook. It has been shown to inhibit mammary tumors in mice. Carnosol and ursolic acid are the major constituents of rosemary, and they both have been shown to inhibit tyrosine protein kinase (TPA), ornithine decarboxylase activity, and tumor promotion. Other compounds found in rosemary, called *diterpenoids*, have antioxidant activity.[102]

Royal Jelly

Royal jelly (a bee product that I consider a mystical food), when fed to a female bee, causes her to become three times larger than other bees. She will then live to be about ten times older than other bees and will produce twice her weight in eggs each day. A rich source of pantothene, about twenty times more so than liver, royal jelly is great for treating anemia. Animal studies have shown that royal jelly can reduce serum cholesterol levels and can be used in preventing and treating hyperlipidemia.[103] It is also an endocrine enhancer, assisting thyroid, adrenal, and reproductive hormones, especially by enhancing progesterone and testosterone levels.

Saffron (*Crocus sativus*)

Saffron is a rich source of carotenoids and is a potent cell oxygenator. Saffron was used in traditional Ayurvedic medicine for circulation, heart, kidney, and liver problems, and as a menstruation promoter. Saffron's carotenoids have been shown to increase the supply of oxygen in the blood, dissolve plaque, and absorb cholesterol. Saffron has also been shown to lower blood pressure because of its artery-cleansing effects.[104,105] Crocetin is believed to be the most active constituent found in saffron. I often prescribe a saffron extract combined with a selenium solution called Selensaff. I think the selenium and saffron complement one another. Selensaff, a product made by Scientific Botanicals (see Resources), is used in cancer therapy to create a redox effect—a process of improving cell function by enhancing both oxygen uptake and the excretion of oxygen waste.

Sage (*Salvia officinalis* and other related species)

Sage possesses estrogenlike hormonal activity. It is specifically indicated for reducing prolactin levels, thus stopping or reducing breast milk production.

Some forms of breast cancer are affected by elevated levels of prolactin. I use sage primarily in breast and prostate cancers. Thujone, which is contained in the volatile oil of sage, is a strong antiseptic and carminative and is believed to be the active compound. Sage, like rosemary, contains rosemarinic acid, a potent anti-inflammatory and antioxidant. It reduces excess sweating, which makes it an excellent herb for the hot flashes that often occur during menopause.

Saw Palmetto (*Serenoa serrulata*)

Saw palmetto has recently gained popularity as a "male" herb because of its beneficial effects on prostate health. It's true that it helps to reduce an enlarged prostate (a condition referred to as benign prostatic hyperplasia—or BPH), but to the surprise of many, I also recommend saw palmetto for female health. It is a great herb for women who have an excess of androgenic hormones. Some of the indications for saw palmetto include hirsutism (excess facial hair), infertility, acne, amnenorrhea, polycystic ovaries, debility, and deficiency. It helps to stimulate breast growth and to bring on menstruation.

Saw palmetto has demonstrated anabolic, antiandrogenic, and estrogenic activity. It is also an immune stimulator. It is the estrogenic and antiandrogenic properties that make this plant useful in prostate cancer therapies. Its healing effects are believed to include the ability to inhibit conversion of testosterone to dihydrotestosterone (DHT) and to help break down and excrete testosterone. High levels of DHT are believed to cause benign prostatic hyperplasia as well as the aggressive hormone-promoter of prostate cancer.[106]

By itself, it is much less effective than when combined with other herbs, such as sage, nettle root, cotton root, andrographis, red clover, cleavers, pygeum, chaste berry, licorice, Chinese skullcap, thuja, and green tea. Saw palmetto's key constituents include volatile oils, fixed oil, saponins, polysaccharides, and tannins. I consider saw palmetto a wonderful tonic herb with a wide range of indications.

Siberian Ginseng (*Eleutherococcus senticosus*)

Siberian ginseng is really not a ginseng at all (it contains no ginsenosides) but was given its name because of its adaptogenic capabilities, which are similar to panax ginseng. Like panax ginseng, Siberian ginseng improves the body's capacity to respond to stress, fatigue, and disease. Siberian ginseng helps to regulate the endocrine system, normalizing the weight of the adrenals, thymus gland, spleen, and liver. It also functions as a plant antioxidant, protecting against harmful radiation while improving oxygen metabolism. In rat studies, Siberian ginseng, as well as panax ginseng, double the life span of rats exposed to prolonged radiation.[107]

I often recommend Siberian ginseng to patients who are undergoing chemotherapy or radiation therapy. The most active compounds in Siberian ginseng are called eleutherosides.

Stephania

This Chinese herb has potent analgesic properties as well as antiedema, diuretic, and anti-inflammatory activity. It is specifically useful for edema in the lower legs, a common problem with cancer patients because cancerous tumors attract sodium, which can cause swelling in the abdomen and lower extremities. Studies with two active constituents found in stephania, fanchinin and demethyltetrandrine, have shown potent pain-relieving effects—sometimes equaling the effects of morphine. Combined with corydalis, stephania has also demonstrated pain relief.[108]

Venus's-Flytrap (*Dioneae muscipula*)

An extract of the carnivorous plant Venus's-flytrap, better known as *carnivora*, has gotten much publicity over the past few years as an anticancer agent used by Dr. Helmut Keller, a German physician. It contains at least three known cancer-inhibiting components, one of which, plumbagin, is reported to enhance phagocytosis of human granulocytes and lymphocytes. Carnivora has been shown to be an effective nontoxic treatment for many different types of cancer. I often use sundew as a substitute for Venus's-flytrap because it contains the same active agents, is easier to find, and is less costly.

Violet (*Viola odorata*)

Viola contains antineoplastic and antiviral activity. Its anti-HIV action has been validated, and it has been used for neoplasms in the breast and alimentary canal. *Viola striata*, another form of *Viola* that possesses the same properties, has shown antitumor effects in murine tests.[109] It is an antiseptic and expectorant that contains glycosides, saponins, flavonoids, carotenoids, and vitamin C.

White Pond Lily (*Nymphaea odorata*)

White pond lily was used primarily in cancers of the uterus and/or cervix by Eclectic physicians and is the chief ingredient of Eli Jones's Compound Nymphaea. This was one of Jones's favorite formulas for female cancers. It also contained poke root and was used both internally and as a douche.

White Willow (*Salix alba*)

White willow contains a glycoside, salacin, which inhibits the production of proinflammatory prostaglandins and increases the immune system's response to fighting cancer.

Wild Indigo (*Baptisia*)

The conditions calling for baptisia are those in which the vital powers are overwhelmed by toxemia and when a low-grade fever is present with a dark, purplish tongue. It has been a favorite remedy for sore throat and sore mouth, particularly in those cases where there is enfeebled capillary circulation and a tendency to ulceration. Baptisia is a specific with this symptomology. It also has a dynamic influence on the intestinal glands, and its actions are enhanced when combined with many other plant medicines. Baptisia is often combined with poke and thuja. This combination of herbs makes up Eli Jones's Cancer Drops formula, a popular combination used by Jones to treat many forms of cancer, particularly breast cancer. Baptisia also has a synergestic effect with echinacea.[110] Baptisia also stimulates white blood-cell production and increases the vitality of tissues threatened with destruction.[111]

Wolfberry (*Lycium*)

Lycium is a popular Chinese tonic herb and, like ho shou wu, is believed to promote long life. *Lycium* protects the liver from damage caused by toxins and has a cooling effect, thereby making it useful in the treatment of fever. It lowers blood pressure, improves vision, stops excess bleeding, soothes a cough, and relieves wheezing. It contains vitamins B_1, B_{12}, and C, as well as betaine, beta-sitosterol, carotene, and physalien. Chinese medicine classifies it as a blood tonic and sometimes calls it the fruit of the matrimony vine.

Yellow Dock (*Rumex crispus*)

Yellow dock contains anthraquinone glycosides, including nepodon and emodin, which are also found in buckthorn and rhubarb. It is an alterative, cholagogue, and laxative, and is employed chiefly in chronic cutaneous disorders with glandular swelling. It is an ingredient in Eli Jones's Scrophularia Compound and in the Hoxsey Formula (see Herbal Formulas for Cancer Treatment, page 163).

Zanthoxylum nitidum

Zanthoxylum nitidum is another variety of prickly ash and possesses the same properties. It promotes the flow of blood and the supply of oxygen and nutrients throughout the body. It contains the alkaloid chelerythrine, lignans, tannins, resins, and volatile oil.

Zedoria (*Curcumin zedoria*)

Zedoria, a relative of ginger and turmeric, has potent immune-enhancing abilities that incude activation of natural killer-cells. Zedoria, like turmeric, has the ability to break down fibrin and expose viral and cancer cells to more effective attack by other agents and immune-fighting chemicals. Its active principals and antitumor agents are believed to be curcumin, curdione, and curcumol. Zedoria has been widely used in China to treat some forms of cancer and has been found to inhibit sarcoma 180. It is used traditionally to treat cervical cancer.[112] Clinical trials in 209 cases of human cervical carcinoma showed a 65 percent effective rate. This herb can improve immunity and protect leukocytes after radiation therapy. Curcumin and curcuminoids are potent inhibitors of mutagenesis and tumor promotion and they also exert an anti-HIV activity. Curcumol is rapidly absorbed by the body and is distributed to all body tissues, including the brain.[113]

Recent clinical studies have also reviewed the effectiveness of elemene, another compound found in zedoria, and found that it exerts potent antitumor activity in human and murine tumor cells *in vitro* and *in vivo*.[114]

I include zedoria as an extract in herbal compounds for internal use, primarily for cervical cancer, or in a diluted mixture to be used as a douche solution. It can also be soaked into gauze or cotton and used as a tampon. I sometimes recommend use of Zedoria Tabs, a traditional Chinese formula, in a dose of 2 to 3 tablets three times a day.

Table 4.5 Major Herbs for Healing

Herb	Compound	Compound Type	Immune Effects
Astragalus (dried root)	Unknown		Antiviral; provides interferon induction, natural killer-cell enhancement, chemo and radiation protection
Celandine	Chelidonine Chelerythrine Protopine Sanguinarine D-limonene Nomilin	Alkaloid	Antitumor, antiviral; increases lymphocytes and natural killer-cells; increases bile flow
Citrus Oils	D-limonene Nomilin	Terpene	Destroys tumors; enhances drug metabolism
Echinacea	Echinacoside Arabinogalactan Echinacin	Glycoside Polysaccharide Pentacadiene Caffeic acid	Antibacterial, antitumor effects; offers nonspecific immune stimulation
Garlic	Allicin Methyl allyl trisulphide	Allyl sulfide	Antitumor effects; kills candida; inhibits cyclo-oxygenase and lipoxygenase; slows tumor growth
Goldenseal	Berberine Hydrastine L-canadine	Alkaloid	Antibiotic, antiviral, antitumor

Mistletoe	Unknown	Alkaloids Lectins Lignans Polysaccharides Polypeptides Viscotoxins	Increases cytotoxicity of lymphocytes; enhances thymus gland function; direct cytostatic action on tumors, nonspecific immunity, and regression of oncogenes
Pau d'Arco	Lapachol Lapachone Alpha and beta xyloidone	Naphthoquinone Quinone	Provides mild antitumor action
Schizandra	Gomisin A-Q Sesquicarene Citral Schizandrol Sterol stigmasterol	Lignan	Antihepatotoxin, antioxidant, nonmutagenic; protects against chemo and radiation
Sundew (carnivorous plant)	Plumbagin Drosren Hydroplumbagin	Napthoquinone	Provides gene repair mechanism; immune activator; cytotoxic, antiviral, antibiotic, antifungal
Turmeric	Curcumin and other oxidant, anticurcuminoids	Phenolic compounds	Antitumor, hepatotoxin; increases lymphocyte production
Uno de Gato	Isopteropodin and other alkaloids, quinovic acid	Alkaloids Glycosides Steroids Triterpenes	Immune system booster, tumor-inhibitor, intestinal antiseptic
Venus's-Flytrap (carnivorous plant)	Plumbagin Drosren Hydroplumbagin	Napthoquinone	Provides gene repair mechanism; immune activator; cytotoxic, antiviral, antiobiotic, antifungal
White Willow	Salicin	Glycoside	Inhibits prostaglandin production; enhances immune response; kills cancer cells

Medicinal Mushrooms

Medicinal mushrooms with immunomodulating activities have been traditionally used as tonics in Traditional Chinese Medicine (TCM). They are now used in cancer treatments to counteract the toxic effects of radiation and chemotherapy. Mushrooms used in cancer therapies are generally processed into liquid or powder in order to obtain the necessary potency. It takes about 15 pounds of reishi mushrooms to produce 1 pound of the powdered concentrate. Medicinal mushrooms make a significant contribution to the healing process by enhancing and stimulating the body's own immune system. This is a very important factor in diseases like cancer and HIV, which have components unique to each individual. In my protocols for people with cancer, I always include one or more medicinal mushroom extract products. Descriptions of some of the more frequently used mushrooms follow.

Maitake (*Grifola frondosus*)

Maitake, literally "dancing mushroom," is indigenous to the northern part of Japan and, although it has been available by cultivation since the mid-1980s, it remains one of the most valuable and expensive mushrooms. Studies have shown it possesses antitumor, anti-HIV, antihypertension, antidiabetes, antiobesity, and antihepatitis activities. Of all the standardized fractions, the maitake D-fraction is one of the most potent for enhancement of the immune system. Studies have also shown that, of all the medicinal mushrooms, it promotes the highest degree of cancer inhibition in oral administration.

Initial research on the anticancer and antitumor actions is being done primarily in Japan, in independent and university laboratories. Some extensive clinical trials are being conducted at various cancer treatment institutes in the United States.

Maitake D-fraction has been shown to complement conventional chemotherapeutic agents. Not only does it seem to improve their positive benefits, it also aids in the amelioration of many of their side effects. Dr. Hiroaki Nanba compared the D-fraction with mitomycin-C (MMC), one of the strongest and most widely used chemotherapeutic drugs used to treat stomach cancer in Japan. With just a small dose, the maitake extract produced approximately 80 percent tumor shrinkage in mice compared to 30 percent with MMC. When D-fraction was combined with MMC in half-doses, tumor shrinkage was brought up to 98 percent, demonstrating a synergistic effect between the maitake D-fraction and MMC.[115]

Reishi (*Ganoderma lucidum*)

The reishi mushroom is traditionally used in Chinese medicine for asthenia-type syndromes, characterized by a deficiency of vital energy and functions of the lower body. Reishi is the perfect remedy for the typical American suffering from constant stress. This type of individual has depressed vital force and is likely to be both deficient and toxic. When a person in such a state develops cancer and is then faced with the toxicities of chemotherapy, the situation calls for reishi. Reishi's overall effects could be described as regulatory and beneficial to the restoration of homeostasis. Its effect on the immune system is total enhancement of immune function: increase of white blood-cell count, platelets, hemoglobin, and various tumor-fighting cells. Reishi also improves both energy and sleep.

One study showed that reishi strongly inhibited the growth of sarcoma 180, with an inhibition rate of 95.6 to 98.6 percent at an interperitonial dosage of 20 mg/kg for ten days in mice.[116] Another study demonstrated that reishi polysaccharides significantly inhibited the proliferation of JTC-26 tumor cells, a human cancer-cell strain. Ganodermic acids U through Z, which are six types of cytotoxic triterpenes found in reishi, showed significant cytotoxicity on hepatoma cells grown *in vitro*.

Due to its stimulating effects on bone marrow, reishi can protect the body during radiation and chemotherapy. Clinical studies have shown reishi to be effective in the treatment of leukopenia induced by radiation, chemical agents, or other factors. Reishi has also improved symptoms of weakness, dizziness, and sleeplessness, and elevated all suppressed blood counts.[117]

Reishi mushrooms, as well as all the medicinal mushrooms mentioned in this chapter, need to be taken in either a purified extract form or brewed as a decoction. Reishi and shiitake mushrooms can also be used in soups.

Shiitake (*Lentinus edodes*)

Shiitake mushrooms have been the subject of many studies since they were discovered to possess cholesterol-lowering properties. The active component responsible was found to be eritadenine, an alkaloid with very low toxicity, which was shown capable of lowering not only serum cholesterol but also phospholipids and triglycerides. In addition, another component, called *lentinan*, which is a beta (1–3) glucan polysaccharide, demonstrated the ability to stimulate helper T-cells and reduce the synthesis of immune-suppressive prostaglandins. Perhaps the most significant finding, however, was the discovery of KS-2, a peptide component, which has been shown to induce interferon production after oral administration, to provide significant protective activity against influenza A2 virus, both prophylactically and chemotherapeutically, and to have an extremely low toxicity level.

Lentinan seems to reverse the depressed enzyme activity associated with cancer, and its antitumor activity is part of the thymus-derived immune mechanism, as shown in tests using laboratory mice. Lentinan inhibits metastasis, prevents chemical and viral oncogenesis, and has minimal side effects. Lentinan has also been shown to inhibit the growth of sarcoma 180 in mice. In addition, follow-up studies on patients with advanced and recurrent stomach and colon/rectal cancers have shown excellent results in using lentinan as part of a combination therapy. KS-2 is not available as a supplement at this time, so I suggest eating shiitake mushrooms frequently either in soups or in any cooked vegetable dish. They're delicious![118,119]

Cloud Fungus (*Coriolus versicolor*)

A polysaccharide preparation from *Coriolus versicolor*, also called PSK, has made this mushroom the focus of much cancer therapy research in Asia and Europe. It is the subject of over two hundred cancer-related articles indexed on Medline, including sixty clinical studies, several of which were multiyear, randomized, double-blind trials involving hundreds of patients. It has been shown to have great promise for other diseases, including herpes, hepatitis, systemic lupus, AIDS, rheumatoid arthritis, and many other viral, fungal, and bacterial conditions.

Over four hundred clinical studies published in Japan since the 1970s have shown that a purified extract from *Coriolus versicolor* has strong benefits to the immune system when given alone or with conventional chemotherapy or radiation treatments for cancer. This mushroom extract was selected as the best out of two hundred that were originally screened by Japanese researchers for antitumor activity in 1971.

Probably the most impressive demonstration of PSK's antitumor function came in 1990, when the results of a ten-year Japanese clinical trial involving colon or gastric cancer patients were announced. In this study, fifty-six patients began taking PSK daily after having undergone surgery for cancer of the colon and rectum. Over a period of thirteen years, the patients returned to the administering clinic (six hospitals were involved) about once every three months for evaluation. The survival rate of these patients was significantly higher than that of the fifty-five patients in the placebo group.[120,121]

The exact mechansim of *Coriolus* extract is unclear. Most likely, its effectiveness is due to an overall activation of the immune system. One thing that is known is that *Coriolus* stimulates both T-killer lymphocytes and macrophages, which are the primary white blood cells responsible for dissolving tumors. It stimulates not only the number of macrophages but the motility of macrophages to the tumor, and at the same time inhibits the tumor cell's motility. It has also been shown to have a beneficial effect on overall T-cell count enhancement and it stimulates spleen and thymic activity.

One Japanese study focused on the effects of PSK once the progression of carcinogenesis had begun. The study demonstrated that PSK influences the steps of cancer metastasis in a number of ways:

- By inhibiting tumor invasion, adhesion, and production of cell matrix-degrading enzymes.
- By suppressing tumor-cell attachment to endothelial cells through the inhibition of tumor-cell-induced platelet aggregation.
- By suppressing tumor-cell migration through the inhibition of tumor cell motility.
- By suppressing tumor growth through the inhibition of angiogenesis.[122]

A recent five-year study of gastric cancer patients reported that PSK was the therapeutic agent responsible for significant improvements in their condition. Studies done by the Japanese government over a period of thirteen years agree with these findings and support evidence that PSK (which is an approved drug in Japan) increases long-term survival and decreases the rate of cancer recurrence.[123] PSK, taken as an adjuvant following surgery for colon cancer, was found to yield an eight-year disease-free survival rate of 30 percent versus a 10 percent rate for patients taking placebo. PSK plus radiation for Stage III non-small cell lung cancer over a five-year period yielded a 22 percent survival versus only a 5 percent rate in those receiving radiation alone.[124] A ten-year study of 227 operable breast cancer patients with histological vascular invasion yielded 58 percent survival in the group receiving postsurgical chemotherapy only versus 75 percent survival in the group that had PSK added to the chemotherapy.[125]

PSK has also been used successfully in conjunction with chemotherapy to produce remissions and extend survival time in cases of leukemia. The average length of complete remission for fourteen people with acute leukemia receiving this combination was thirty-six weeks compared to twenty-five weeks for those who received chemotherapy only. The average survival time from diagnosis for the group receiving the combination was twenty-one months compared to only twelve months for those on chemotherapy alone.

Coriolus, sometimes called turkey tail, is beneficial by itself and also in conjunction with other cancer therapeutics. It has been shown to diminish the immune suppression of some other forms of therapy. The vast majority of *Coriolus* (about 70 percent) is excreted through the lungs, which makes it very effective when kidney or liver function is impaired.[126]

It is important to note that these studies used PSK as a single agent. I use PSK along with other herbal and natural agents. The dose recommended is 5 capsules daily before or between meals. In my practice, *Coriolus versicolor* extract, along with other mushroom extracts, such as the maitake D-fraction, are a regular part of my arsenal against cancer.

Poria cocos

Poria cocos, also called tuckahoe or China root, contains polysaccharides that have been shown to increase the curative effects of antitumor compounds, namely chemotherapy, and have also demonstrated immunostimulating action as well as radiation-protective effects. It is classified as a spleen tonic and has diuretic properties and immune-stimulating activity. Animal studies have demonstrated it inhibits tumor growth and invasion.[127]

Reishi 5, made by New Chapter (see Resources), is a supplement that I recommend often. It is a combination of several different mushroom supplements and it contains *Poria cocos*.

Table 4.6 Mushrooms, Immunity, and Cancer

Mushroom	Compound	Compound Type	Immune Effects
All medicinal mushrooms listed below	Beta-glucans	Triterpenes	Adaptogenic, antitumor, immunostimulant
Reishi	Ganodermic acid	Triterpenes Ganoderma polysaccharide (GPS)	Antitumor, immunostimulant
Shiitake	Lentinan; viruslike double pachymaran	Polysaccharide Stranded DNA	Stimulates T-helper cells, interferon, natural killer-cells, macrophages
Maitake	Beta-glucans	Polysaccharide	Antitumor, immunostimulant
Cloud fungus (*Coriolus versicolor*)	PSK	Polysaccharide	Immune enhancer, antioxidant, antiviral
Poria cocos	Pachymanese	Polysaccharide	Tumor inhibitor, antimutagenic

Sea Herbs

Often forgotten or overlooked in our culture, sea herbs offer unparalleled healing and nutritive value. They hide beneath the surface of the vast oceans and are usually considered persistent nuisances, clouding the waters and feeling slimy if we happen to touch them while swimming.

Sea herbs actually contain many nutrients, including all essential minerals and trace minerals. They are rich in plant iron and contain carotenoids, vitamin C, and all the B vitamins, including vitamin B_{12} (one of the only vegetable sources of this vitamin). They are the best source of calcium in its organic form, but they are most impressive as antitoxins. Sea herbs are specific for detoxifying and healing from radiation exposure. The brown sea herb wakame, which is thought to have the strongest cancer-inhibiting activity of all sea herbs, was used in miso soup to protect those who survived the atomic blast at Nagasaki against the effects of radiation.

Perhaps the most important essential nutrient found in sea herbs, and one that is frequently missing from our modern diet, is iodine. Iodine is required for the normal function of the thyroid gland, and a deficiency can cause a cascade of metabolic events, resulting in serious endocrine-related imbalances. The most obvious manifestation of this condition is hypothyroidism (low thyroid function), which, when severe, can lead to goiter or enlargement of the thyroid gland.

I believe that an insufficient intake of organic iodine in today's modern diet has led to a serious and chronic form of low-grade hypothyroidism, a major contributing factor to breast and ovarian cancers. Even a mild low thyroid function can cause an imbalance of other hormones, such as estrogen, progesterone, and androgen, hormones that play a pivotal role in reproductive health as well as in the prevention of cancerous and noncancerous tumors, such as fibroids and fibrocystic breast disease. Low thyroid function frequently coincides with low adrenal function—what I call a "hypo-overall endocrine system"; it's just not working up to speed. This condition manifests itself in many ways, including fatigue, low energy during the day, insomnia, low body temperature, very low blood pressure, low-grade depression, dry skin, dry hair, pear-shaped figure, weight gain, infertility, PMS, sensitivity to cold (particularly the extremities), calcification buildup, hardening of the arteries, cystic breasts and/or ovaries, and cancers of the breast and ovaries.

Unfortunately, a thyroid blood test does not always pick up this condition, particularly if it is not severe.

The thyroid itself regulates body temperature, energy production, growth, and metabolism. Many common health problems can be treated (or perhaps avoided completely) by including sea herbs in the diet, taking them in supplement form, or taking iodine in the form of Atomidine, an iodine solution made popular by Edgar Cayce.

The only supplemental form of sea herbs that I recommend is Ocean Herbs by New Chapter (see Resources). It is hand-harvested in clean waters. I do not trust commercial kelp tablets because they are machine-harvested and often contain undesirable substances. A common brand of edible sea herbs that I do recommend is Maine Coast Seaweeds (see Resources), available in most health food stores. This product is organic and contains all the natural constituents.

Since the composition of seawater is similar to most of our body's fluids, sea herbs are extremely compatible with the human body. Unlike iodized salt, which is not well utilized by the body, natural sea herb nutrients are readily absorbed and contain natural and well-balanced constituents. For instance, although they contain sodium, sea herbs can actually help remove excess water and lower blood pressure in cases of hypertension because they are also an excellent source of potassium.

Sea herbs also contain alginates, a unique substance that has the ability to bond to and chelate out heavy metals such as mercury, lead, excess iron, and copper. For anyone undergoing radiation therapy, I normally recommend three to four capsules of Ocean Herbs daily for the duration of therapy, and for one to two months thereafter.

Sea herbs can also buffer excess acidity in the digestive system and can be helpful in a weight-loss program when included in the diet. The intake by Japanese women of naturally occurring iodine in the form of sea herbs and fish is apparently the reason why they are seldom overweight and rarely have pear-shaped figures. It is also one of the reasons why they have a lower incidence of breast and ovarian cancers. Japanese men have a lower incidence of prostate cancer for the same reason.

Including sea herbs in the diet not only supplies a wide range of vital nutrients, it will also provide the body with an excellent source of protection from cancer and heart disease.

Table 4.7 **Sea Herbs, Immunity, and Cancer**

Seaweed	Compound	Compound Type	Immune Effects
Laminaria	Fucoidan	Polysaccharide Fatty acids	Antiviral and immunostimulant
Chlorella	Chlorellin	Glycolipid	Anti-HIV and immunostimulant; increases interferon production
Spirulina	GLA	Cartenoids Phycocyanin	Liver- and kidney-protective; inhibits cancer colony formation

Bladderwrack (*Fucus vesiculosus*)

Bladderwrack is a seaweed that was often used by the Eclectics as a medicinal plant. It is a gentle but stimulating alterative, suited for people (usually women) with cold and fatty conditions. My specific indications would be hypothyroidism, particularly in large, pear-shaped women with breast or ovarian cancer who tend to be cold and have subnormal body temperatures. Bladderwrack improves lymphatic and thyroid function. It improves nutrition and supplies an organic source of trace elements, iodine, and minerals. When I use bladderwrack in a tonic, I usually recommend it be used in a 5 to 10 percent ratio to the tonic. It's best to start with a small dose and work up gradually, checking the body temperature as an indicator. I sometimes recommend Atomidine (see Resources), a pure iodine solution. Each drop supplies 150 mcg of iodine; I usually recommend 1 to 6 drops per day, depending upon the person.

Spirulina

Spirulina is a blue-green microalga that is rich in chlorophyll. Its nutrients are easy to digest and absorb, making it an excellent source of energy for those who are weak and suffer from poor assimilation. Studies have rated spirulina's protein digestibility at 85 percent versus approximately 20 percent for beef.

It offers an effective nutrient treatment for severe liver damage resulting from malnutrition, alcoholism, or the consumption of nutrient-destroying foods or drugs. It also offers protection to the kidneys when taking strong medications. Spirulina's pure protein, which arrives within the context of massive amounts of beta-carotene, chlorophyll, fatty-acid GLA, and other nutrients, is especially helpful to those who have eaten too many animal products and refined foods—usually those who are overweight, diabetic, hypoglycemic, or suffering from cancer, arthritis, or other degenerative diseases.

Spirulina contains the blue pigment *phycocyanin*, a biliprotein that has been shown to inhibit cancer colony formation.[128]

HERBAL FORMULAS FOR CANCER TREATMENT

The longer I work with cancer patients, the more likely I am to create a custom formula for each individual I see. I use my knowledge of herbs, my observations of each individual, plus prayer and intuition to select the herbal remedy or remedies appropriate for each person I treat. Nevertheless, I occasionally use general formulas in my practice, and many of them have proven to be useful, even curative, for cancer. I have included some of these formulas on the following pages.

Hoxsey (Trifolium) Formula
(with a few changes and modifications)

The Hoxsey Formula is a classic alterative compound best prepared by an herbalist that has been used for over one hundred years. Its primary action is to increase the body's ability to remove metabolic waste, which leads to overall enhancement in the assimilation of nutrients. In my own version of this formula, I have added celandine (*Cheladonium*) because of its anticancer and liver-protective effects. For more information about each herb, consult the Index to locate the herb's description in this chapter.

Ingredients:
- Red clover
- Celandine
- Uno de gato
- Licorice
- Burdock
- Queen's root

- Poke root
- Goldenseal
- Buckthorn bark
- Thuja
- Yellow dock
- Bloodroot
- Prickly ash
- Mayapple
- Potassium iodide

Compound Scrophularia

(Eli Jones's Cancer Syrup)

Although Eli Jones believed in creating an individualized formula for each patient, after many years of testing different remedies for the internal treatment of cancer, he did eventually form a combination, which he named "Cancer Syrup." Eli Jones wrote:

> It has been the earnest study of my life to find such a combination which I could leave as a help to my brother and sister physicians in their efforts to cure the more desperate forms of cancer. I have the utmost faith in the curative power of this combination. I never mentioned this remedy to anyone . . . until I had thoroughly tested it in many difficult cases of genuine cancer, so that I could conscientiously recommend it . . .

Jones makes it a point to mention that great care should be taken to use fresh herbs to make this formula, which should be compounded by an herbalist.

Ingredients:
- Figwort (leaves and root)
- Poke root
- Yellow dock
- False bittersweet (bark and root)
- Turkey corn (root)
- Mayapple (root)
- Juniper berries
- Prickly ash berries
- Guaiacum wood

SPES

SPES, which means "hope" in Latin, is a concentrated and highly purified Chinese herbal preparation that can, at the very least, greatly improve the quality of life for people with terminal cancer. All of the following SPES products are made by Botaniclab (see Resources). The benefits of SPES as an effective herbal formula for those with cancer include the following:

1. Provides fast (twenty-four to forty-eight hours) and effective relief from cancer-associated pain and is more effective than morphine, which often elicits many adverse side effects, such as drug dependency, respiratory depression, decreased mental alertness, constipation, and, most of all, a suppression of the vital force. SPES is able to relieve pain by reducing B-endorphinlike substances in cerebrospinal fluid and serum, decreasing monamines, and increasing ACT levels. Results obtained from a clinical trial carried out in Shanghai Hospital and involving twenty-two terminally ill patients with various diseases confirmed that SPES significantly reduces the discomfort caused by cancer without having any adverse effects.[129]

2. Relieves other cancer-associated symptoms by improving gastrointestinal function and sleep, and increasing appetite and energy levels.

3. Minimizes side effects while working synergistically with chemotherapy and radiation therapy, improving both white and red blood counts, hemoglobin, and platelet counts.

4. Suppresses further cancer metastasis.

5. Is cytotoxic to many cancer-cell lines, in particular, liver tumors. Suppression of the oncogene N-ras mRNA may completely reverse the cancerous condition. Hepatoma cells are known to overexpress N-ras mRNA. SPES can suppress the transcription of the N-ras gene and effectively enter into the nucleus and cause hepatoma cell lysis, the process of disintegration or dissolution of cells.

Ingredients:

- Agrimony
- Cheng-min chou
- Cervus nippon temmininck
- Corydalis bulbosa
- Ganoderma japonicum

- Glycyrrhiza uralensis fisch
- Lycoris radiata
- Mou-hui tou
- Panax ginseng
- Pyrola rotundifolia
- Rabdosia rubescens
- Stephania sinica diels
- Stephania delavayi diels
- Zanthoxylum nitidum
- Soy milk

Both animal and human clinical trials have demonstrated the high potency and low toxicity of SPES. The usual dose is 2 to 6 capsules taken on an empty stomach.

I find it interesting that one of the main herbs in SPES, corydalis, was one of the most popular herbs used by Eli Jones to treat cancer over a hundred years ago in the United States.

What makes SPES so effective is not only the combination of herbs, but its processing and concentration as well. I am presently recommending SPES for many of the people I see and am extremely impressed with its effectiveness as a cancer pain reliever and anticancer agent.

SPES I

SPES I is an herbal compound similar to SPES in its ability to inhibit cancer growth, but it is not as effective for pain. I recommend this compound very often for those undergoing conventional cancer treatments, such as chemotherapy and radiation therapy, and have found it to be most effective for specific types of cancer, including some leukemias and lymphomas. It is sometimes questionable whether SPES or SPES I will be the most effective for solid tumors.

Ingredients:
- Psuedoginseng
- Corydalis
- Agrimony

- Isatidis
- White peony root
- Licorice
- Reishi

SPES M

SPES M is an herbal formula that increases immune functions, counteracts carcinomas, retards the progression of carcinomas, inhibits metastasis, and reverses the division of carcinoma.

The herbs in SPES M are specially processed and concentrated. In Chinese medicine, SPES M is listed as a tonic to be used to support the body for chronic deficiency.

Ingredients:

- Pseudoginseng
- Astragalus
- Agrimony
- White peony root
- Licorice
- Reishi
- Royal jelly
- Isatidis

These are the pharmacological actions of SPES M:

1. Inhibits tumor growth at a rate of about 133 percent.

2. Enters into a cancer cell's nucleus, where it inhibits DNA replication, reduces the growth of cancer, and increases phagocytosis.

3. Reverses the internal and exterior cellular structures of the carcinoma to inhibit abnormal gene expression.

4. Increases cAMP level in the plasma, in cerebrospinal fluids, and in tissues. It also increases SOD levels, activates natural killer-cells, increases the adhesion of antitumoral cells, boosts the antitumoral ability, and inhibits metastasis.

5. Enhances immunity, T-cell counts, and the formation of antibodies.

6. Increases all blood counts and platelet counts, thereby counteracting the bone marrow suppression of chemotherapy and/or radiation therapy.

7. Increases gastrointestinal functions, appetite, and overall vitality, and improves sleep.

PC SPES: Prostate Cancer Hope

International Medical Research, Inc., has been doing research on prostate cancer for over ten years and, in that time, has become convinced that this disease is the product of the dysfunction of multiple genes and cellular pathways that cannot be easily addressed by a single chemical.

After studying the effect of various herbal combinations on immune enhancement and cancer suppression, the company recently developed a proprietary herbal compound that has shown some positive results for metastatic prostate carcinoma. PC SPES contains eight herbs known to produce benefits to the immune system and, in the case of saw palmetto, to the prostate specifically.

Ingredients:

- Reishi
- Rabdosia rubescens
- Chinese skullcap
- Isaditis
- Chrysanthemum
- Licorice
- Saw palmetto

This herbal composition was studied at the laboratory of Zbigniew Darzynkiewicz, M.D., Ph.D., at the Cancer Research Institute, New York Medical College in Valhalla, New York. The extract from these herbs was found to exert potent cytostatic and cytotoxic activity on several tumor-cell lines, including prostatic carcinoma. The *in vitro* activity was observed at concentrations that are achievable in patient tissues. The activity centers around arresting tumor cells in the G1 phase of their reproductive cycle, thereby causing active cell death (apoptosis).[130] It was noted that one of the essential genes (the bcl-2 gene), which would normally protect cells from apoptosis, thereby promoting their survival, is down-regulated by treatment with this herbal extract, suggesting that cells treated with this herbal extract may be more sensitive to other antitumor agents. This is being further investigated at the Cancer Research Institute.

I personally have been working with PC SPES and SPES for the last few years and I believe that they are the two most exciting products for the treatment of cancer I have ever seen. PC SPES, along with a few other supplements and some diet modifications, can be, I believe, a complete cure for prostate cancer, at least for the majority of men.

Mainstream treatments for prostate cancer at this time center around prostatectomy, radiation therapy, or androgen deprivation. I am not convinced that prostatectomy or radiation are curative in metastatic or local prostate cancer. Androgen deprivation, which involves giving combination hormone therapy (CHT) to block the production of testosterone, is partially successful at controlling, not curing, prostate cancer in a significant number of cases.

PC SPES can induce programmed cell death from a number of directions, including an androgen-antagonist effect brought about by certain plantlike hormones found in the formula.

PC SPES can be taken without CHT treatment, or in addition to CHT treatment, especially if CHT is no longer controlling the cancer. I would prefer it to be tried without CHT, resorting to the use of CHT only after all natural treatments have stopped working (which, according to my experience, is highly unlikely).

Hepastat

Hepastat, also made by Botaniclab (see Resources), is a concentrated herbal preparation similar to the traditional Chinese formula Minor Bupleurum (Xiao Chai Hu Tang). This formula has been found extremely effective in treating hepatitis C. It is also effective at inhibiting cancer by enhancing the immune system, by inducing apoptosis, and by inhibiting angiogenesis. It has been shown to increase the effectiveness of the standard chemotherapeutic drug 5-fluorouracil (5-FU). It is most useful in breast and liver cancers but can also be used to treat colon cancer. I sometimes use this formula to detox chemotherapy; for example, cisplatin causes oxidative stress and can cause glutathione depletion. I usually suggest 3 capsules one to two times daily.

I always recommend taking at least one dose before bed because the liver does most of its detoxifying during the night. This time is called the *anabolic time* because it is during the night, while we are resting, that enzyme systems Phase I and II kick in and go to work, rebuilding and repairing any damage that's been done.

Ingredients:

- Bupleurum
- Chinese skullcap
- White peony root
- Isatidis
- Astragalus
- Milk thistle
- Royal jelly
- Licorice

Marrow Plus

(Milletia—Chinese Herbal Formula)

This formula may be taken for symptoms of bone marrow suppression caused by chemotherapy or radiation therapy. While on chemotherapy, white and red blood-cell counts and platelet counts tend to drop dramatically, and this herbal combination helps to support a person's immune system. It also helps to build blood and is therefore useful after a blood transfusion. The usual dose is 3 to 4 tablets given three to four times daily.

Ingredients:

- Milletia
- Ho shou wu
- Salvia
- Codonopsis
- Astragalus
- Ligusticum
- Rehmannia
- Lycium

- Dong quai
- Lotus seed
- Citrus
- Red date extract
- Oryza
- Gelatinum

Milletia, the main herb in this formula, is commonly used during cancer therapy to stimulate bone marrow function when it is suppressed by radiation or chemotherapy. This herb increases white blood-cell count. Codonopsis, in particular, is used in China to treat patients with low white blood-cell counts due to radiation or chemotherapy, and is also administered to increase red blood-cell counts. Rehmannia nourishes and strengthens the kidneys, which are necessary for blood regeneration. Dong quai is a strong blood tonic and helps increase the body's folic acid and vitamin B_{12} concentrations so that anemia is alleviated in many cases.

Super-Tonic

An excellent overall cancer-inhibiting compound of herbs that I recommend frequently, Super-Tonic is especially good for people who have had surgery or are undergoing radiation therapy. (See Resources.)

Ingredients:

- Siberian ginseng
- Schizandra
- Green tea
- Ginkgo biloba
- Milk thistle
- Ashwaganda
- Turmeric
- Amla
- Triphalia extract
- Boswellia extract
- Black pepper

TOPICAL TREATMENTS

Recently, I have been recommending more and more external/transdermal mixtures that have a wide range of applications for various cancers. I am excited about the use of transdermal essential oils that are mixed with other plant oils and DMSO (dimethyl sulfoxide, an anti-inflammatory agent). Essential oils are some of the most potent cancer fighters found in nature, and we've only just begun to scratch the surface of their potential use in cancer treatment. I am currently working with many variations of these mixtures that can be applied to any soft tissue area of skin, the soles of the feet, the scalp, or the area of skin that is directly over an organ, such as the liver. Some can also be used as additions to bathwater. The following are external formulas that are currently available.

Lavender Poke Oil

This is my own formula, which has several variations, depending on the specifics of the condition. One of the main uses for this remedy is in breast cancer following a lumpectomy. After the initial healing is done, usually two to three weeks after surgery, I recommend using this oil on the breast and/or lymph nodes two to three times daily. It could also be used following radiation therapy or as part of a treatment for cystic breasts.

Ingredients:
- Poke oil
- Hypericum oil
- DMSO
- Organic essential oils of lavender, rosemary, and rose geranium
- Vitamin E oil

Azelaic Acid

Azelaic acid is a naturally occurring, nontoxic dicarboxylic acid that has been widely studied in Europe over the last decade. Studies have shown that this fatty acid possesses significant properties that offer therapeutic applications in the field of dermatology. It is a known competitive inhibitor of tyrosinase, with its main target being the mitochondria. Cell culture studies in melanoma, lymphoma, and leukemia-derived cell lines have shown an inhibitory effect by azelaic acid. Melanoma cells exposed to azelaic acid, for instance, show an inhibitory effect on DNA synthesis and on plasminogen activator activity. This cytotoxic effect is due to the antimitochondrial action, which exhibits itself as degeneration of mitochondria, eventually leading to cell death. Adjacent normal cells, however, remain unaffected, which demonstrates azelaic acid's affinity to abnormal cells. In other studies, it has also been shown that nontoxic concentrations of azelaic acid reduced DNA synthesis of cultured melanoma cells but had no overt effect on the protein synthesis of these same cells.

Still other studies have shown that basal cell carcinoma responds dramatically to a mixture of azelaic acid and other standard dermatological agents such as 5-FU.[131–133]

I recommend Melazepam, a brand of azelaic acid produced by Emerson Ecologics (see Resources). This cream, which contains other ingredients as well, is helpful when applied to pre-basal cell cancerous skin growths.

Bloodroot, Turmeric, and Zinc Chloride Escharotic Paste

This is the most popular external herbal skin cancer remedy. It is used for basal cell cancers and will work most satisfactorily on small skin tumors of the nose or forehead. I usually recommend my own variation, in which I include bloodroot and zinc chloride, azelaic acid cream, and a powder or fluid extract of turmeric. Be very careful with these ingredients, particularly the zinc chloride, because it burns and could be very painful. Before using the remedy, it is best to cover the surrounding area with adhesive strips for protection. Apply with a piece of cloth and keep on for twenty-four hours. Then remove and clean with warm water. You may or may not need to apply a second time, but never use more than two applications and do not exceed a total of forty-eight hours because it may then work too deeply and cause tissue damage. This formula is not commercially made but can be compounded for you by an herbalist or naturopathic doctor.

Poultice Powder

This is a simple drawing poultice powder (not available commercially) that is used to remove cancerous pus from a tumor.

Ingredients:

- 1 to 2 tablespoons flaxseeds, freshly ground to a powder
- 1 to 2 tablespoons slippery elm powder
- 1 tablespoon lobelia seeds, freshly ground to a powder
- 1 teaspoon bayberry or goldenseal powder

Mix 1 to 2 teaspoons of the poultice powder with enough boiled water to make a paste. Stir until all lumps dissolve. Then spread on a soft white cloth big enough to cover the growth and the red inflamed skin around it. Do this every two hours until no more pus forms. Clean the area between each application with an herbal antiseptic solution such as calendula succus, distilled witch hazel, or colloidal silver.

Bentonite clay or plain white cabbage may also be used for the same purposes. If using cabbage, it should be raw and macerated to a pulp and then applied, covered, and left on for a few hours or overnight.

Yellow Healing Salve

This is one of Eli Jones's cancer-healing salves that will heal all tissue in the area from which a cancerous growth has been removed while allowing any pus to be drawn out. It can be used following a poultice.

Ingredients:

- Burgundy pitch
- White pine turpentine
- Beeswax
- Mutton tallow
- Olive oil

Melt, stir, and cool ingredients. Store in glass jars. Spread on soft white cloth and apply to sore three times a day until completely healed.

This product is not made commercially. It may be compounded for you by an herbalist or naturopathic doctor. I also recommend Herbal Ed's Salve or any of the other good over-the-counter healing herbal salves (see Resources).

5

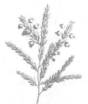

Useful Supplements in Cancer Therapy

Nothing is rich but the inexhaustible wealth of nature.
She shows us only surfaces, but she is millions of
fathoms deep.

—*Ralph Waldo Emerson*

VITAMINS AND MINERALS

Due to their particular mechanisms of action, vitamins, minerals, and many other natural compounds offer a hopeful new approach to cancer therapy that is quite different from standard therapies such as chemotherapy, radiation, surgery, and immunotherapy. (See table 5.1, Major Supplements for Cancer Prevention and Treatment, on pages 214 to 217.) Experimental, epidemiological, and clinical studies are accumulating that reveal vitamins as a new class of compounds with remarkable prophylactic and therapeutic activities for both the person with cancer and for those who want to prevent cancer.

175

Vitamins, minerals, and other phytonutrients influence many cellular functions that are important in the induction and promotion of cancer, such as cell growth and cell differentiation, antioxidation, DNA synthesis, and cell membrane alterations. They protect against excessive oxidative stress, suppressing free-radical damage when cells are stressed by chemical or radiation-enhanced cell transformation. Protective systems affected by these antioxidants include enzyme induction (e.g., catalase, peroxidase, dismutase), supply of thiols, and interference with free-radical mechanisms in the initiation and promotion stages of malignant transformation.[1,2]

The biological mechanisms for cancer inhibition and regression through the use of antioxidant nutrients are gradually becoming understood and appear to act through four types of pathways:

1. Tumor inhibition by immune cytokine activation or modulation and through an anti-inflammatory mechanism.

2. Stimulation of cancer-suppression genes and down-regulation of oncogenes.

3. Inhibition of tumor angiogenesis.

4. Stimulation of cellular differentiation and the resultant apoptosis of neoplastic cells.

Combinations of antioxidant nutrients and herbs produce a synergistic effect that results in an overall cancer-inhibiting action. Uniquely, these nutrients are also able to selectively act upon cancer cells while allowing healthy cells to function normally.

A combination of beta-carotene, vitamin E, and selenium reduced the risk of dying from cancer and other diseases in a National Cancer Institute–sponsored study in Linxian, China. Of the nearly thirty thousand men and women ages forty to sixty-nine who took part in the study, those who took this combination over five years had a 13 percent reduction in cancer death rate and a 9 percent reduction in total death. "This is a hopeful sign that vitamins and minerals may help prevent the onset of cancer in healthy individuals," said William J. Blot of NCI's biostatistics branch and one of the principal investigators of this study.[3]

Recently, because of a few negative studies that have shown the possibility that certain vitamins may protect a mutated cell from apoptosis (programmed cell death), it is now theorized that certain antioxidants could interfere with the body's normal oxidative process of removing damaged cells. However, the studies were done with synthetic isolated beta-carotene, which bears no resemblance to the nutrient supplied to us by nature, and is certainly not a formulation that I would recommend to my patients as a supplement.

For optimal health, we need to take in oxygen through the air we breathe and the foods we eat; we need essential fatty acids; and we need cell-protective agents to assist in the removal of waste. An inadequate amount of oxygen allows cancer cells, viruses, fungi, and bacteria to flourish; on the other hand, too much oxygen may cause free radicals to proliferate and become oxidative waste. When oxygen reacts with rancid fats, heavy metals, steroid hormones, or chemical carcinogens, it causes healthy cells to become damaged and then to mutate. These mutated cells do not die off through normal apoptosis and can, therefore, become cancerous cells. To prevent this deadly scenario, we need a careful balance between oxygenation and oxygen waste protection. This is where proper supplementation comes in. By using our knowledge of the synergistic effects that vitamins have upon each other, we can regulate this important balance within the body. For example, the synergy between vitamins E, A, and C enhances the effects of chemotherapeutic drugs and radiation therapy, and reduces their systemic toxic effects.

However, before taking supplements as part of a preventive or treatment plan for cancer, it is important to be very selective about the type, the combination, the quality, and the dosage. For example, the only beta-carotene supplement I recommend is a liquid called Beta-Plex by Scientific Botanicals (see Resources), which is derived from food and contains all the known and unknown carotenoids balanced together just as they are in nature. Many of the popular over-the-counter brands of vitamins are not worth taking and may actually be harmful. Seek the advice of an expert in this field before purchasing vitamin supplements.

For cancer patients undergoing conventional treatments, I recommend starting nutritional supplementation at least one week prior to surgery, radiation, or chemotherapy. The benefits of supplement use will be described more fully throughout this chapter and include the following:

1. *Supplements can decrease short-term toxic side effects.* Nutrients can help lessen hair loss and nausea and provide extra energy and faster recovery from immune suppression. In addition to helping restore proper levels of platelets and white and red blood-cell counts, they also protect healthy cells from chemotherapy without interfering with the cytotoxic effects upon cancer cells (a particular benefit of N-acetyl cysteine).

2. Supplements can decrease long-term toxic side effects. Certain nutrients can protect organs from long-term damage. For example, studies have shown that coenzyme Q10 (CoQ10) reduces the cardiac damage caused by adriamycin, a frequently used chemotherapeutic drug.[4] The serious side effects of many other drugs (methotrexate and cytoxan, to name just two) can also be significantly reduced by appropriate nutrient supplementation.

3. *Supplements have positive synergistic effects.* Many nutrients exhibit a synergistic effect when used with chemotherapeutic drugs. Others, by inhibiting mutation of cancer, allow the body to experience the longer-lasting cytotoxic effects of chemotherapy and radiation. Examples of this are the positive effects of combining folic acid and beta-glucan with 5-FU and also the use of quercetin with Adriamycin.

4. *Supplements can inhibit cancer.* All supplements synergistically assist the body's defense mechanisms as they inhibit metastatic cancer and prevent recurrences.

I customize a nutritional supplement regime for each cancer patient I see, recommending particular supplements and directing the dosage and method of use. Some supplements are more effective when taken with meals, while others, such as enzymes, are best taken on an empty stomach. Whenever possible, I have included directives such as those in the individual nutrient descriptions that follow.

Two general supplements that I often recommend are Cyto-Redoxin by Tyler Encapsulations (includes vitamin C, E, selenium, N-acetyl cysteine, CoQ10, alpha-lipoic acid, carotene complex, zinc, grape seed extract, and green tea extract) and Clinical Nutrients Antioxidant by Phyto Pharmica, which has similar ingredients. Many times general supplements like these (and others listed in Resources) are the foundation of a protocol I recommend, and I add other specific nutrients and supplements based on the individual's immediate needs.

Vitamin A

The National Research Council reported that vitamin A was able to suppress chemically induced tumors in lab animals, and numerous other researchers have shown its anticarcinogenic effect.[5] Vitamin A may interfere with the mutation of cells that have been exposed to carcinogens, either by inhibiting enzymes that activate chemicals to their carcinogenic form or by stimulating immune responses.

On the basis of epidemiologic and experimental evidence of the anti-cancer activity of vitamin A when used in high doses, a clinical trial was conducted at the National Cancer Institute in Milan to determine whether vitamin A administration could reduce the occurrence of cancer relapses within three years and/or the occurrence of new primary tumors beyond three years. In this study, postsurgical lung cancer patients were given vitamin A in doses of 300,000 IU daily for a period of fourteen months. At the time of analysis, there was a relapse rate of 18 percent in the treated group and 28 percent in the control group. The largest difference between the groups was observed for bone metastases (two versus seven) and brain metastases (three versus six), and only two new cases of primary cancer were detected, both in the control group.[6]

A randomized study of 307 surgically cured lung cancer patients receiving 300,000 IU of vitamin A daily for twelve months versus a group taking no supplements, found that 37 percent of the supplemented group and 48 percent of the control group developed new primary tumors. The tumor-free interval was significantly longer in the group receiving vitamin A. Further, primary tumors developed in eighteen supplemented patients and twenty-nine control patients. This study confirms that high doses and prolonged administration of vitamin A can effectively reduce the incidence of new primary tumors and increase the tumor-free interval in heavy smokers surgically cured of lung cancer.[7,8] *Note:* Dosages over 50,000 IU should be taken only under the supervision of a health care professional.

I usually recommend vitamin A in mycellized form. When the body is fighting an illness, is under stress, or is simply aging, it loses its ability to manufacture its own mycelles, the basic unit of absorption for vitamins A, D, E, and K, beta-carotene, essential fatty acids, and lecithin. Mycellization is a natural process of manufacturing water-soluble fat for easy absorption.

Carotenoids

Carotenoids can protect phagocytic cells from auto-oxidative damage, enhance T- and B-lymphocyte proliferate responses, and enhance macrophage, cytotoxic T-cell, and natural killer-cell tumoricidal capacities, as well as increase the production of certain interleukins. Carotenoids protect the body, especially the lipids and organ walls in the cell, from oxidative damage.

The carotenoid family contains over eight hundred different members, each with a slightly different molecular structure and physical properties. It is best to consume a full spectrum of carotenoid pigments. There are two main types of carotenoids. One type contains no oxygen and has provitamin A abilities, which means that it can remain in the body as carotene but can be converted into vitamin A upon demand. Examples of this type of carotenoid, such as beta-carotene and the recently popular lycopene found abundantly in tomatoes, are typically orange/red in color.

The other type of carotenoid, called xanthophyll, has no provitamin A conversion abilities. Xanthophyll-rich carotenoids are primarily yellow in color and include many flowers, such as calendula, as well as the spice saffron. The color changes we see in ripening fruit or the leaves turning in the fall is the result of carotenoid pigments emerging after being masked by green chlorophyll pigments. Lutein, found in green leafy vegetables, capsanthin, and canthaxanthin are other examples of xanthophyll carotenoids. Carotenoids protect the epithelial tissue (skin, stomach, and lungs) from becoming cancerous. The carotenoid lycopene has been shown to be useful in treating pancreatic cancer[9] and in reducing the risk of prostate cancer.[10]

Beta-carotene and canthaxanthin have been shown to protect animals against three types of tumors: UV-induced skin tumors, carcinogen-induced skin tumors, and UV plus carcinogen-induced skin tumors.[11] Evidence continues to accumulate that carotenoids may possess intrinsic chemopreventive action with respect to damage of the nucleus, malignant transformation, and tumor formation.

Recent studies have also shown that beta-carotene and canthaxanthin can inhibit neoplastic transformation by enhancing normal cellular communication. This mode of action is referred to as *gap junctional communication*. Enhanced communication leads to decreased proliferation, whereas a low level of communication is associated with high proliferation rates. Junctional communication has many similarities to the effects of tumor-suppressor genes.[12]

Another study measured beta-carotene levels in both healthy women and women with cervical cancer. Significantly lower levels of this carotenoid were found in the cancer group. The same study demonstrated a marked increase in beta-carotene levels in cervicovaginal cells for all subjects after oral supplementation. The findings support a previous hypothesis that beta-carotene deficiency may have an etiologic role in the development of cervical cancer.[13]

It has been demonstrated both in experimental and clinical applications that carotenoids and retinoids (the form of vitamin A released from the liver) inhibit carcinogenesis in the promotional stage. One form of retinoid (13-cis-retinoic acid) is being tested in various cancers and is showing promise. Some of these cancers include squamous cell carcinoma cell lines, both acute and chronic myelocytic leukemia, ovarian cancer, small-cell lung cancer, neuroblastoma, and multiple myeloma. This treatment does cause immune suppression, but vitamin E reduces the toxicity and permits prolonged drug delivery.

Recently there have been some studies using carotenoids, in particular beta-carotene, along with certain chemotherapeutic agents, to see what effect they might have upon each other. The result of these studies indicates that carotenoids could have a synergistic effect with some chemotherapeutic agents.[14]

A case-controlled study in Melbourne, Australia, of eighty-eight consecutive males admitted for the surgical removal of nonmelanocytic skin cancer and eighty-eight male controls admitted for small elective surgeries has shown that those who developed skin cancer had lower levels of beta-carotene and vitamin A than the controls. The incidence of skin cancer was inversely related to the level of serum beta-carotene.[15]

As mentioned earlier, I recommend one carotenoid supplement only: Beta-Plex by Scientific Botanicals. This is a liquid solution of naturally occurring full-spectrum carotenoids from vegetables. Until very recently, most of the research on carotenoids has been done with synthetic beta-carotene only. If a full-spectrum carotenoid supplement, such as Beta-Plex, were to be used in clinical trials, I believe we would see consistently impressive results both for cancer prevention and treatment.

Vitamin E Succinate

Vitamin E's most characterized function is as a lipid-soluble antioxidant within the cell membranes, functioning as a free-radical scavenger to prevent lipid peroxidation of polyunsaturated fats. Vitamin E also increases the effective-ness of selenium, detoxifies nitrates, and protects against cancer, especially prostate cancer. Studies on the antiproliferation activities of vitamin E show that the succinate ester (the dry form) is the most effective form and that tumor cell growth inhibition is probably more than just antioxidant functions.

Vitamin E and selenium act alone and in synergy to protect against the effects of radiation and chemotherapeutic agents. Vitamin E appears to confer its protection in an alternate complementary mechanism by reducing cellular lipid peroxidation products. Selenium confers protection in part by inducing or acti-vating cellular free-radical scavenging systems and by enhancing peroxide break-down, thus increasing the capacity of the cell to cope with oxidative stress.

Retrovirus-induced immune dysfunctions can, through a multistage process, cause tumorigenesis. Vitamin E can inhibit or reverse this process by several mechanisms, some of which include:

- Enhancing mitogen-mediated T-cells
- Regulating T-suppressor cells
- Affecting the arachidonic acid cascade by reducing the regulation of prostaglandin E2 and increasing the regulation of interleukin-2[16]

While vitamin E closely interacts with selenium, it also interacts with vi-tamin C. Vitamin C has been shown to preserve the antioxidant action of vi-tamin E by reducing oxidized vitamin E.[17]

An Arizona Cancer Center researcher reported at a national conference on cancer and nutrition that vitamin E oil applied directly to the skin of lab-oratory mice exposed to ultraviolet-B light, the most cancer-causing rays of the sun, protected them against developing skin cancer.[18]

A recent study showed that 50 mg of alpha-tocopherol per day (a modest intake of vitamin E) reduced prostate cancer incidence by 32 percent and prostate cancer deaths by 41 percent in a group of male smokers in Finland.[19]

Vitamin E, when taken at 200 IU per day, reduced the risk of developing colon cancer by 57 percent, according to a recent study from the University of Washington School of Medicine.[20]

In summary, vitamin E inhibits cancer development and management by:

- Inhibiting neoplastic cell growth
- Serving as a strong antioxidant and free-radical scavenger

- Inhibiting mutagenic activity
- Influencing cell integrity and cell membrane maintenance
- Taking part in DNA synthesis and chromosomal breakage induced by carcinogenesis
  - Stimulating immune system activity
  - Preventing platelet aggregation
  - Modulating prostaglandin biosynthesis[21]

Vitamin C

The form of vitamin C that I recommend is the ascorbate form mixed with a multitude of flavonoids. Vitamin C ascorbate is nonacidic, better assimilated, and, therefore, does not cause gastric acidity.

Consumption of foods high in vitamin C is clearly associated with a decreased risk of certain cancers. The most convincing evidence concerns cancers of the bladder, larynx, esophagus, stomach, and pancreas. This effect could be the result of antioxidation, immune enhancement, or a blockage of the conversion of nitrates and nitrogen-containing compounds to carcinogens. Other cancers upon which vitamin C seems to have a protective effect include cancers of the rectum, cervix, lung, and oral cavity.[22]

Vitamin C is important in collagen synthesis, the biochemical basis of healthy tissue such as the gums, skin, and teeth. Vitamin C is also involved in peptide hormones and neurotransmitters, the production of norepinephrine, cartilage maturation, maintenance of cytochrome P-450, carnitine synthesis, and the epiphyseal growth plate, cartilage that is the site of longitudinal bone growth. This vitamin is a potent antioxidant and free-radical scavenger and the first line of defense for free-radical scavenging in cigarette smokers. Vitamin C, within the plasma, is a more effective free-radical scavenger than beta-carotene, vitamin E, and glutathione. Vitamin C is concentrated in neutrophils and lymphocytes to a very high degree. There is an inverse correlation between neutrophil glucose concentration and vitamin C levels. This may be a potential reason why uncontrolled diabetics are susceptible to bacterial and other infections. Animals deficient in vitamin C have had reduced antibacterial action. Vitamin C ascorbate has an antiviral effect on the Rhus sarcoma virus and human immunodeficiency virus. It is possible that vitamin C has an effect on virus production in infected cells and also extracellularly.

A review of seventy-five epidemiological studies showed significant evidence of reduced risk for cancer in those with a higher dietary intake of vitamin C. There may be other factors involved, since this was a dietary study and many other nutrients were involved. Vitamin C has also been shown to inhibit the development of estrogen-induced kidney tumors in hamsters. Large doses of vitamin C reduced the severity and incidence of mammary tumors in RIII mice and ultraviolet light-induced skin tumors in hairless mice. Isomers and metabolites of vitamin C may also have therapeutic benefit in different cancer sites in experimental models.[23]

Vitamin C ascorbate, in conjunction with other nutrients such as zinc, vitamin B_{12}, and other cancer-inhibiting agents, has a synergistic antitumor effect. Vitamin C enhances traditional cancer therapies and reduces their toxicity. Adriamycin and radiation toxicity were reduced in animal models receiving vitamin C. The amount needed to prevent deficiency may not be the optimal amount. Ascorbate's superior activity against peroxyl radicals in human plasma marrow, but not tumor tissues, protects the skin and bones from the effects of radiation treatments.[24,25]

Even though scurvy is rare in the United States, marginal vitamin C deficiency may be common. At-risk populations are smokers, those with chronic problems, including cancer and dialysis, those eating marginal diets (especially the elderly and indigent), and those who abuse alcohol and drugs. Within the next decade, optimal vitamin C levels should be known.

Vitamin C does not kill cancer cells but restrains them. The hypothesis is that cancer cells release enzymes, such as hyaluronidase and collagenase, that modify the properties of the ground substance (the intracellular cement in which all cells are embedded), allowing the malignant cells to penetrate and invade the surrounding tissues. Vitamin C, along with flavonoids, acts to strengthen the ground substance and to restrain the invasiveness of cancer cells by neutralizing hyaluronidase and enhancing the synthesis of collagen fibrils. In addition, vitamin C plays a role in the stimulation and modification of the immune system.

I believe that vitamin C is overrated as an anticancer agent. In a few studies involving some leukemia cell lines, high amounts of vitamin C appeared to cause an acceleration of the cancer. I do recommend vitamin C ascorbate in conjunction with other more important supplements, particularly flavonoids, such as quercetin and/or PCOs (see page 210). I do not usually recommend more than 3,000 mg per day, which is best taken in small, frequent doses: 500 to 1,000 mg three to four times daily along with a complex of flavonoids that include quercetin.

Vitamin D

Vitamin D helps to prevent colon and breast cancers. It is theorized that vitamin D binds with calcium and reduces the turnover rate of the cells that line the colon. Cells that don't turn over are very resistant to carcinogens.

Vitamin D has an inhibitory effect on episomes, submicroscopic circular DNA molecules that carry amplified oncogenes as well as amplified drug-resistant genes. Vitamin D_3 is reported to inhibit the incorporation of messages at chromosomal sites, thereby providing a strategy that might make some episomes more susceptible to elimination.[26]

Vitamin D may have the ability to inhibit the proliferative activity of hormones, such as estrogen in breast cancer, and has been shown to suppress breast and prostate cancer growth. Sunlight exposure, which leads to an increased level of vitamin D, correlates with a reduced risk of breast cancer. I usually recommend small amounts of vitamin D (400 to 1,000 IU) for those people without sunlight exposure, especially during the winter. I also occasionally recommend cod liver oil during the winter months as a source of vitamin D and omega-3 fatty acids. Vitamin D deficiency is very common in the elderly and in people who live in parts of the world with little sunlight; it is also one of the major contributing factors to osteoporosis.

Vitamin K

Vitamin K is a fat-soluble antihemorrhagic agent comprising three similar compounds:

- Vitamin K_1 (phylloquinone), found naturally in all green plants
- Vitamin K_2 (menaquinone), products of bacteria
- Vitamin K_3 (menadione), a synthetic derivative

Researchers at the UCLA School of Medicine discovered that vitamin K is a very effective cancer-cell fighter. Tests have shown that vitamin K can stop and sometimes shrink tumor growth. It also acts as a tumor analgesic.[27] Vitamin K_3 has been widely researched in cancer studies. A significant inhibition by vitamin K_3 was observed in several human cancer-cell lines, including breast, ovary, colon, stomach, and kidney cancers, as well as primary and squamous cell carcinomas of the lungs. The inhibition of cancer cells is a dose-dependent phenomenon. Clinical trials using vitamin K_3 and 5-FU for patients with metastatic adenocarcinoma of the breast and colon showed some objective responses that have lasted more than twelve months in four responding patients. It has also been suggested that vitamin K_3 is a radiosensitizing agent. The addition of vitamin K_3 to radiation therapy in patients with cancer of the mouth area increased the survival rate at five years to 39 percent as compared to 20 percent in patients treated with radiation alone.[28,29] Vitamin K_1 is derived from vegetable sources and is therefore nontoxic. I recommend a form of vitamin K_1 created by Scientific Botanicals (see Resources).

Vitamin B_6

Many human enzyme systems that involve protein metabolism, catabolism, anabolism, or enzyme production require vitamin B_6 in order to function properly. Vitamin B_6 also improves immune function.[30] Pyridoxal-5-phosphate (P5P), the biologically active coenzyme form of vitamin B_6, has been shown to reduce cell growth and kill a number of cell types in culture. The most substantial inhibiting effect was found with metastatic melanoma cells.[31]

Folic Acid and Vitamin B_{12}

Folic acid and vitamin B_{12} appear to aid in a process that turns cancer genes off by helping transfer methyl groups and their metabolism. When the process, called methylation, doesn't work, as is the case in alcohol abuse, or if the person is on the chemo drug methotrexate, cancer genes produce proteins that may cause cells to proliferate. A methyl-group-deficient diet leading to hypomethylation of DNA and RNA can promote cancer in the liver. A significant body of information suggests that a deficiency of vitamin B_{12} can enhance the activity of various carcinogens. Other studies also indicate a link between alterations of the intracellular metabolism of cobalamin (B_{12}) and the increased growth of melanoma. There is a strong association between folate deficiency and cervical dysplasia, cervical and uterine cancers, cancers of the gastrointestinal tract, squamous cancers of the respiratory tract, and bone marrow cancers.[32] A recent study carried out at the Harvard Medical School has shown that long-term use of multivitamins may substantially reduce the risk of colon cancer. The study points to folic acid as the nutrient responsible for this benefit.[33]

The onset of folate deficiency in tumor cells is accompanied by changes in the adhesive properties of the cells. Growth of murine melanoma cells in a low-folate medium for longer than two-and-a-half days resulted in tumor cells that adhered more rapidly and in higher percentages to plastic dishes coated with laminin or fibronectin. Because folate deficiency affects several important characteristics of tumor cells, inadequate levels of this vitamin may contribute to the progression of malignancies. Studies in mice indicate that folate-deficient B_{16} melanoma cells produce more metastases than folate-replete control cells.[34]

It is increasingly apparent that methylation, the process of methyl metabolism, plays a central role in chemical carcinogenesis. Methyl groups are supplied in the diet (eggs and any green vegetables) principally by methionine and choline, and normal methyl metabolism requires, in addition, the nutrients folate and B_{12}. Deficiencies of choline, methionine, B_{12}, or folate are of widely varying importance in humans, with folate deficiency being by far the most important. Vitamin B_{12} is found in seaweed, some seafood, and meat, and is therefore difficult to get in a vegetarian diet. Subclinical or borderline definiency of these nutrients is now thought to be a risk factor for cancer as well as heart disease. Testing for elevated levels of homocysteine in the blood is an effective way to evaluate methylation efficiency, as well as to determine the need for folic acid and/or vitamin B_{12} supplementation.

Methotrexate, a standard chemotherapuetic agent used to treat various cancers, interferes with the activation of folate, therefore disrupting DNA replication for cancer and other cells. While it is generally accepted that folate supplementation must be avoided while a patient is on this drug, 1 mg of folate can reduce the side effects of methotrexate without interfering with its therapeutic effect. Methotrexate also negatively affects the metabolism of methyl compounds by causing a deficiency of methionine, choline, and vita-min B_{12}.[35]

I usually recommend Hydroxy Folate, a liquid B_{12} and folic acid solution made by Scientific Botanicals (see Resources), in doses of 2 to 4 drops orally once a day for patients using methotrexate. Each drop contains 200 mcg of B_{12} and folic acid.

In a recent study, folic acid, along with vitamin B_{12} supplementation, reduced cellular atypia squamous metaplasia in heavy smokers.[36] Recent evidence also suggests that folic acid and derivatives contribute to the protective effect of fruits and vegetables against the risk of large bowel cancers.[37]

Vitamin B_{12} and folic acid offer significant help in many areas of distress that plague cancer patients, such as anemia, fatigue, neuropathy and other nerve damage, liver weakness, and digestion. Vitamin B_{12} is required for the production of hydrochloric acid, which in turn is needed for protein digestion, and both supplements improve appetite and help with sleep disturbances.

I often recommend Folirinse, a liquid folic acid supplement also made by Scientific Botanicals, for cervical dysplasia. I have found it extremely effective at reversing this precancerous condition. Each drop of Folirinse contains 5 mg of folic acid. I usually recommend 1 to 2 drops daily until there has been a reversal of the dysplasia and a normal Pap smear. Thereafter, I recommend a lower dose (1 to 2 mg daily) as a prophylactic measure. Any dose over 800 mcg requires a doctor's prescription.

Calcium

I usually recommend calcium orotate for cancer patients with bone metastases. Calcium orotate is far superior to any other form of calcium in recalcifying bone that has been lost because of metastatic cancer. Along with vitamin K_1, it also helps to diminish pain. A new drug called Aredia (or pamadronate) also appears to be very promising for recalcifying bone and reducing pain due to bone cancer. I have recommended Aredia therapy to many of my clients who have bone metastasis. It has been been nothing short of miraculous for that condition when taken along with other treatments I recommend.

Calcium is under active clinical study in colon carcinogenesis. Studies suggest that dietary calcium significantly reduces the incidence of colon cancer in animals by significantly reducing hyperproliferation in colonic epithelium induced by bile salts and fatty acids.[38] A recent study evaluating calcium as a possible inhibitor of colon cancer involved 175 patients with adenomatous colon polyps and 50 patients with colorectal cancer who received calcium supplementation. It showed that calcium supplementation can prevent the recurrence of polyps and can prolong survival in patients with colorectal cancer.[39]

There have been several other epidemiological reports showing the inverse relationship between dietary calcium and the incidence of colon cancer.[40] One study evaluated 2,591 Dutch civil servants, forty to sixty-five years of age, during a twenty-eight-year follow-up for the relationship between calcium intake and the risk of gastrointestinal cancer. Woman who had the lowest calcium intake had an increased risk of gastrointestinal cancer. Men and women with a lower than average calcium intake had an increased colorectal cancer mortality. These results were significant for women.[41,42]

Potassium and Magnesium

Potassium and magnesium aspartate activate the formation of ATP that is needed to insure the optimal functioning of the host's defense system. Magnesium improves the activity of white granulocytic blood cells and increases the production of immune-defensive substances, including antibodies and other complementary factors that activate specific antibodies.

Increased potassium intake is associated with decreased cancer risk, whereas increased sodium intake is associated with increased cancer risk. The ratio of potassium to sodium appears to be more important than the levels of individual electrolytes. Generally, intracellular potassium concentrations are higher in noncancerous tissues than in cancerous tissues. Conversely, intracellular sodium is higher in tumor cells than in normal cells.

In potassium-depleted patients, villous tumors of the large bowel are prone to become malignant at an earlier stage than in patients whose potassium is not depleted. This suggests that potassium depletion plays a role in the loss of the growth control leading to malignant transformation of the tumor.[43]

An increase of cancer has been found worldwide in areas where magnesium levels are lowest. This is also true of selenium. In rat studies, magnesium deficiency caused neoplastic growths of both lymphomas and leukemias. Many people with cancer have low levels of magnesium to begin with, and when they undergo chemotherapy and/or radiation therapy, their need for magnesium, as well as potassium, can become crucial. The drugs cisplatin, cyclophosphamide, vinblastine, bleomycin, cyclosporin, and taxol cause hypomagnesemia. Magnesium supplementation (magnesium orotate is preferred), with or without potassium, is important when taking these drugs and for some time afterward as well. Magnesium also works as a natural laxative. Low magnesium levels are also clearly related with increased risk of heart disease mortality.

Cisplatin and Hypomagnesemia

Cisplatin therapy may cause hypomagnesemia through renal tubular magnesium wasting, which may in turn cause neuromuscular irritability, weakness, confusion, seizures, and ventricular arrhythmias. In one study, twenty-three patients being treated with a cisplatin-based adjuvant chemotherapeutic regimen were randomly given either magnesium aspartate hydrochloride through all cycles of chemotherapy or intermittently, whenever their serum magnesium levels dropped. Of the intermittent magnesium-supplemented patients, 89 percent had to receive magnesium supplementation by the third cycle of chemotherapy, when similar dosages of magnesium were given to both groups. These results confirm that there is a high incidence of hypomagnesemia in cisplatin-treated patients. By the fourth cycle of chemotherapy, all patients had had episodes of hypomagnesemia. I recommend a continual supplementation of magnesium aspartate hydrochloride during cisplatin therapy.[44]

Potassium Iodide and Tumor Growth

In a mice model, animals receiving potassium iodide orally to block the thyroid gland against radioactive iodine displayed slower tumor growth than mice not receiving potassium iodide. It is thought that potassium iodide has an effect on pituitary function mediated through the thyroid gland. This leads to decreased estrogen production in the body due to the inhibition of follicle-stimulating function and stimulation of luteinizing function of the pituitary. The iodine may also change hormonal actions within the tumor.[45]

Potassium iodide was used by the Eclectic physicians for a wide range of ailments involving glandular swelling such as swollen spleen or liver, large lymphatic glands, goiter, or syphilis. The specific indication for potassium iodide is pale coloring of the mucous membranes of the mouth.[46] Potassium iodide is an ingredient in the Hoxsey Formula, a traditional treatment for many types of cancer.

Iodine

Low intake of iodine (a common deficiency in the United States and Europe) can lead to low thyroid function (hypothyroidism), a very important correlating factor in breast, ovarian, and endometrial cancers. Low iodine levels may allow an imbalance of estrogens, and this altered endocrine state may be the factor responsible for increased risk of these cancers.[47]

At least 75 percent of the breast and ovarian cancer patients that I see have this condition. Some external signs of low thyroid function include low body temperature, dry hair and skin, hormone imbalances, depression, excess weight in the lower part of the body (pear-shaped body type), and low energy levels. I recommend eating foods naturally rich in iodine, which include seaweed, eggs, apricots, and blackstrap molasses. I also supplement diets with a high-quality hand-harvested seaweed supplement called Ocean Herbs (see Resources). I recommend 2 to 6 capsules daily. Seaweed, in addition to being rich in natural iodine, is also rich in all minerals and trace minerals, including calcium and potassium. It also contains alginates and lignans, both great detoxifiers and anticancer compounds.

Another product I recommend is Atomidine (see Resources), an iodine solution that is helpful in cases of enlarged glands, tonsillitis, fibrocystic breast disease, fibroid tumors, and congestion of the ovaries accompanied by pain. It may be used both internally and externally. I normally recommend 1 to 6 drops daily, but this supplement should be monitored by a health care practitioner who can check basal metabolic temperature and adjust the dosage accordingly.

Selenium

Selenium is the best-documented anticancer mineral. Selenium functions as an antioxidant in the enzyme glutathione peroxidase and stimulates both cellular and humoral immunity. It is a potent enhancer of cell-mediated immunity.

Colon cancer studies show that selenium works by inhibiting lipid peroxidation. Selenium has been found to decrease the binding of various chemical carcinogens to DNA. This process takes place in the membranes of the liver and kidney where enzymes function as drug metabolizers.[48]

Selenium's main function in the body is to convert hydrogen peroxide to water, which is important for cellular health. Blood levels of this trace mineral are usually depressed in cancer patients. The cancer prevention component of the National Cancer Institute has compiled information showing that there are fewer cancer deaths in areas containing high levels of selenium in the soil than in areas with low levels of this important trace mineral.

Epidemiological studies show that high selenium intake is associated with a reduction in tumors at various sites, including mammary tissue. Numerous studies also document the ability of dietary selenium to reduce the incidence and total number of tumors induced by a variety of carcinogens. The ability of selenium to alter the metabolism of some carcinogens (including the mammary carcinogen DMBA) indicates that this trace element can be effective in inhibiting the initiation phase of carcinogens. Alterations in DMBA-DNA adducts resulting from dietary selenium supplementation were found to correlate with final tumor incidence and tumor number. Although the mechanism is unknown, several lines of evidence also point to the ability of selenium to effectively inhibit the promotional stage of carcinogenesis. Selenium supplements are also effective in depressing the incidence of virally induced mammary tumors. The efficacy by which selenium inhibits chemically induced, virally induced, and transplantable tumors makes it a unique dietary nutrient.

The December 1996 issue of the *Journal of the American Medical Association* reported the results of a clinical trial in which half the subjects received 200 mcg of selenium-containing yeast per day along with their normal diets, and the other half received normal diets only. The results are quite striking: the incidence of cancers of the lung, colon, and prostate were more than 50 percent lower among those taking the selenium-containing yeast.[49]

A study done with rats that were given the mammary carcinogen DMBA concluded that administration of the dietary supplement selenium in the form of sodium selenite markedly decreased the binding of DMBA to mammary cell DNA. Increasing the dietary content of selenium resulted in a proportional decrease in the binding of DMBA to DNA.[50]

Studies have shown that the higher the level of selenium, the lower the incidence of tumor formation. The ability of selenium to effectively inhibit the incidence of chemically and virally induced tumors and to depress the growth of some transplantable tumors was strongly supported by this study.[51] Selenium, a trace mineral, must be used judiciously. Safe dosages can range from 50 to 400 mcg. Higher doses should be used only under the supervision of a qualified health care professional.

Selenium Therapy and Various Cancers

Oral cancer. Baseline selenium levels were evaluated in twenty-seven patients with precancerous lesions and nineteen patients with malignant oral cavity lesions as well as thirteen healthy controls. Mean serum selenium levels were 105, 101, and 77.03 mg/ml in the precancerous, control, and malignant groups, respectively. There was a statistically significant difference between the neoplastic, precancerous, and control groups. After clinical evaluation, precancerous patients received three four-week cycles of selenium in either the organic or the inorganic form at 300 mcg per day. Of the twenty-two precancerous patients entering the study, eighteen were available for evaluation for clinical response. Selenium levels tended to increase after the first and second cycles and then gradually returned to baseline values. At the end of the therapy there were two complete responses, five partial responses, six minor responses, and five stable diseases with an objective response of 38.8 percent. Progression after the therapy occurred in seven out of eighteen patients. Patients with malignant neoplasms had low selenium levels, whereas healthy controls and those with precancerous lesions both had higher selenium levels. These results suggest the need for longer treatment periods with selenium. Steady supplementation with selenium-enriched yeast may have allowed for a more rapid increase in maintenance of higher selenium levels. I conclude that these are encouraging results demonstrating the effect of selenium therapy in the treatment of precancerous dysplastic lesions of the oral cavity.[52]

Ovarian cancer. A study published in the January 1996 issue of the *Journal of the National Cancer Institute* stated that serum selenium was associated with a decreased risk of ovarian cancer and that selenium may have a protective role against the development of ovarian cancer.[53]

Skin cancer. Selenium has been found to have a protective effect against skin cancers, which are on the rise in the United States. Selenium appears to protect the skin from the damages of ultraviolet radiation by maintaining or enhancing the antioxidant enzyme systems, superoxide dismutase, catalase, and glutathione peroxidase.[54] In a study evaluating two hundred melanoma cases in Stages I, II, and III and fifty-one epidemotrophic cutaneous T-cell lymphomas in Stages I through IV for the relationship to selenium levels, it was shown that there were decreased serum selenium concentrations in patients with melanoma and lymphoma relative to disease severity. The concentration was significantly lower in melanomas (at Stages I and II) that recurred within two years compared to those without recurrence. Before treatment, serum selenium levels were higher in the cutaneous T-cell lymphoma group, with good response to treatment compared with those without response. These results show the prognostic value of selenium assays in the follow-up of melanoma and cutaneous T-cell lymphoma patients.[55]

Bowel cancer. Another study has shown that the low selenium serum levels in patients with large bowel cancer were significantly increased after selenium supplementation and actually demonstrated the promotion of cell-mediated immunity as shown by tumor and normal tissue samples taken before and after surgery. This study indicates a close relationship between low selenium levels and carcinogenesis of the colon and rectum.[56]

Selenium and Chemotherapy

Selenium has a protective effect against cisplatin-induced nephrotoxicity and bone marrow suppression. Twenty patients received selenium in the first cycle of cisplatin chemotherapy and were compared to twenty-one patients who did not take selenium. The patients were crossed over for the second chemotherapy cycle. The selenium was given for a period of time from four days before to four days after chemotherapy. Serum selenium doubled in those receiving selenium supplementation. On day fourteen after the initiation of chemotherapy, the peripheral white blood-cell counts were significantly higher in the selenium-treated subjects than in the controls. There was significant reduction in the blood transfusion volume for the treated group compared to the controls. Nephrotoxicity from cisplatin was significantly lower in the selenium-treated patients. There were no toxic effects from the selenium supplementation. This suggests that selenium, which is a very low-cost supplement, can reduce the nephrotoxicity and bone marrow suppression induced by cisplatin. The kinds of cancers being treated included lung, breast, stomach, esophagus, and colon.[57]

I often recommend selenium in liquid form in combination with saffron, which is rich in aqueous carotenoids. The product is called Selensaff, made by Scientific Botanicals (see Resources).

Molybdenum

Molybdenum, another trace mineral, has been shown to inhibit and reduce the incidence of esophageal cancer.[58] I often recommend a supplement that combines glutathione and molybdenum, called Chem-Defense (see Resources). The anticancer effects of molybdenum are presumably due to its role in the detoxification of cancer-causing chemicals. Another beneficial effect of molybdenum is its ability to help the liver chelate and excrete excess copper. A low uric acid count can sometimes indicate a need for molybdenum.

Cesium Chloride

Another trace mineral that is becoming popular as part of the nutritional arsenal against cancer is cesium chloride. It belongs to a class of alkali metals that include lithium, potassium, and sodium. Cesium most resembles potassium, and lithium most resembles sodium. Administration of these metals can alter the intracellular environment.

Cesium chloride taken in high doses (3 to 6 grams daily) can temporarily raise the pH of certain tissues, tumor cells in particular. When the pH is elevated enough in a tumor cell, necrosis will follow. Cesium, when given to cancer patients in dosages of 6 grams per day, will raise the intracellular pH in tumor cells to eight units, a level incompatible with the life of a tumor. This elevation in pH will also buffer the acids, such as lipoic acid, produced by the tumor and reduce pain because of the reduction in acid waste being produced by the tumor.

In a number of tumor-cell lines, cesium has been shown to inhibit tumor cell proliferation. Even high doses of cesium produce little, if any, side effects other than creating a greater need for potassium and magnesium. If you or your doctor are considering high pH cesium therapy, be sure to supplement this with potassium and magnesium aspartate or orotate.

Zinc

Zinc is found in virtually every cell of the body. It is a component in over two hundred enzymes and in many functions of the immune system. Studies reported by Dr. Xu Huibi of China have shown that zinc levels in cancer patients tend to be lower than in healthy individuals. The elderly, in particular, have low zinc status. A low level of zinc can lead to a decrease in T-cell, granulocyte, and natural killer-cell functions. Zinc's effects on the immune system include stimulation of polymorphonuclear neutrophils to produce more reactive oxygen species, which are bactericidal and have an antitumor effect. Zinc combines with the phosphate radical of the cell membrane, phospholipid, and sulphydryl groups of protein that in turn can form stable complexes and decrease lipid peroxidation of the cell membrane. Zinc apparently induces human endogenous a-interferon. Recently, zinc supplementation was shown to reduce lipid peroxide levels.[59]

It has been noted in animal models that spleen and lymph node T-cell ratios are low when zinc is deficient. Oral zinc sulfate intake can increase helper/suppressor ratios in the peripheral blood of aged individuals, and zinc is important in strengthening cellular immune function in cancer patients.[60]

Zinc can also accelerate healing following an operation and can be an aid to improving appetite. A recent study has demonstrated that zinc supplementation can prevent or correct taste abnormalities caused by radiation therapy to the head or neck.[61]

I usually supplement zinc with a combination formula, not as a single mineral. It is important to avoid taking large amounts of zinc. If I do recommend it as a single nutrient, I suggest a food form of zinc (Whole Food Complex, see Resources) and specify a dose of 1 to 2 tablets daily, not to exceed 50 mg of total zinc per day. Whole food supplements are those that are produced by a natural growth process using yeast. Supplements created in this way have less potential for toxicity or side effects such as nausea.

Coenzyme Q10 (CoQ10)

Among health care practitioners, the treatment of cardiovascular disease with CoQ10 has become well established in Japan and in the United States. In fact, I consider CoQ10 to be one of the top five supplements for any type of heart disease. I have seen it make a dramatic difference time and time again. The use of CoQ10 for cancer patients is relatively new, but some studies demonstrate that its use in cancer therapies is warranted.

In a clinical protocol, thirty-two patients with high-risk breast cancer were treated with antioxidants, essential fatty acids, and 90 mg of CoQ10. Six of the thirty-two patients showed tumor regression. In one of these six patients the dosage of CoQ10 was increased to 390 mg. In one month, that patient's tumor was no longer palpable; in another month, mammography confirmed the absence of the tumor. Encouraged, another case of verified breast cancer, after nonradical surgery and with verified residual tumor within the tumor bed, was then treated with 300 mg CoQ10. After three months, the patient was in excellent clinical condition and there was no residual tumor tissue. The bioenergetic activity of CoQ10, expressed as hematological or immunological activity, may be dominant but not the sole molecular mechanism causing the regression of breast cancer.[62]

CoQ10 enhances the removal of foreign material twice as fast among individuals using the supplement as compared to those who do not. This is particularly important for people with cancer because toxin removal is crucial to healing. Remember, cancer itself causes toxins to accumulate, but chemo and radiation cause even more stress to the detoxifying systems of the body. Animals treated with CoQ10 developed tumors 31 percent slower than nontreated animals. Further, mice that had been inoculated with cancer and treated with CoQ10 had more than double the life span of mice not given the CoQ10.[63]

CoQ10 is recommended for anyone with cancer who is on the chemotherapeutic drug Adriamycin. Adriamycin depletes CoQ10 levels in the heart muscle, which can lead to heart damage (this is a serious side effect of this drug). When CoQ10 is administered in conjunction with this drug, heart damage does not occur.

CoQ10 is a vital constituent of the mitochondrial electron transport function. Most healthy young individuals produce adequate quantities of CoQ10 to meet their bodies' needs. However, when mitochondrial bioenergetics are inhibited (for example, in those receiving chemotherapy) or when the need for CoQ10 levels is high (the stress of having cancer produces such a need), CoQ10 becomes an essential nutrient.

I recommend 30 to 400 mg per day of CoQ10, taken after a meal with some type of fat such as the EPA-rich Eskimo Oil, made by Tyler Encapsulations (see Resources) for better absorbability. More positive research will be available soon that demonstrates the beneficial effects of CoQ10 in cancer treatments.

Lipoic Acid

Lipoic acid (alpha-lipoic acid), also referred to as thiotic acid, is one of my favorite and most frequently prescribed supplements. It has several beneficial effects on the whole body, in particular, the liver. Its list of functions is impressive. As a coenzyme, lipoic acid is essential for ATP production and cell efficiency. As an antioxidant, it works with glutathione to protect the cell and increase glutathione even more, perhaps, than NAC (N-acetyl cysteine). It is an antitoxin and has radiation-protective properties.

Lipoic acid can protect the liver from the deadly poisoning of the amanita mushroom. It provides better results than milk thistle, another specific remedy for this use. In a Czechoslovakian study, thirty-nine of forty people afflicted by this deadly poison were saved by taking lipoic acid.[64]

In a 1995 European conference, several speakers described the reversal of diabetic neuropathies using lipoic acid. Lipoic acid can actually regenerate not only the liver but also nerve tissue. It is used primarily for idiopathic liver enzyme elevation, hepatitis, and drug-induced liver injury.[65]

Lipoic acid is an excellent treatment for chemotherapy-induced neuropathy as well as many other problems caused by chemotherapy. I have found lipoic acid is the most useful supplement in treating all liver disorders, both acute and chronic. Lipoic acid is the ideal antioxidant, with the following biochemical properties:

1. It quenches free radicals.
2. It is easily absorbed and is readily bioavailable.
3. It concentrates in tissues, cells, and extracellular fluid.
4. It interacts with other antioxidants, such as vitamins C and E and NAC, enhancing their beneficial effects and increasing cellular glutathione more effectively than any other supplement available.
5. It has positive effects on gene expression.

Like CoQ10 and NAC, lipoic acid functions as an antioxidant, scavenging oxidative waste, and also as a pro-oxidant. It enhances oxygen and energy levels and acts as an anti-inflammatory agent. It also plays a pivotal role as a catalyst during photosynthesis when electromagnetic energy is transformed into chemical energy. It is used to treat hypoxia, a state characterized by poor oxygen uptake leading to fatigued muscles. People with cancer are often in a state of hypoxia and, because of this, would benefit greatly from lipoic acid supplementation.

One of the many benefits of lipoic acid in relation to cancer treatment is its ability to reduce lactic and pyruvic acids. Cancer cells produce an excess of lactic acid, which helps the cancer to multiply, metastasize, and create angiogenic factors.

German research shows that lipoic acid activates T-cell function, regenerates glutathione, and prevents oncogene activation.[66]

Free radicals and other cell-regulating enzymes can influence gene expression by activating a protein complex called nuclear factor kappa-B (NF-kappa-B). This activator can bind to DNA in genes and cause changes in the rate of gene expression and activation. As we age, the level of NF-kappa-B increases, making it more likely that gene defects will occur and accelerate the aging process.

Other protein subunits (called I-kappa-B) keep NF-kappa-B in check by inhibiting gene damage, but constant stress caused by free radicals, peroxides, and ultraviolet energy eventually allows NK-kappa-B to penetrate into the nucleus and damage DNA. One of the many unique actions of lipoic acid is its ability to terminate free radicals in the bloodstream, in the liver, on cell membranes, and in the cell interior (the cytosol). Lipoic acid protects both the cytosol and the DNA in the cell's nucleus from NF-kappa-B. Basically, this demonstrates the capability of lipoic acid to suppress proto-oncogene expression.[67]

Cancer, being a sugar-lover, causes an increase in glycation, the modification of a protein by the action of a sugar molecule. Lipoic acid protects against and reduces glycation, another reason why this supplement is so valuable at every level of treatment and why it is also so useful as a form of protection against cancer and other chronic diseases. In addition, lipoic acid can increase immune surveillance and protect the bone marrow, the liver, and the kidneys from chemotherapy-induced toxicity.[68]

Results of another recent study have shown that lipoic acid is a key element in enhancing glutathione synthesis, a finding that demonstrates the importance of lipoic acid in restoration of severely glutathione-deficient cells.[69]

The effects of lipoic acid can be dramatic, and I have seen them clinically. I believe lipoic acid works so well because nature, instead of adding a hydroxal group to form a monophenol nutrient like vitamin E or adding several hydroxal groups similar to bioflavonoids, adds two sulfur atoms and links them together. These sulfur atoms have a lot to do with the way lipoic acid works as an enzyme, antioxidant, and pro-oxidant. I believe it works synergistically with omega-3 fatty acids and sulfur-rich proteins. The fact that the body's natural stores of lipoic acid diminish with age could be one of the many reasons why cancer incidence increases with age.

Studies have also shown that lipoic acid protects and enhances glutathione S-transferase (GST). Therefore, as lipoic acid diminishes, GST can suffer a loss of function or alteration; this decreases the body's ability to detoxify certain carcinogenic compounds and may increase the risk of developing and/or promoting cancer.[70]

Glutathione (GSH)

Glutathione (GSH) is a cysteine-containing tripeptide amino acid. It is the most abundant nonprotein thiol in mammals, evolving as a molecule that protects cells against oxidation. It maintains many important enzyme functions and other cellular components in a reduced state. Part of GSH's uniqueness is that it functions as a detoxifying agent both intracellularly and extracellularly, with the liver and lungs containing the highest levels.

Supplementing the diet with lipoic acid, NAC, and glutathione itself (in the reduced form), as well as herbs such as milk thistle and turmeric, will protect, maintain, and enhance glutathione levels. Enhancement of glutathione is a critical part to any successful program for both preventing and treating cancer. Cancer, by its very nature, depletes GSH. Chemotherapy and radiation therapy also deplete GSH, making these supplements critical when cancer patients are undergoing such therapies.

Necrosis and apoptosis are two distinct mechanisms of cell death that may be distinguished morphologically as well as biochemically. Apoptosis is a physiological suicide of sorts, a programmed death, while necrosis describes the death of tissue which has been affected by local injury. Several cell lines were tested with GSH against either 5-FU, a frequently used chemotherapy, or a control group. The cell lines tested consisted of one small-cell carcinoma, one colon carcinoma, one neuroblastoma, one mammary carcinoma, and one acute myeloic leukemia line. The results showed that apoptosis is induced in tumor cells after ten days of incubation and four applications of GSH. The cell lines treated with 5-FU did not show any apoptosis.[71]

An animal study conducted in 1993 demonstrated the ability of reduced glutathione to inhibit the development of oral carcinogenesis. In that study, hamsters were given oral supplementation of reduced glutathione after exposure to DMBA. The control group was untreated. After fourteen weeks, the glutathione group demonstrated significantly fewer and smaller tumors.[72]

A more recent study involved ovarian cancer patients being treated with cisplatin, a chemotherapeutic agent. The study demonstrated that by adding glutathione to the cisplatin, more cycles of the cisplatin treatment could be administered because less toxicity occurred. The glutathione also produced a statistically significant improvement in depression, nausea, peripheral neurotoxicity, hair loss, and shortness of breath.[73]

One of my key goals in supplementation is the enhancement of glutathione by adding nutrients such as lipoic acid and cysteine, and flavonoids, such as milk thistle, schizandra, turmeric, and whey protein to individual protocols.

Glutathione and the Detoxification of Cisplatin

The toxicity of cisplatin, an effective drug in the treatment of solid tumors, is a major obstacle to its use. GSH, a safe compound that prevents cisplatin-induced nephrotoxicity without affecting its antitumor activity, is a promising antidote. The protective effects of GSH allow higher doses of cisplatin to be used safely, improving its efficacy against certain tumors. In one study, glutathione was given fifteen minutes before each cisplatin treatment in fifty-one patients with a total of 229 courses of therapy. The high-dose regimen was tolerable, and no patient developed toxicity. Nephrotoxicity was minimal. The most frequent side effects were slight damage to ear nerves and surrounding nerve endings. In the thirty patients with ovarian cancer, 59 percent achieved complete clinical remission. Twenty-two out of twenty-six were negative on a second laparoscopy. The advantage of using N-acetyl cysteine together with high doses of cisplatin to raise glutathione was demonstrated by the impressive response rate in the treatment of ovarian cancer.[74]

N-Acetyl Cysteine

N-acetyl cysteine (NAC) is an endogenous product of the sulphur-containing amino acid cysteine that can act as a precursor to glutathione (GSH). Without cysteine, glutathione cannot be synthesized. Dietary cystine converts to cysteine in the intestinal tract and is more stable than cysteine itself. GSH is one of the most important antioxidants and is a significant anticarcinogen, especially in the lungs and liver where the highest level of GSH is found. GSH also plays a role in protecting the nervous system. Intracellular GSH is necessary for the multiplication of lymphocytes and antibody production, an essential part of the immune response process. Using NAC, lipoic acid, and vitamin C will raise intracellular glutathione levels more effectively than by simply using oral glutathione because oral glutathione is poorly absorbed.

NAC is a potent cancer-preventive agent. Some of the ways in which NAC aids in the prevention and treatment of cancer are:

- It protects against extracellular mutagenic agents from exogenous and endogenous sources.
- It inhibits genotoxicity of reactive oxygen species.
- It blocks reactive oxygen species.
- It protects DNA and nuclear enzymes.
- It prevents the formation of carcinogen-DNA adducts.[75]

One example of NAC's ability to protect the liver is its use as an antidote to acetaminophen (Tylenol™) overdose. Another one of NAC's uses, clinically practiced for a number of years, is its ability to thin the viscosity of mucus, making it a mucolytic agent. I have been using NAC for many years to thin mucus in many conditions, including bronchitis, sinusitis, and otitis media, and have found it extremely effective. NAC disrupts disulphide bonds within mucus, clearing disulfide bridges between glycoproteins.

NAC has been shown to enhance the antitumor effects of IL (interleukin)-2 primarily because of its ability to increase intracellular glutathione. IL-2, when given as a treatment for cancer, induces marked oxidative stress via reactive oxygen and nitrogen intermediates. NAC reduces the toxicity of IL-2, demonstrating its synergistic effect as an antitumor treatment.[76]

A large five-year study on the use of NAC as a cancer-inhibiting supplement is currently in progress. In this study, conducted by a European group called EORTC (European Organization for Research in the Treatment of Cancer), patients who were treated for their carcinomas and showed no detectable cancer following their standard treatments, were given NAC, 600 mg daily for two years.[77] Other studies have demonstrated an average increase of 38 percent in blood plasma glutathione levels due to the administration of NAC. No other supplement, including glutathione itself, can claim this.[78]

Taurine

While taurine is not an essential amino acid, its value as a nutritional supplement is quite significant, especially during chemotherapy, which lowers taurine. Following are some of the benefits of taurine as a nutritional supplement:

• It is an effective and key component to the detoxification of chemicals and heavy metals and, like NAC, can help the body manufacture glutathione when under free-radical stress.

• Along with magnesium, it can act as a natural calcium channel-blocking agent and help regulate blood pressure. Taurine has a protective effect on cardiovascular function.

• It is extremely helpful at inhibiting seizures, and therefore can help people with brain tumors who are on dilantin and suffering from many side effects. By adding taurine and magnesium, dilantin and its side effects can be reduced. It can also help expel sodium and reduce edema.

• A key component of bile, taurine assists in liver function.

• It influences blood glucose and insulin levels and increases glycogen synthesis. Taurine plays a role in the proper functioning of the pancreas.[79]

Glutamine

Glutamine is the most abundant amino acid in the blood and is a free amino acid in the human body. It has multiple functions.

Glutamine levels decline markedly during periods of injury, illness, trauma, radiation therapy, and stress, leading to muscle wasting. Glutamine supplementation prevents immunosuppression and muscle atrophy during periods of stress and heals gastric and peptic ulcers.[80]

Glutamine is best taken sublingually (under the tongue) for maximum absorption, or as part of a good low-temperature whey protein supplement such as Country Life, available in most health food stores.

There are several reasons why I might suggest glutamine to cancer patients. Human studies have shown that L-glutamine is an essential nutrient for the cells of the small intestine and is the primary metabolic fuel for enterocytes. It plays an important role in the prevention of mucosal atrophy during total parenteral nutrition (TPN). L-glutamine can prevent many of the health problems associated with the administration of TPN to cancer patients, which can result in villous atrophy and a breakdown of the gut mucosal barrier, promoting translocation of gut bacteria into the bloodstream and lymph nodes. By supplementing TPN with glutamine, the gut mucosa can be protected from becoming too permeable, damaged, and leaky.

Glutamine may be second only to glucose as a source of fuel for the body, but while glucose feeds tumor growth, glutamine does not. The body makes glutamine very slowly, and it is considered an essential amino acid for sick people. Cancer patients who are in a catabolic state, causing them to lose vital muscle tissue, are deficient in both blood and tissue concentrations of glutamine. These people, especially, will benefit from taking L-glutamine.[81]

In addition, glutamine is very important for the maintenance of immune function, particularly when the body is under stress and not getting the nutrition and fuel it needs. When a person is sick, the body will pull glutamine from vital muscle tissue and use it to produce lymphocytes and macrophages. These cells consume glutamine at a high rate under normal conditions, but this process is greatly accelerated when the body is working to destroy pathogens. Glutamine assists in the production of NK cells and glutathione. Glutamine can also enhance the amino acid cysteine. When glutamine availability is below par, it will not only cause important muscle loss, but it could also compromise glutathione synthesis. Studies show that when patients received a TPN formulation to which glutamine has been added, their glutathione plasma levels were raised significantly. Furthermore, liver glutathione levels are maintained by including glutamine in the diet. Foods such as spinach, kale, and parsley are rich in constituents that form glutathione precursors.[82,83]

Patients who are receiving glutamine and are recovering from surgery, wound healing, or radiation therapy experience less weight loss and speedier recoveries than those who do not receive glutamine. Prophylactic glutamine protects the intestinal mucosa from radiation injury. Glutamine also enhances chemotherapy and reduces toxicity. In animal models glutamine supplementation protects the host from methotrexate-induced enterocolitis and enhances the tumoricidal effectiveness of methotrexate while reducing morbidity and mortality.[84] Other studies have demonstrated decreased mortality following radiation and chemotherapy. One study in particular demonstrated glutamine's efficacy in accelerating healing after radiation treatment. Animals treated with glutamine had a 100 percent survival rate as compared to the control group's rate of 45 percent. Increased healing of radiated intestines and decreased systemic infections resulting from bacterial translocation were also demonstrated.[85]

Glutamine therapy appears to be extremely beneficial to people undergoing chemotherapy. In a recent report, glutamine was given to people with myelogenous leukemia. The dose was 6 grams dissolved in water three days prior to chemotherapy. Glutamine offered protection to the gastrointestinal tract by reducing the duration and severity of diarrhea.[86]

I usually prefer to administer glutamine as a powder. I recommend 1 to 2 teaspoons one to three times daily.

Calcium D-Glucarate

Calcium D-glucarate (CDG) is an effective cancer-inhibiting supplement, particularly in hormonal-driven cancers such as breast cancer. CDG is the calcium salt of D-glucaric acid, a naturally occurring substance found in humans and many plants that is an important detoxifying agent because of its effects on glucuronidation.

CDG works by metabolizing an excess of estrogen in the body. Normally, estrogen is metabolized in the liver and the body rids itself of estrogen by passing it through the liver, where it hooks onto a conjugate called glucuronic acid and passes out with the stool. This process, called *glucoronidation*, is the way the body detoxifies and cleans house.

Under normal healthy conditions, which must include low levels of liver stress and good sleep patterns, the glucuronide conjugate passes from the liver into the bile and then into the gut, where it is dispersed and ultimately eliminated through the bowel. Sometimes there are high levels of an enzyme called beta-glucuronidase that rip the glucuronide conjugate off the estrogen. Then the estrogen is free to be reabsorbed back into the bloodstream in a more oxidized, reactive, cancer-promoting form. CDG stops the glucuronidase from freeing the estrogen for reabsorption—a very important step in stopping this dangerous process.

Glucuronidation is part of the Phase II conjugation pathway of the liver, which detoxifies and excretes not only estrogen but xenobiotics, lipid-soluble toxins, and other steroid hormones, all of which can act as promoting agents to cancer.

One important effect of taking CDG orally is that it reduces serum estrogen levels, which in turn inhibits breast tumors. In addition to preventing breast cancer (as well as other hormone-related cancers), CDG can inhibit the recurrence of cancer and be part of a protocol for the treatment of cancer.[87,88]

I presently suggest doses of 2 to 4 capsules (500 mg each) two to three times daily.

FLAVONOIDS

Flavonoids are brightly colored substances commonly found in most plants. They account for a significant percentage of the chemical constituents of those plants and are usually found alongside vitamin C in nature. Both substances were discovered by Albert Szent-Gyorgyi and isolated from paprika in the 1930s. Szent-Gyorgyi himself called bioflavonoids "vitamin P" and suggested they were crucial for the integrity of the small blood vessels and as treatment for the skin disease purpura. Scientists refused to acknowledge the value of flavonoids, however, and they have existed in a kind of nutritional limbo ever since.

Flavonoids, referred to as "biological response modifiers," possess anti-inflammatory, antiallergic, antiviral, and anticarcinogenic properties. The potent antioxidant activity of flavonoids may be their most important healing aspect.

Flavonoids can be found in a wide variety of fruits, vegetables, and many, many herbs. Some of the best-known flavonoids are citrin, hesperidin, and rutin; they are abundantly found in the white pulp of citrus fruits and in grapes, plums, black currants, apricots, buckwheat, cherries, blackberries, and rose hips. They remove toxic copper from the body and protect vitamin C from the destructive action of some copper-containing enzymes. There is a synergy between flavonoids and vitamin C that may play a role in promoting vitamin C's anticancer effects.

There are five categories of flavonoids:

1. *Anthocyanins, anthochlors.* Anthocyanins are red-blue pigments in plants (such as plums and cherries). Anthochlors are yellow and are found primarily in flowers (such as calendula) in abundance.

2. *Minor flavonoids.* Minor flavonoids include flavonons, flavon-3-ols, dihydroflavones, and dihydrochalcones. Some flavon-3-ols include catechin and epigallocatechin 3-gallate, which is found in green tea, and proanthocyanidin oligomers (PCOs). Pycnogenols include a group of PCOs.

3. *Flavones and flavonols.* Flavones and flavonols are the most widely occurring flavonoids and they include quercetin, a major flavonoid I often recommend as a supplement.

4. *Isoflavonoids.* Isoflavonoids, found primarily in legumes, include genistein, which is found in soybeans.

5. *Tannins.* Tannins include proanthocyanidins, anthocyanides, and gallic acid phenolics (this is what gives red wine some of its health benefits). When supplementing with PCOs or pycnogenol, be sure to get the real thing. Look for the name of the French researcher Jack Masquelier on the bottle. Another supplement that I often recommend is PCO Phytosome by Phyto Pharmica (see Resources).[89]

Flavonoids are being evaluated by themselves, and together with other substances, in the treatment of cancer. A synthetic relative of bioflavonoids, flavone acetic acid (FAA), is an immune booster, although not a very useful drug by itself. FAA increases natural killer-cell activity in mice. In Italian laboratory tests, FAA produced mixed results. Some transplanted human tumors were unaffected, but those grown under the skin and in the liver of test animals were significantly inhibited. Italian scientists said this test demonstrated the "great importance of the site of tumor growth for FAA efficacy."[90]

FAA was also clinically evaluated in cancer patients. Fifty-four patients were given large infusions for up to six hours. No objective responses were seen in this trial, however. Scientists are puzzling over why this drug works much better in mice than in people. Some have concluded that there is "a clear immunological component in the mechanism of action of FAA."[91,92]

However, FAA does seem to have one powerful effect. When FAA is combined with interleukin-2 (IL-2), the combination is very powerful. As an added benefit, IL-2 taken with FAA does not have its usual severe toxicity. In mice, kidney cancer treated with FAA and IL-2 resulted in "up to 80 percent long-term survival" whereas either substance alone was "unable to induce any long-term survivors." The two substances appeared to work by stimulating natural killer-cells and the production of natural tumor-necrosis factor. Used together in humans, there were nearly 60 percent more long-term survivors than when either drug was used alone.[93–95]

Because flavonoids inhibit carcinogenesis by several mechanisms, my protocols always include flavonoid supplements, usually more than one, and in fairly high doses; for example, POCs: 100 to 200 mg two to six times daily or quercetin: 500 to 1,000 mg three times daily.

The Anticancer Actions of Flavonoids

Flavonoids have the following anticancer actions:

1. *Inhibition of mitosis.* They reduce the rate of uncontrolled cell division caused by cancer.

2. *Blocking or competing for cell-surface receptor sites.* By occupying these receptor sites, cancer-cell-surface enzymes have nowhere to dock on the surface of healthy cells and therefore cannot transform healthy cells.

3. *Stabilization of collagen.* The base membrane that surrounds capillaries protects against tumor growth and invasion. Flavonoids, by strengthening this membrane, inhibit collagen breakdown, which can therefore inhibit tumor invasion and metastasis.

4. *Binding with laminin.* Laminin is a glycoprotein in the extracellular matrix that regulates invasion. Laminin accumulates between invading cells and host tissue and can bind to tissue-type plasminogen activators and reduce tumor activation and tumor invasion.

5. *Anti-inflammatory, antiallergenic, and antioxidant.* Flavonoids are perhaps the best inhibitors and scavengers of free radicals; they are also the best anti-inflammatory agents. By acting as anti-inflammatory agents, flavonoids regulate eicosanoid-mediated inflammation and reduce tumor-promoting prostaglandin E2.

6. *Inducing the production of transforming growth factor (TGF) beta-1.* TGF beta-1 is a cytokeine that can regulate or down-regulate some growth factors, particularly in cancer promotion and initiation.

7. *Altering gene expression.* Flavonoid mechanisms are capable of inhibiting genetic viral and chemically induced damage to cells.

8. *Inhibition of angiogenesis.* Flavonoids inhibit the transfer of blood supply to the tumor through hyaluronidase inhibition. Hyaluronidase is an enzyme that takes part in the inflammation process; it triggers the release of mast cells and histamines. PCOs contain a group of flavonoids that inhibit this process.[96]

Anthocyanidins and Proanthocyanidins

These flavonoids give certain plants their dark purple and blue color, such as grapes, hawthorn, bilberry, and cherries. Their free-radical scavenging effects are twenty to fifty times greater than vitamins C or E. They also reinforce the natural cross-linking of collagen that forms the matrix of connective tissue, a very important function during any postsurgical healing. They are also anti-inflammatory, preventing the release and synthesis of compounds that promote inflammation, such as histamines, serine proteases, prostaglandins, and leukotrienes.

Oligomeric Proanthocyanidins (OPCs)

The bark of conifers is rich in flavonoids called OPCs, particularly the bark of the maritime pine, *Pinus maritima*. OPCs are also found in grape seeds. OPCs are useful as an anti-inflammatory in adjunctive nutritional support for primary treatment of hemorrhoids, swollen joints, athletic injuries, postsurgical edema, and postsurgical lymphedema in women with breast cancer who have had lymph node dissections.[97]

In vitro tests demonstrate OPCs are twenty times more powerful than ascorbic acid and fifty times more powerful than vitamin E as free-radical scavengers. OPCs have been defined as the natural stable form of the vitamin P substance found in numerous vegetables. PCOs (proanthocyanidin oligomers) are very similar to OPCs, but OPCs are the patented product with which most of the research and documented studies have been done.[98]

Quercetin

Terrence Leighton, chairman of microbiology and immunology at the University of Berkeley, believes that quercetin, a flavone found in onions, broccoli, eucalyptus, and blue-green algae, is one of the most powerful anti-cancer agents present in nature.

By blocking proflammatory reactions in the body that release arachidonic acid into the cells, quercetin acts as a powerful inhibitor of the tumor-promoting PGE-2. It also stabilizes mast cell walls by prolonging the health of lipids, by blocking lipoxygenase activity, and by stabilizing capillary beds, decreasing capillary fragility.

Quercetin has been shown to inhibit the growth of several human cancer-cell lines, including breast (estrogen-receptor [ER] positive and ER-negative), ovarian, squamous cell, cervical, bladder, and gastric cancers, plus acute myeloid and acute lymphoid leukemia, Moloney murine leukemia (by inhibiting reverse transcriptase), and some lymphomas.[99–101]

Quercetin also inhibits multidrug resistance within the tumor-cell line. Multidrug resistance is associated with overexpression of a membrane protein called *P-glycoprotein*. Heat shock factor (HSF) is produced within the cell in response to heat or various forms of stress (for example, chemotherapy). HSF can cause P-glycoprotein to be overexpressed, which can then lead to chemotherapy resistance within the tumor cell. The result is that an effective cytotoxic drug is no longer doing its job. Quercetin can inhibit this process in a variety of neoplastic cell lines as well as in many chemotherapeutic agents that might be used to treat that particular cancer. Quercetin enhances the cytotoxic effects of many chemotherapeutic drugs, including Adriamycin and Cytoxan. It also potentiates the cytotoxicity of Adriamycin against Adriamycin-resistant human breast cancer cells.[102–105]

Quercetin binds to type II estrogen-binding sites more effectively than the antiestrogen drug tamoxifen, which is used so often to treat and inhibit the recurrence of estrogen-positive breast cancer. Type II estrogen-binding sites differ from true estrogen-binding sites because their actual purpose is to bind an endogenous isoflavonoid, or ligand, that has growth-inhibitory rather than estrogen-binding activity. By securing these binding sites with weak plant estrogens, the true estrogens have nowhere to bind, which stops the promotion of cancer growth. Type II estrogen-binding sites are present in a variety of human cancers, including breast cancer and melanoma.[106]

Another mechanism by which quercetin shows its antitumor effects is by inhibiting the expression of certain gene mutations. Quercetin inhibits the mutation of the tumor-suppressor protein gene p53. The mutation, or defect, of this suppressor is involved in more than half of all cancer-cell lines including breast, ovarian, and prostate cancers.[107]

There is no supplement that I recommend more often than quercetin. There are claims that quercetin is poorly absorbed, but based on my years of clinical experience with this supplement, I choose to disagree. Taking quercetin with bromelain on an empty stomach thirty minutes before a meal results in a very high degree of bioavailability. I usually recommend between 1 and 3 grams per day in divided doses taken with vitamin C and bromelain.

Other Flavonoids

Apigenin is a nontoxic, nonmutagenic flavonoid found in certain vegetables. It has a significant potential for being a cancer-preventive agent. In one study it produced a 43 to 62 percent inhibition of mutagenicity and a 67 to 80 percent reduction of tumor-promotion activity. Apigenin also has a chemoprotective effect and has been shown to be as effective as cromoglycate in inhibiting basophil histamine release. The flavonoids luteolin and amentoflavone exhibit an even higher inhibitory effect. Chamomile is a rich source of apigenin.[108]

Robinetin is a flavonoid that produced an 87 percent reduction in muta-genicity and a 67 to 80 percent reduction in tumor-promotion activity in one study. The anticancer effects of the flavonoids robinetin and apigenin were assessed in a study published in the journal *Carcinogenesis*. The research was conducted at the University of Nebraska Medical Center.[109]

A recent study evaluated the potential anticarcinogenic flavonoids quercetin, kaempferol, myricetin, apigenin, and luteolin in 4,112 adults. The average intake of all flavonoids was 23 mg per day. The most important flavonoid was quercetin, with a mean intake of 16 mg per day. The major sources of flavonoids were green tea, onions, and apples. The evaluation of this study concluded that the antioxidant effects of these flavonoids exceeds that of beta-carotene and vitamin E.[110]

ESSENTIAL FATTY ACIDS (EFAs) AND OTHER IMPORTANT FATS

Currently, supermarkets offer mostly toxic processed oils or, just as bad, food with all the fat removed. Food that has been altered to become fat-free, the big rage in health food these days, is really not healthy food at all. It is gener-ally food in which fat has been replaced with chemicals and sugar.

Recently, in the race to lower cholesterol, there has been much misinfor-mation disseminated about fats. Contrary to popular opinion, healthy fats should make up a large part of our diet, about 25 to 30 percent. Most Americans are seriously deficient in the essential fatty acids.

The Role of EFAs

The life processes of plants, animals, and humans are greatly dependent on sunlight and its transformation into photons, electrons, and pi-electrons. Unsaturated fatty acids play a major role in this transfer of electrons and therefore in the effect that respiratory enzymes and auto-oxidation have on maintaining or restoring normal metabolism.

Here's how the transfer works. The energy the sun gives off is called pho-ton energy. Electrons that orbit every atom in the universe are made up of two photons. Electrons absorb photons through vibration, and this leads to energy. Electrons can also emit photons, which involves a great expenditure of energy. This is where essential fatty acids come in. Alpha-linolenic acid and linoleic acid possess the ability to transfer immense amounts of energy. The transferral of energy brought about by these particular fatty acids plays an important role in the functions of all cellular membranes. They are involved in the assimilation and transportation of oxygen, assisting in cell energy production. They are equally involved in the cell's detoxification of cellular waste products and poisons, including the detoxification of chemotherapeutic drugs and radiation.

The brain itself, as well as the nervous system, is primarily composed of unsaturated lipids or fats. To effectively utilize protein, we need fat. In creating the bridge between fats and proteins, hydrogen, the lightest of all atoms, boosts its energy level by absorbing photons, transferring and releasing electrons. Sulfur, mostly sulfur-rich protein, also plays a vital role in this process. The interaction of lipids with sulfur-rich proteins is the key to the successful nutrition protocol of Dr. Johanna Budwig, who has cured so many people of cancer.

A defect in the metabolism of EFAs can lead to a wide variety of illnesses, including cancer. EFAs are essential, just as their name implies. They are required components of all membranes within the body and, like vitamins and minerals, can only be obtained by diet. There are two groups of EFAs, omega-6 and omega-3. The parent compounds of these two groups are linoleic acid (LA), from the omega-6 group, and alpha-linolenic acid (ALA), from the omega-3 group. LA and ALA are metabolized in the body by a series of alternating desaturations in which a new carbon bond is introduced. This process leads EFAs to biological pathways that alter eicosanoids and/or prostaglandins, thromboxanes, leukotrienes, and hydroxy fatty acids. If there are disturbances in this process, the delicate balance of prostaglandin formation and utilization will be altered.

There are two important enzymes involved in the conversion of essential fatty acids into the preferred anti-inflammatory and tumor-inhibiting Series I eicosanoids. (Do not confuse these with the Series II eicosanoids, which are formed from arachidonic acid [AA] and are tumor-promoting.) The first enzyme is delta-6 desaturase and the second is delta-5 desaturase. Delta-6 converts linoleic acid into gamma-linolenic acid (GLA), which is then converted into dihomo-gamma linolenic acid (DGLA). Delta-5 is involved in the formation of DGLA to form either Series I eicosanoids or AA, the precursor of Series II eicosanoids.

Table 5.1 Major Supplements for Cancer Prevention and Treatment

Supplement	Summary of Actions	Specific Uses and Interactions	General Daily Range
Vitamin A	Anticarcinogenic; immunostimulating	Protects against lung and throat cancer	10,000–25,000 IU
Carotenoids	Antioxidant; inhibits carcinogenesis	Protects against leukemia, myeloma, and cervical, breast, lung, prostate, pancreatic, throat, and colon cancers	15,000–50,000 IU
Vitamin E	Antioxidant; reduces cellular lipid peroxidation; stimulates immune system	Protects against skin, prostate, and colon cancers	200–800 IU
Vitamin C ascorbate	Antioxidant; inhibits carcinogen formation; important in collagen synthesis and glutathione activity	Protects against cancers of lung, larynx, esophagus, stomach, pancreas; protects skin and bones from effects of radiation	500–2,000 mg
Vitamin D	Inhibits/reduces proliferative effects of estrogen in breast cancer and testosterone in prostate cancer	Prevents colon, breast, and prostate cancer	400–1,000 IU
Vitamin K (nontoxic form)	Antihemorrhagic; tumor analgesic; cancer inhibitor	Fights cancer cells	5–20 mg
Coenzyme B_6 (pyridoxal-5-phosphate)	Reduces cell growth; inhibits protein tyrosine kinase	Prevents melanoma and neuropathy	50–100 mg

Folic acid and Vitamin B$_{12}$	Turns cancer genes off; improves appetite and sleep; aids in methyl metabolism	Treats cervical dysplasia, squamous metaplasia, cancers of gastro-intestinal tract	400–2,000 mcg each
Calcium oratate	Recalcifies bone; inhibits colon cancer	Inhibits bone metastases; reduces pain; helps in colon cancer	100–300 mg
Potassium	Provides immune-defensive actions	Decreases cancer risk; activates ATP	200–400 mg
Magnesium	Provides immune defensive actions	Natural laxative	200–600 mg
Coenzyme Q10	Removes toxins from body; is vital to body's mitochondrial electron transport system	Prevents heart disease; specific for anyone using Adriamycin, a chemo-therapeutic drug; a cytotoxic anticancer agent	100–600 mg
Lipoic acid	Pro-oxidant/antioxidant; increases cell efficiency; antitoxin, has radiation-protective properties; reduces lactic and pyruvic acids; activates T-cell functions; increases glutathione levels	Provides liver and kidney protection; immune surveillance; enhances intercellular glutathione; inhibits oncogene transformation	200–600 mg
Glutathione	Protects cells against oxidation; a detoxifying agent both intracellularly and extracellularly; induces tumor-cell death	Critical to prevent and treat cancer	50–400 mg

(Continued)

Table 5.1 Continued

Supplement	Summary of Actions	Specific Uses and Interactions	General Daily Range
Selenium	Antioxidant; stimulates cellular immunity; inhibits lipid peroxidation; converts hydrogen peroxide to water in body	Anticancer mineral; protects against skin, breast, colon and throat cancers; protects immune system from chemotherapy	100–800 mg
Molybdenum	Detoxifier; helps liver excrete copper	Inhibits esophageal cancer	200–400 mcg
Zinc	Stimulates immune system; strengthens cellular immune function	Accelerates healing after surgery; improves appetite; prevents loss of taste	10–50 mg
N-acetyl cysteine	Helps to synthesize glutathione; antioxidant; anticarcinogenic; protects DNA	Provides liver, heart, and lung protection from chemotherapy-induced damage	500–3,000 mg
Taurine	Detoxifies heavy metals; helps liver, kidneys, and heart	Inhibits seizures; regulates blood pressure	1,000–6,000 mg
Glutamine	Regulates protein synthesis; removes renal ammonia; maintains immune function	Heals gastric and peptic ulcers; an essential nutrient for cells of small intestine	2,000–6,000 mg
Calcium D-glucarate	Detoxifies; metabolizes excess estrogen	Inhibits hormonal-driven cancers	1,000–6,000 mg
Quercetin	Anticancer activity; anti-inflammatory; stabilizes mast cells; inhibits mutation of suppressor p53 gene	Inhibits breast, ovarian, and prostate cancers; works synergistically with many chemotherapies	1,000–2,000 mg

Anthocyanins and related flavonoids (grape seed, pinebark, hawthorn, bilberry extracts)	Anti-inflammatory, antiallergic, antiviral, anticancer	Protects heart, nerves, vascular system; works synergistically with NAC and lipoic acid	100–600 mg
Catechins (green tea polyphenols)	Anticancer agent; induces apoptosis in many cancer lines	Antiviral, immunomodulating, antioxidant; protects heart and liver; accelerates healing after surgery	50–2,000 mg

A note about dosages: Dosages noted here are general daily range guidelines. In most cases, the lower dosages are for prevention and the higher ones are for treatment. Individual protocols for treating specific conditions should be supervised by a qualified health care professional.

Supplementing the diet with GLA supplements becomes important if there is a deficiency of delta-6 desaturase. Many things influence delta-6 and can cause a deficiency or underactivity. For example, a diet high in refined sugars, starches, and hydrogenated fats will completely alter this pathway and lead to eicosanoid imbalance favorable for tumor growth. The resulting high blood insulin levels cause more damaging Series II eicosanoids to form.

Many cancer-cell lines are known to be totally devoid of delta-6 desaturase, and many viral infections, such as the Epstein-Barr virus, are known to have significant inhibitor effects on this important enzyme. Omega-3 essential fatty acids and eicosapentaenoic acids (EPA) also play a pivotal role in eicosanoid formation, a potent inhibitor of AA. (See table 5.2).

Omega-3 Fatty Acids

Flaxseed oil is rich in essential fatty acids, particularly ALA, which, when taken in combination with sulfur-rich proteins, actually works to create a new food. This was first discovered and made famous by Johanna Budwig, a West German physician who had done a great deal of research on the oil-protein combination. She discovered that EFAs need to bind to sulfur-rich proteins (she used low-fat cottage cheese) before the body can properly assimilate them. Budwig found that by feeding people with terminal cancer this oil-protein combination, the yellowish-green substance in their blood was replaced by the healthy red pigment, hemaglobin. The phosphatides returned and the lipoproteins reappeared.

Of all the deficiencies that may exist in people with cancer, perhaps those that are most important and totally ignored are EFAs, which, when taken with protein, enhance our albumin levels. Albumin is a blood protein of immense importance to good health. When flaxseed oil and sulfur-rich protein are combined, the ALA and the EFAs in the flaxseed oil become water-soluble and electron-rich; this causes the cell membrane to become more stable by making it more flexible and fluidlike. The electron-rich fatty acids now allow for efficient transport of materials and energy between the inner and outer cell membrane. This is important to the health of all cells and to the entire immune system.

A simple recipe for achieving these cellular benefits is to add 1 to 2 teaspoons of flaxseed oil or ground flaxseeds to 1 cup of organic yogurt (preferably goat or soy yogurt).

Table 5.2 Actions of Essential Fatty Acids

Fatty Acid	Source	Action	Daily Range
Omega-3 fatty acids:		Source of ALA and EPA	
Alpha-linolenic acid (ALA)	Flaxseed oil, purslane, hemp oil	Antitumor; anticachexic; inhibits metastasis; anti-inflammatory; prostaglandin regulating	1–2 teaspoons
Eicosapentaenoic acid (EPA) and DHA	Fish oils, Eskimo Oil		1–4 tablespoons
Gamma-linolenic acid (GLA)	Evening primrose oil, borage oil, black currant oil	Suppresses tumor growth; regulates hormones	3,000–6,000 IU
Squalene	Shark liver oil	Useful in cancers of viral origin, such as cervical cancer; increases cytotoxicity of many chemotherapy drugs	1,000–3,000 IU
Alkylglycerols	Bone marrow, shark liver oil, mother's milk	Protects bone marrow during chemotherapy; inhibits white blood-cell suppression; helps with low platelet counts	1,000–3,000 IU
Medium-chain triglycerides	Coconut and coconut oil	Promotes healthy weight gain; is source of easily absorbable energy; resists opportunistic infections	1–2 tablespoons
Lecithin	Soybeans, egg yolks	Lowers serum cholesterol; reduces platelet aggregation; reverses psoriasis; helps to excrete toxins; protects the liver	1–2 tablespoons
Butyric acid	Cottage cheese, Parmesan cheese, butter	Cancer inhibiting	2–6 tablets (300 mg each)
Conjugated linoleic acid (CLA)	Dairy products	Cancer inhibiting	2,000–3,000 mg

Omega-3 fatty acids are extremely important because they modulate prostaglandins, which are very active biological substances important to nearly every bodily function. They suppress tumor-promoting prostaglandin E2 by increasing prostaglandin E3 and suppressing AA. They also inhibit cancer wasting. EPA and ALA, as well as other related omega-3 fatty acids, plus GLA from evening primrose oil, have been found to kill a number of tumor-cell lines and cause a significant reduction in tumor growth in animal studies.[111]

Good sources of omega-3 fatty acids include salmon and rainbow trout from clean waters. Include them in your diet two to four times weekly. I also recommend Eskimo Oil (see Resources), a stable fish oil that includes lemon oil for stability and long shelf life and is free of the contaminants sometimes found in other fish oil supplements. Fish oil that is rich in EPA/DHA oils seems, in some cases, to require fewer enzymatic pathways to form and modulate prostaglandin regulation compared to flaxseed oil, although flaxseed oil certainly serves most people very well. Hemp oil and purslane are also rich omega-3 sources. Purslane can also be used as a salad green.

Gamma-Linolenic Acid

Gamma-linolenic acid (GLA) has been shown to prevent the proliferation of numerous malignant cell lines in culture. Evening primrose oil (EPO) containing 9 percent GLA reduced the growth rate of transplanted breast cancer in rats. A study of twenty-one patients with advanced hepatocellular carcinoma who failed with all conventional therapies showed marked subjective improvement while receiving 18 to 36 EPO caps a day.[112]

GLA and EPA, or ALA, have been shown to have a synergistic effect as they work together to regulate prostaglandins. This in turn causes an increase in fluidity and flexibility on cell membranes that not only controls primary tumor proliferation but potentiates the response to chemotherapy, radiotherapy, and hyperthermic treatments.[113]

Squalene

Squalene, found mainly in shark liver oil and olive oil, enhances the polarization of cell membranes and thus intensifies the docking of defensive cells onto cancerous cells, restoring the cell's electrostatic order and activating the formation of surveillance steroids. Squalene is especially indicated for those cancers of a herpes virus origin—for example, cervical cancer. Squalene possesses antiviral as well as anticancer activity.

Even in cases where sharks are exposed to aflatoxin B1, the most potent naturally occuring liver-cancer-causing agent known, squalene protects them against cancer. Squalene is an individually resolved component of shark liver oil. This ubiquitous compound is a metabolite of sterol synthesis and is also found in human tissues and plasma. Squalene also activates the key antioxidant enzyme, glutathione transferase. Squalene has been examined for its ability to potentiate the cytotoxicity and antitumor activity of anticancer therapies, such as Adriamycin, 5-FU, and cis-platinum, *in vivo* and *in vitro*. The antitumor activities of these anticancer agents combined with squalene were tested against sarcoma 180 ascite cells. This combination of anticancer agents with membrane-active agents is useful because it can overcome drug resistance and inhibit the development of drug-resistant tumors.

Studies have reported antitumor activity of highly purified squalene in murine transplantable tumor systems. In cancer immunotherapy, augmentation of tumor-specific (as well as nonspecific) immunity is critically important. Olive oil is also very rich in squalene, and, in fact, most commercial squalene products are derived from olive oil.[114]

Squalene has an enhancing effect on cellular oxygen uptake, which produces a more efficient metabolism at the cellular level. By inhibiting fatty acid lipid peroxidation, it offers protection from the sun when used externally. Squalene and shea butter are two of the best fatty acids to use for protecting skin from aging, sun damage, and skin cancer. Using these fatty acids externally and at the same time taking plant antioxidants internally, such as green tea, turmeric, hawthorn, St. John's wort, lavender, or rosemary along with a full-spectrum carotenoid supplement, ascorbate vitamin C, dry vitamin E, and selenium, supplies the body with nutrients that are protection against skin cancer as well as other cancers and chronic illnesses.

Another recent study has demonstrated that squalamine, a steroid derived from shark liver, inhibits angiogenesis and tumor growth in multiple animal models and may be well suited for treatment of tumors and other diseases characterized by neovascularization in humans.[115]

Alkylglycerols

Alkylglycerols are found abundantly in animals, chiefly in bone marrow, but also in mother's milk (ten times more than in cow's milk), as well as in shark liver oil, from which they are extracted for oral consumption. Alkylglycerols have been shown to be powerful protectors of bone marrow function during chemotherapy and radiation therapy. Alkylglycerols are particularly helpful for the production of granulocytes and thrombocytes in the bone marrow and can inhibit leucopenia (white blood-cell suppression), thrombocytopenia (low platelet count), and to a lesser extent, anemia.

In a vast research project at Radiumhemmet in Stockholm, Sweden, Astrid Brohult was able to demonstrate that patients with carcinoma of the uterine cervix who received alkylglycerols both before their first radiation treatment and throughout the course of external radiation, had a significantly better survival rate than patients who were not given alkylglycerols.[116]

Medium-Chain Triglycerides

Medium-chain triglycerides (MCTs) are used to induce the body's energy source to derive from fats rather than sugar (glucose).

Elevated blood glucose can divert prostaglandin pathways toward tumor-promoting PGE-2, which is immune suppressive, aggregatory, and vaso-constrictive, and inhibits the biosynthetic pathways of estrogen binders. Maintaining low levels of blood glucose selectively starves tumors while also causing lower insulin output; this helps regulate prostaglandin synthesis. MCT oil can aid in keeping blood glucose levels low. It is also a very easily absorbable source of energy.

Cancer cells gobble up sugar ten to fifteen times more than normal cells do. Tumors of the central nervous system seem to be the most sensitive to glucose, but all cancerous growth is fed by glucose. This is what leads to cancer-caused cachexia (wasting syndrome). Cancer cells steal glucose from the liver by converting lactic acid into glucose. Inhibiting cancer-cell gluconeogenesis without interfering with normal cell metabolism may be one important aspect to slowing or stopping tumor growth and inhibiting cachexia. Cachexia, not the cancer itself, is what makes some cancers fatal.

Lecithin

Lecithin is an important dietary source of phosphatidylcholine and has been shown to completely prevent disruption of the mucosal barrier due to bile injury.

Choline, a component of lecithin, is involved in methyl metabolism and lipid transport. It is essential for normal liver function. Lecithin can assist the liver by correcting phospholipid and phosphatidylcholine depletion. Many chemo drugs, for example methotrexate, cause disruptions in methyl metabolism. Lecithin may also enhance the proper utilization of EFAs, such as the conversion of the ALA present in flaxseed oil into PG3.[117]

Lecithin is a recommended supplement for people with methylation problems, such as elevated homocysteine levels. It is also recommended for those using methotrexate as a cancer therapy or for those who need a fat emulsifier to help with a weak gallbladder or liver. The dosage varies according to the individual situation.

Butyric Acid

Foods rich in butyric acid are cottage cheese, yogurt (both should be made from organic whole milk), butter, and Parmesan cheese. The primary mechanism of butyric acid appears to be the initiation of differentiation of undifferentiated cells by the unmasking of the genetic material of the cell. It is thought that the primary effect of butyric acid is on the cell membrane.

Dr. Jonathan Wright explains it this way:

> Based on numerous studies, it appears highly probable that butyrate is a major cancer-inhibiting metabolite. Butyrate has been shown to suppress the neoplastic state *in vitro* of Syrian hamster cells. It induces differentiation in mouse leukemia cells, human carcinoma, and colon carcinoma cell lines. . . . When fiber is exposed to colonic flora, butyrate is the major metabolite. It has therefore been postulated that a possible mechanism for the anticancer action of fiber in the colon is due to increased fermentation of fiber to butyrate by the bacteria residing there.

As a practitioner, Dr. Wright relies on the relatively inexpensive stool butyrate test as an important risk factor marker for colon cancer. He has found that the colon cancer risk is high when the butyrate is low.[118]

It has also been suggested that butyrate be used as an anticancer agent. This has proven to be effective from several biochemical standpoints. In rat ascites hepatomas, butyrate treatment led to loss of contact inhibition, which lessens the tendency for cancer cells to metastasize or break away from a primary tumor and travel to other parts of the body.

In addition, while cancer cells are in a state of rapid DNA replication compared to normal cells, HeLa cells (a type of human cell) treated with butyrate undergo extensive acetylation with the inhibition of both DNA synthesis and cell replication. Borenfreund et al. have also deomonstrated the reversal of tumorigenicity in hepatoma cells treated with butyrate. In rat hepatoma cells induced by a chemical carcinogen, large aggregates of filaments are seen interspersed with microtubules, polyribosomes, and membranous structures. Treatment with butyrate resulted in a progressive return to the appearance of normal hepatocyte morphology and the disintegration of the abnormal filament aggregates.[119–123]

Conjugated Linoleic Acid

Conjugated linoleic acid (CLA) is a collective term that refers to a mixture of positional and geometric isomers of linoleic acid. Believe it or not, this is a fatty acid that is naturally present in dairy products and meat.

A 1991 study published in *Cancer Research* showed that 1 percent of CLA in the diet suppressed mammary carcinogenesis in rats given a high dose of DMBA, a known carcinogen. The same journal published another more recent study demonstrating that dietary CLA at a much lower dose produced a dose-dependent inhibition in mammary tumor yield when fed to rats treated with a lower dose of the same carcinogen.[124]

CLA is a unique anticarcinogen because it is present in foods from animal sources. Its efficacy in cancer protection occurs at levels that are normally consumed by humans. This is one reason why not all people on a cancer-inhibiting diet need to be on a strict vegetarian diet. I must stress, however, that dairy products and meat have become so polluted with chemicals and growth hormones that, in spite of their CLA content, they have become carcinogenic. For this reason, all animal products in the diet must be organic.

ENZYMES

Enzymes not only play a major role in digestion but also act as anti-inflammatory, fibrinolytic, and thrombolytic agents in the body. The use of enzymes in cancer therapy began in 1902 with John Beard, the leading embryologist of that time, whose book, *The Enzyme Treatment of Cancer,* became a classic. Since then the use of a wide range of enzyme preparations for the treatment of cancer has grown.

The main mechanism by which enzymes appear to inhibit cancer has to do with their fibrinolytic effects. Fibrinogen is four to fifteen times higher in cancerous tissue as compared to healthy tissue; the protective fibrin net that surrounds cancer cells helps to protect them from our own immune system. Enzyme preparations, taken in combination with specific herbs and mushroom extracts, work synergistically to break down fibrin. Thus, many of my protocols combine enzymes with herbs and mushroom extracts; they should be taken together between meals to enhance their effectiveness.

Proteolytic Enzymes

Wobenzym

Proteolytic enzymes, such as trypsin, chymotrypsin, bromelain, papain, serratio-peptase, SOD (superoxide dismutase), amylase, protease, and lipase, all make up Wobenzym, called Wobe-Mucos in Germany where it is manufactured (see Resources). This oral preparation, which also comes in suppository form, is indicated for the treatment of many disorders, including pancreatic insufficiency, chronic pancreatitis, cystic fibrosis, multiple sclerosis, herpes zoster, and chronic inflammatory diseases. It is also used as an adjunct to radiation therapy and to inhibit mestastatic cancer. These enzymes are strong modulators of the immune system because they activate macrophages that induce phagocytosis and release tumor necrosis factor-alpha (TNF-alpha), TNF-beta, IL-1, and IL-2. They also activate cytotoxic lymphocytes and natural killer-cells. In addition, they cleave to certain immunologic-active proteins, which in turn stimulate lymphocytes to infiltrate tumor sites.

Circulating immune complexes (CIC) are known to be present in people with cancer and are responsible for much of the cancer-associated immuno-suppression. Removal or modulation of these blocking factors can reverse this condition. This is part of the theory behind proteolytic enzyme therapy in cancer. Through this mechanism, proteolytic enzymes can also down-regulate an overactive immune system, thereby making them useful in treating autoimmune diseases as well.

A great deal of research on proteolytic enzymes is currently going on in many laboratories and cancer research centers around the world. One study of the use of enzymes combined with radiation therapy showed that those taking enzymes had a greater sense of general well-being, were better able to tolerate radiation, and required fewer drugs to offset the side effects of radiation treatments.[125]

An important part of my protocols for inhibiting cancer involves the combination of either Wobenzym supplementation or bromelain, a proteolytic enzyme derived from pineapple, with turmeric extract tablets containing 95 percent curcumin, quercetin, and sometimes one or more medical mushroom extract capsules (reishi, maitake, shiitake). Besides turmeric's anticancer, antioxidant, anti-inflammatory, fibrinolytic, and liver-protective properties, I believe it has a synergistic effect with enzyme therapy, particularly bromelain.

Cancer cells produce excessive amounts of fibrin, and therefore people who have cancer are more likely to develop blood clots, emboli, phlebitis, and thromboses. Fibrin is used by the cancer cells as a form of camouflage called *glycoprotein shield*. This protects the cancer cells from the immune system. Proteolytic enzymes, along with turmeric (which acts as an anticoagulant and fibrolytic agent), unmask the fibrin coating of cancer cells, thereby allowing attack from the immune system. This removes the stickiness of the cancer cell and helps to reduce the spread of cancer.

Proteolytic enzymes may also benefit patients undergoing radiation/chemotherapy by reducing side effects and exposing cancer cells to the cytotoxic agents, allowing for better effectiveness.

L-asparaginase, another enzyme preparation produced from yeast, is a valuable therapeutic modality for the treatment of both acute lymphoblastic leukemia and acute nonlymphoblastic leukemia.[126]

Bromelain

Bromelain causes interference with the growth of malignant cells by inhibiting the production of a mucus substance that protects the surface of the cancer cell from identification and docking by the lymph cells. This is one of the ways cancer cells elude the body's defenses. Bromelain inactivates prostaglandin E2 and thromboxanes. Oncogenic prostaglandin E2 inhibits the tumor-killing function of macrophages, while thromboxanes lead to platelet aggregation and favor the development of castaway tumor cells.

The enzymatic deshielding effects of bromelain are also necessary to prevent metastasis. Bromelain has been shown to inhibit the metastasis of breast and ovarian cancer. It also delays the development of UV light-induced skin cancer in mice and inhibits metastasis of the Lewis lung cancer in mice. The bromelain used must be crude and undiluted (a GDU rating of 2,000 is best).

Bromelain has also been shown to enhance the cytotoxic effects of many chemotherapies, including 5-FU and vincristine. Bromelain also enhances the absorption and usability of both quercetin and the curcuminoids found in turmeric. This is why I often recommend that bromelain, quercetin, and turmeric be taken together thirty minutes before meals. Their combined action is very powerful. I recommend bromelain more often than Wobenzym, although I use them both.[127–129] (See table 5.3.)

GLANDULAR SUPPLEMENTS

Spleen Extract

The only spleen extract product I use in my practice is SP500, which consists of an extract of polypeptide spleen fractions. The small molecular-weight spleen peptides found in SP500 contain two important active ingredients, tuftsin and splenopentin. Tuftsin increases macrophage activity against infection and/or cancer cells; and splenopentin increases white blood-cell production, only if suppressed, as well as other immune-regulating compounds, including interleukin-3 and macrophage colony-stimulating factors. SP500 has shown a significant positive effect on the immune system, including substantially increasing phagocytic function and T- and B-cells in bone marrow. It inhibits the spreading of tumor metastases, reduces the damaging effect from radiation, and induces interferon production.[130]

The indications for use of SP500 would include:

- Low white blood-cell count
- As an adjunct to medical treatments for cancer

Table 5.3 Actions of Enzymes in Cancer Treatment

Enzyme	Summary of Actions	Specific Uses and Interaction	General Daily Range
Wobenzym	Moderates immune system; activates natural killer-cells	Helpful for disorders of the pancreas; cystic fibrosis; multiple sclerosis; useful adjunct to radiation therapy; inhibits metastases	2–4 tablets 3–4 times daily between meals
L-asparaginase	Anti-inflammatory; immune regulating; fibrinolytic	Helpful in acute lymphoblastic leukemia and nonlymphoblastic leukemia	500–1,000 mg 3 times a day under supervision
Bromelain	Inhibits metastases; enhances cytotoxic effects of many chemotherapies; anti-inflammatory; immune regulating; fibrinolytic	Helpful in breast and ovarian cancers; helpful in postsurgical healing	1,000–6,000 mg

- Bacterial or viral infections
- Low tuftsin levels, postspleenectomy
- Autoimmune disorders associated with a low platelet count

Thymus Extract

Thymus gland extract increases the activity and the number of T-lymphocytes and boosts the gland's level of tumosterone, a steroid occurring in the thymus gland and in all the body's lymph cells. Tumosterone seems to migrate directly into the nucleus of the cancer cell, where its natural gene-repairing factor erases its erroneous genetic programming; this either kills the cancer cell or causes it to revert to normal. Tumosterone repairs and prevents gene defects and also seems to block the tumor cell's ability to fatten itself.

In Germany, thymus and spleen extracts are some of the most important biological response modifiers (BRMs) used in cancer treatment. A study in Germany of small-cell bronchial carcinoma patients showed that those who used BRMs with their standard cancer therapy had a success rate twice that of those who did not.[131]

Thymic Protein A is a new specialized "intact" thymic protein that contains the complete 500-amino chain that fits the receptor site on the T-4 cell. The T-4 cell is the key to regulating the immune system. Chemotherapy and radiation therapy damage the immune system, including the T-4 cells. The protein in Thymic Protein A acts as a software program that turns on the immune system's computer system. No other thymus product is processed in a manner that contains intact thymic protein, not even thymosin, a patented thymic fraction containing fragments of the whole protein.

Many people who undergo chemotherapy and radiation therapy die of opportunistic infections because of the weakening effects these therapies have on the immune system. Thymic Protein A is one of the more valuable supplements available to enhance the immune system.

Thymic Protein A, marketed as Bio Pro Protein A, is sold as a powder in sealed individual-dose packets (see Resources). It should be taken under the tongue, where it is rapidly absorbed. Each box contains thirty packets. The recommended dose is 1 to 3 packets daily.

Aqueous Liver Extract

The liver in this product (see Resources) is derived from raw organic liver that has been enzymatically hydrolyzed and made into an extract containing liquefied protein fractions. I recommend this supplement to cancer patients and have found it helpful in strengthening not only the liver but the entire body. It is also very useful in treating the anemia caused by the cancer itself or by chemotherapy or hormone therapy. Flutamine, a drug used to treat prostate cancer, for example, is known to cause anemia. Iron supplementation is not an option for anemic cancer patients because iron can react with hydroxal radicals and become carcinogenic. Fresh liver is used as a food in the Gerson Therapy. I feel that for very weak or anemic patients, eating organic liver two times a week can be helpful in lieu of the capsules. One capsule is equal to one ounce of liver.

OTHER USEFUL SUPPLEMENTS

Chlorella

Chlorella is a one-celled green algae food product that is highly nutritive. It contains high-quality protein (58 percent protein), vitamins (all the B vitamins plus vitamins C and E), minerals, including many important trace minerals, omega-3 fatty acids, and mucopolysaccharides. Chlorella has been shown to improve immune function in people undergoing chemotherapy and/or radiation therapy. Chlorella increases macrophage activity, activates both T-cells and B-cells, and has shown antitumor effects. In addition, chlorellan, a substance found in chlorella, stimulates interferon production.

Chlorella is a whole food rich in many phytochemicals, some of which have been identified but many of which are still unknown. A group of elements referred to as chlorella growth factor, or CGF, are believed to be one group of compounds in chlorella that give it its health-promoting ability. Chlorella stimulates the growth of friendly bacteria, which in turn has the probiotic effect of strengthening gut flora and resisting disease.

Chlorella helps protect the body in its fight against both viruses and cancer. A series of studies during the 1980s showed that tumor growth in mice could be reduced or stopped by injecting a water solution of chlorella around the neoplastic growth. Even tumor regrowth was cut down significantly. In another study by the same researchers, tumor cells were killed completely by the chlorella injection. The researchers then began to give chlorella in oral form, and the antitumor effect was still significant.[132,133]

A study on chlorella published in Japan in 1992 showed that chlorella has impressive effects on blood chemistry. It increased red blood cells, white blood cells, platelets, and albumin. The ability of chlorella to increase albumin is vitally important because so many people with cancer have a decreased level of albumin. This decreased level correlates with a poor prognosis; chlorella is a truly important supplement for anyone whose albumin level is low.[134]

There have been dozens of animal studies on chlorella and chlorella extracts involving immune response to cancer. One such study involved mice given chlorella prior to transplantation of mammary carcinoma. The results were a 70 percent sixty-day survival of the chlorella group versus no survival in the control group. Mice in the control group were also transplanted with tumors but did not receive chlorella.[135]

In 1990, a study on chlorella was performed at the Medical College of Virginia. Fifteen glioblastoma patients were administered 20 grams of powdered chlorella and 150 ml of liquid chlorella, in some cases combined with standard chemotherapy and/or radiation therapy. There was a significant increase in health and immune status immediately, and a striking 40 percent two-year survival rate was reflected in follow-up studies. This is extremely rare for this type of tumor, which normally might yield a 10 percent survival rate after two years.[136]

There are other beneficial algaes, such as spirulina, a blue-green alga, and other super green foods, but I believe chlorella is the best, particularly for people with cancer and/or a weak constitution.

Greens Plus

Greens Plus is a synergistic blend of enzymatically alive, nutrient-rich foods that provide optimum alkaline pH for every cell in the body. It is a whole, living food containing concentrated sources of vitamins, organic covalent minerals, essential amino acids, phytochemicals, enzymes, coenzymes, cell salts, chlorophyll, standardized herbal extracts, unique botanical extracts, and soluble and insoluble plant fibers from high-quality, organic, nutrient-rich foods (see Resources). Its actual components are chlorella; milk thistle; echinacea; probiotic cultures; European bilberry; organically and hydroponically grown soy sprouts; acerola berry juice powder; ultra lecithin; Hawaiian spirulina; organically grown alfalfa, barley, wheat grass, and red beet juice powder; royal jelly; Montana bee pollen; grape seed; green tea; licorice root; Siberian ginseng; dunaliela salina (a type of seaweed); astragalus; natural vitamin E; Nova Scotia dulse; and pharmaceutical-grade ginkgo biloba.

Greens Plus in a blender drink is quite tasty. I frequently recommend it as part of a shake recipe in various doses, ranging from 1 teaspoon to 2 tablespoons daily. (See the recipe for Flaxseed and Chlorella Shake on page 382.)

Inositol Hexaphosphate

Inositol hexaphosphate (IP-6), found abundantly in cereals and legumes, has recently been the subject of many studies that have demonstrated its ability to inhibit cell proliferation and act as a chemopreventive and chemotherapeutic agent for human cancers.

One study has shown that IP-6 not only decreases cellular proliferation but also causes differentiation of malignant cells, which can result in a reversion to normal phenotype. This study strongly indicates that IP-6 works in a number of ways—by being involved in the signal transduction pathways, cell cycle regulatory genes, differentiation genes, oncogenes, and even tumor-suppressor genes.[137]

Another study compared the effects of pure IP-6 versus a high-bran diet in the prevention of DMBA-induced rat mammary carcinogenesis. This study found a significant reduction in tumor number, incidence, and multiplicity when using the pure IP-6, suggesting that IP-6 is a better cancer prophylactic than large quantities of fiber.[138,139]

Yet another current study has demonstrated the significant interaction of phytic acid and green tea. While the use of green tea alone produced marginal results in experiments designed to suppress colonic preneoplastic lesions in rats, there were significant and positive results when it was combined with phytic acid.[140] Other studies have shown the antitumor activity of phytic acid in subcutaneously transplanted fibrosarcomas in mice and the induced enhancement of natural killer-cell activity.[141,142]

In addition, IP-6, which is soluble and can be administered in drinking water, is rapidly absorbed through the stomach and upper small intestine, where it becomes quickly dephosphorylated within the mucosal cells and is distributed to various organs.[143] Another important study has shown IP-6's ability to exert its antineoplastic effects by significantly reducing large intestinal cancer in rats even though treatment was begun five months after carcinogenic induction. This demonstrates IP-6's potential use as an important chemointervention agent.[144]

Lactobacillus Brevis

Lactobacillus brevis, also referred to as Lacto Brev, is a concentrated extract of a Japanese pickle called the *suguki*. Experts at the Pasteur Institute of Kyoto found that this extract boosted interferon production 65 percent in four weeks and increased natural killer-cell activity by 57 percent.

Studies have shown that interferon capability is lower in people with cancer as well as in those with diabetes and pulmonary tuberculosis. Studies have also shown that an effective cure rate and the ability to prevent cancer can be greatly enhanced by raising the natural production of interferon. The administration of interferon as an immune-activating agent has been used to treat chronic hepatitis and has recently been approved as a treatment for various cancers, including chronic myeloid leukemia and some low-grade lymphomas. The problem with this therapy is that it is not extremely effective and causes many unwanted side effects, such as flulike symptoms, gastrointestinal disturbances, fatigue, and bone marrow suppression. Moreover, the long-term side effects of interferon are unknown because it has not yet been used for an extended period of time. Dr. Tsunataro Kishida of the Pasteur Institute of Kyoto has shown that taking Lacto Brev orally increases the body's natural production of interferon. Lacto Brev has also been shown to significantly enhance natural killer-cell production.[145]

I have found Lacto Brev very effective at boosting interferon levels; however, some people have complained it makes them feel like they have a low-grade fever. I recommend Lacto Brev for a number of cancers, including lymphomas, leukemias, and brain tumors. I usually suggest taking it in doses of 3 capsules three times daily, every other day. On the nights when Lacto Brev is taken, I recommend drinking 2 to 3 cups of a diaphoretic tea, such as yarrow, peppermint, elder, or boneset, and taking a hot Espom salt bath. I believe that following this regimen enhances the effectiveness of the Lacto Brev. I also recommend its use along with conventional alpha interferon administration, but in this case, I recommend using the Lacto Brev and interferon on alternate days.

Beta 1,3 Glucan

Beta-glucans are polysaccharides that are synthesized by a variety of plants, including the fruiting body of edible mushrooms. This explains why these mushrooms benefit the immune system. Extensive investigation of a beta 1,3 glucan extracted from a common yeast has shown it contributes potent diverse overall enhancements to the immune system. Considered a biological response modifier of the immune system, beta 1,3 glucan has been shown to stimulate both humoral and cell-mediated immunity as well as to activate macrophages more effectively than any other agent known. Activating macrophages strengthens the immune system significantly and protects against various pathogens. One example of the result of macrophage activation is the appearance of gamma interferon, which increases the production of nitric oxide and superoxide, directly leading to an immunological war on microorganisms.[146]

Studies have shown that administration of beta 1,3 glucan to people with AIDS increases IL-1 and IL-2 levels. Mild fevers were seen in many of these people one hour after taking beta 1,3 glucan. The onset of fever was associated with a peak in IL-1 activity, suggesting a fever-producing response from the beta 1,3 glucan.[147]

Beta 1,3 glucan is recommended before and after cancer surgery to enhance healing, reduce the chance of infection, and inhibit recurring and/or metastatic cancer. I recommend beta 1,3 glucan (94 percent pure) as part of a combined protocol for many cancer patients and believe it to be of great benefit. I usually recommend 3 to 6 capsules (500 mg each) daily. Except for the mild fever experienced by some, beta-glucan has no known side effects or contraindications.

Resveratrol

Resveratrol, a stilbene derivative and polyphenol found abundantly in grape leaves and red wine, possesses chemopreventative properties and functions as a plant defense molecule.

Resveratrol inhibits cancer by many mechanisms, including anti-inflammatory activity, antioxidant activity, and induction of Phase II detoxifying enzymes.[148] It has been found to inhibit the development of promyelocytic leukemia in mice given a carcinogen that induces this type of cancer. When incubated with hepatoma cells, resveratrol induced Phase II detoxifying enzymes that detoxified and inhibited the proliferation of these cells. Resveratrol also inhibited the development of preneoplastic lesions when mice were exposed to tumor initiators and promoters.[149]

Grape skins, leaves, juice and red wine are all good sources of resveratrol. Source Naturals (see Resources) packages resveratrol as a supplement.

Modified Citrus Pectin

Modified citrus pectin (MCP) is a specially prepared (pH modified) complex carbohydrate fiber that appears to block, or jam up, the metastatic process of cancer development. Carbohydrate lectins foster a cancer cell's adhesion to the blood vessel wall of any organ it attempts to colonize. By binding these lectins to a specially processed pH-modified pectin instead, the hope is to keep cancer cells circulating in the bloodstream until they either die or are eliminated. MCP is rich in galactosyl, a specific lectin that competes with cancer cells for the receptor site, thereby interfering with the cancer cell's interaction with metastatic target sites.

In a number of human cancers, the amount of galectin (one particular lectin used by cancer cells) produced increases proportionally as the cancer grows from the earliest to the most advanced stages. It is reasonable to theorize that higher galectin levels permit greater adhesion of cancer cells as well as increase the ability of these cells to bind to noncancerous cells at a target site. The lectin receptors that bind to cell-surface carbohydrates and glycoproteins may serve as the cement that allows cancer cells to clump together and form metastatic tumors.

MCP has been shown to significantly inhibit the adhesion of a number of cancers to the endothelium, including human prostate adenocarcinoma cells, human breast carcinoma cells, human melanoma cells, and human laryngeal epidermoid carcinoma cells. MCP also appears to inhibit lung and kidney cancers. The antiadhesive effects of MCP extend to a variety of different malignant cell lines. This means that MCP is able to inhibit the metastatic cascade through a nontumor-specific mechanism.[150]

In 1995, the *Journal of the National Cancer Institute* reported a study that showed the inhibition of metastasis of prostate cancer in rats by oral administration of MCP. The author showed that MCP bound to the surface of prostate cancer cells and protected the animals in the study from metastatic cancer. MCP prevents free-floating cancer cells from anchoring to other tissues; thus they are then eventually eliminated by a healthy immune system.[151]

There have been a number of published papers showing that MCP inhibits cancer cells and assists the immune response by enhancing the cytotoxicity of natural killer-cells and T-cells.[152]

I recommend MCP in doses of 1 teaspoon to 1 tablespoon daily, added either to juice or water or as an ingredient in a shake recipe that I specifically develop for the individual.

Low-Temperature Whey Protein

Whey protein has the highest biological value of any protein source available and should be incorporated into specialized foods for patients with impaired gastrointestinal function, including those with cancer.[153] Low-temperature whey protein is rich in immunoglobins, vital to the health of the immune system and to the digestive system, and is the highest quality protein obtainable.

Immunocal, one concentrated whey product, is a patented product that is a unique source of glutathione precursors. It is used in many hepatitis, AIDS, and cancer studies. In a study being done at Brooklyn Hospital in New York, Immunocal is given as a cancer-inhibiting therapy, as well as a protection therapy to women with recurring breast cancer who have undergone intense radiation therapy.

Probioplex, made by Metagenics (see Resources), is also a patented whey protein composed of a lactalbumin, eighteen amino acids, calcium, iron-binding protein, various cellular components, and other nutrients. Immunocal is richer in cysteine than Probioplex; otherwise they are very similar. I also recommend Protein 290 by Country Life (see Resources), a 100 percent cross-flow microfiltration whey protein product.

If these products are unavailable and you must select another whey protein powder product, make sure it is a cross-flow microfiltration (CFM) whey isolate. CFM whey protein uses membrane technology that results in a 98 percent pure undenatured whey protein.

The health benefits of low-temperature whey protein are many:

• It provides high concentrations of biologically active globulin proteins similar to those found in colostrum.

• It causes opsonization, the ability to coat pathogens, such as bacteria and viruses. This assists the immune system in the identification and removal of the pathogens, thereby improving the chemotoxic activity of white blood cells toward many bacteria and viruses.

• It enhances the gastrointestinal tract's ability to colonize acidophilus and bifidus, the healthy bacteria that are vital to the immune system and to the flora of our digestive tract.

• It acts as a barrier to further bowel invasion in incidences of colon cancer.

• It neutralizes bacterial toxins, such as *E. coli.*

• It is antiviral, antibacterial, antifungal, and antiparasitic.

• It helps combat diarrhea and many digestive tract disorders, including overall poor digestion, irritable bowel syndrome, and digestive problems brought on by antibiotic use.

• It inhibits tumor growth.

Lactoferrin

Lactoferrin, lipoic acid, and chlorella are the three best supplements I have found for enhancing the nutritional status and raising the albumin level of those with cancer or any chronic illness. Lactoferrin, an iron-binding protein, is a vital element to the human body. It retrieves iron from the foods we eat and delivers it to areas of the body where it is needed. Many people, particularly those with cancer, become anemic because their body is not assimilating iron properly. Symptoms of iron deficiency appear even though plenty of iron is being ingested. Many doctors will then tell their patients to take iron supplements when what they really need is lactoferrin and/or vitamin B_{12} and folic acid, which will assist them to assimilate iron from their food and nutrients.

Unless a person is specifically iron deficient and not just generally anemic, iron supplements should be avoided. Taking iron supplements usually provides no help and can actually do some harm by creating free-radical damage.

The body struggles to remove excess iron, which can support the growth of infectious organisms, including bacteria, viruses, yeast, and other parasites. Excess iron can catalyze the production of oxygen radicals and increase the chance for cancer cells to survive and flourish.[154]

Lactoferrin can also assist the body by helping to produce alpha-interferon, which has profound immune-stimulating action. For patients who are anemic, I usually recommend 4 capsules before bed.

Soy Supplements

Soybean consumption is associated with a reduced rate of breast, prostate, and colon cancer. This is most likely related to the presence of isoflavones that are weakly estrogenic and anticarcinogenic. Diets rich in soy phytoestrogens can reduce circulating ovarian steroids and adrenal androgens, an effect that may account, at least in part, for the decreased risk of breast cancer in women whose diets are rich in legumes.[155]

Isoflavonoid glycosides found in soy, as well as in other legumes, are converted by intestinal bacteria to hormonelike compounds. These compounds can inhibit cancer through several pathways. By acting as weak estrogen-mimicking molecules, soy isoflavonoids can affect sex-hormone production, metabolism, and biological activity; intracellular enzymes; protein synthesis; growth factor action; malignant cell proliferation; cell adhesion and differentiation—all of which have a profound inhibiting effect on cancer development and growth.

These substances can also reduce hot flashes, vaginal dryness, and other menopausal symptoms. Thus, they are the perfect solution for menopausal or postmenopausal women with breast cancer. Soy foods are also beneficial to well women who want a natural alternative to hormone replacement therapy as well as protection from breast cancer, heart disease, and osteoporosis. Studies have shown that soy consumption can prevent the oxidation of LDL cholesterol.[156,157]

Two isoflavone-rich supplements I often recommend, both made by Nutritional Therapeutics, are Harmonizer and Soy Power (see Resources). I suggest 2 to 4 tablets one to three times daily.

Another new whole food supplement that I recommend is Breast Basics by New Chapter (see Resources). Full-spectrum nutrients such as this formula offer a range of important natural constituents, not just one isolated active compound. There is strong evidence in the research community that such a whole-food supplement presents antioxidants and nutrients in their safest and most biologically active form. The activated soy in Breast Basics is produced using an active nutritional yeast culture that is an abundant source of B vitamins, glutathione, beta-glucans, and enzymes such as superoxide dismutase. When this yeast culture interacts with soybeans, the isoflavones become converted into genistein, a very biologically active form, thereby aiding in the digestive and assimilation process.

Genistein

Genistein, an isoflavone that is presently being investigated for its anticancer activity, has an antiangiogenesis effect on tumors. Angiogenesis, as previously explained, is the process of generating new capillary blood vessels, a critical step in the growth and proliferation of solid tumors. Cancer needs food and oxygen as it grows. The cancer forms new blood vessels to satisfy these needs. When cancer cannot form new blood vessels, its growth will stop. Genistein inhibits angiogenesis by neutralizing vascular endothelial growth factor (VEGF), the substance put out by tumors to encourage blood vessel nourishment. Genistein has additional anticancer actions:

• It inhibits cancer-promoting forms of sex hormones from binding to receptor sites.

• It inhibits some inflammatory processes that promote cancer, such as leukotriene production.

• It inhibits certain cancer-signaling enzymes, one of which is tyrosine kinase, which can cause cancer cells to differentiate.

• It inhibits mitosis of cancer cells.

Soy isoflavones, which include genistein and daidzin, as well as the soy saponins (also referred to as *glycophospholipids*), all have a beneficial effect on hormonal receptor-type cancers, such as breast cancer and prostate cancer. In breast cancer, isoflavones block the entry of estrogen into the cell, thereby causing cancer cells to lose their ability to function. Isoflavones cause cancer cells to dedifferentiate and turn more primitive, less specialized, and less deadly.

Genistein is generally more available in fermented soy products, such as tempeh and miso, rather than soy milk or tofu. Supro is a patented soy protein product that has been used in many clinical trials for lowering cholesterol and blood lipids. It contains high amounts of genistein. Many of the soy protein products sold in natural food stores contain supro soy protein. Although there are some encouraging reports on the use of benistein as an anticancer agent, I recommend using whole soy food concentrates rather than isolates such as genistein.

Bovine Cartilage and Shark Cartilage

Both bovine and shark cartilage inhibit angiogenesis when placed in close proximity with cancer cells; they do not prevent angiogenesis in healthy cells.[158,159]

As an antitumor and anticancer agent, shark cartilage has received more publicity than any other supplement I can remember. Although I believe it may have some beneficial effects in a few cases, its benefits are limited to inhibiting angiogenesis (and thus metastasis), and I feel at this time that it is overrated. In fact, based on a recent study, Cartilage Technologies, Inc., the manufacturer of a leading brand of shark cartilage, has discontinued the sponsorship of an FDA-supervised clinical trial that was designed to evaluate shark cartilage as a treatment for cancer. One of its spokesmen has stated that the company is "unable to find meaningful scientific data to support further investment in pursuing drug status for shark cartilage."[160]

Although I am not enthusiastic about either bovine or shark cartilage, if I had to choose between the two, I would look to bovine since there have been studies showing its benefits as a cancer inhibitor. So far, there has been no such documentation for shark cartilage.

DHEA

DHEA (dehydroepiandrosterone) is an adrenal steroid hormone that functions as a reservoir for other hormones from which the body can draw. It is represented in relatively important amounts in the blood plasma and works from outside the cell. This steroid inhibits enzymes, namely glucose-6-phosphate-dehydrogenase, which plays a pivotal role in the manifestation of cancer metabolism. This anticancer surveillance hormone may inhibit the metabolism of cancer cells. For various reasons, the cancer cell fails to become an immunological alien to the host and will, therefore, be more easily rejected. DHEA may also play a role in the prevention of other diseases including diabetes, heart disease, and osteoporosis, as well as autoimmune diseases, such as lupus, AIDS, Alzheimer's, and other age-related disorders. DHEA has also been shown to prevent chemically induced colon, liver, and skin papillomas in mice.

Many *pre*menopausal women with breast cancer have abnormally low DHEA levels in their blood and, for that group, DHEA may offer protection against cancer. Symptoms that indicate a low level of DHEA include lack of decisiveness and latent depression. However, women who are *post*menopausal with breast cancer sometimes exhibit an elevated DHEA level and, therefore, DHEA is counterindicated for them.[161]

7-Keto is a relatively new natural form of DHEA that has been shown in clinical trials to deliver the beneficial effects of DHEA without many of the risks. It has a variety of therapeutic effects on the endocrine system by way of the adrenal gland and it has shown an ability to enhance T-cells and IL-2 production.[162]

In my practice, I occasionally recommend DHEA after testing shows low levels of the hormone, when I feel it will be of benefit to the person for both the short and long term. I use DHEA with caution. I recommend a low dose (usually 5 to 10 mg and generally no more than 25 mg). DHEA is not for everyone. I prefer to use herbs like licorice to modulate adrenal function and increase DHEA and ACTH levels in a more natural way. Recently I have been recommending more 7-Keto and pregnenolone than DHEA, particularly for women.

Pregnenolone

Pregnenolone is a steroid precursor made from cholesterol. From pregnenolone, the body produces other hormones, including DHEA and progesterone. Inside the cytoplasm, enzymes convert pregnenolone into either progesterone or DHEA, depending on the tissues' needs.

I have found low-dose pregnenolone to be very helpful for many people, particularly woman with hormone-endocrine imbalances. It recharges the entire endocrine system including thyroid, adrenal, and reproductive hormones, and even the pancreas, thus helping regulate blood sugar. Pregnenolone can help restore impaired memory and enhance mood. It does this by acting on DMDA

(N-methyl-D-aspartate) receptors, which affect learning and memory by regulating the function of the synapses on neurons. Pregnenolone may be the best inhibitor of dementia.

Pregnenolone can also help protect the body from cortisone toxicity. Cortisone, as well as other steroids, are often used as part of a protocol to treat cancer. Pregnenolone can repair enzymes within the liver—cytochrome P-450 in particular—that are important to detoxifying hormones and carcinogens. Pregnenolone is indicated for women approaching menopause who are at high risk for breast or ovarian cancer or who are having difficulty with the change of life and want to avoid hormone replacement therapy.[163] In cases of women who have had breast cancer, however, I prefer to begin treating their symptoms using herbal and dietary means.

When pregnenolone is indicated, I usually recommend a low dose of 10 mg, taken sublingually.

Melatonin

Melatonin, a hormone produced by the pineal gland, has gained popularity as a natural sleep aid without side effects. Melatonin levels are low during the day because light inhibits its production, but at night the pineal gland produces melatonin and levels may go up as much as five to fifteen times. As a sleeping aid, it works well for some, but does nothing for others. The key element is to avoid exposure to light during the night because light exposure during sleeping time greatly diminishes melatonin levels.

People with cancer who are not sleeping well may indeed have low levels of melatonin and may benefit in at least two ways from taking it as a supplement. First, melatonin supplementation may help a person to sleep longer and more soundly and second, it aids in immune function and is an anticarcinogen. It is an important antioxidant, possibly five times better than glutathione at scavenging free radicals, particularly hydroxal radicals, and better than vitamin E at scavenging lipid peroxidation. Melatonin, due to its lipophilic structure, is readily diffused into all tissues of the body, including intracellular membranes. There it protects against free-radical damage.

The melatonin-cancer relationship started with a study published in the early 1980s by the National Institutes of Health. That study found that women with estrogen-positive breast cancer had lower nighttime melatonin levels than women who did not have breast cancer. Melatonin appears to have not only antioxidant protection against breast cancer but also an antiestrogenic effect. Melatonin also inhibits melanoma cell lines, perhaps in a similar manner, by an antiestrogen mechanism.[164]

Certain immune functions are stimulated by melatonin, as shown by a recent Italian study that used a combination of melatonin (40 mg per day) and IL-2 to treat people with advanced colorectal cancer. IL-2 alone did nothing at all, but the addition of melatonin with IL-2 produced a significant reduction in the proliferation of neoplastic cells.[165]

Some people with late-stage metastatic cancer have been reported to stabilize as a result of melatonin supplementation. Remarkable results have been seen in metastatic renal cell cancer.[166] In addition, recent research has shown that melatonin can prevent and suppress the severe nephrotoxicity that can be induced by treatment with Adriamycin, a commonly used chemotherapeutic drug.[167]

Melatonin has been shown to inhibit the growth of some cancer-cell lines, including prostate cancer, either by exerting a direct cytostatic action or by decreasing the endogenous production of some tumor growth factors. A recent study involving men with metastatic prostate cancer who were on hormone therapy showed melatonin to have an anticancer effect by decreasing PSA serum levels by an average of 57 percent compared to men on hormone therapy but not taking melatonin. Melatonin was also shown to normalize platelet counts in 914 men with persistent thrombocytopenia. Melatonin appears to overcome the clinical resistance to hormone therapy, or at least delay the resistance in men with metastatic prostate cancer.[168]

I strongly believe that cancer patients must get quality sleep if they are to get well. Benzodiazepine drugs and other sleeping medications used to treat sleep disorders do not help a person to get the deep sleep they really need. They also tend to become less and less effective the longer they are used. I think these drugs are misused and overprescribed today, especially among the elderly. Melatonin supplementation works better for the elderly than it does for middle-aged or younger people. In one study that compared melatonin to Restoril, a common sleep medication, melatonin was shown to be better tolerated and to improve the quality of sleep.[169]

If I believe that melatonin supplementation may be beneficial as a sleep aid, an immune enhancer, and a possible cancer inhibitor, I start the patient with a low dosage (1 mg before bed, sublingually). Sublingual melatonin is absorbed by the body more efficiently. If this does not help bring on sleep, the dose may be slowly increased to 5 mg (or occasionally as high as 10 mg). If the sleep patterns do no improve, the melatonin should be discontinued. I do not recommend melatonin as a supplement unless there is a sleep problem. Those who do take melatonin should take it before bed at night, never during the day.

Other Natural Approaches to Insomnia

Many people with cancer suffer from anxiety and insomnia. I believe this must be addressed in as natural a way as possible. This is an important aspect to healing that is very often overlooked. I recommend developing a sleeping pattern that is in harmony with an individual's circadian rhythm. Besides trying melatonin, I recommend not sleeping during the day and getting some natural sun exposure. Taking a hot Epsom salt bath with lavender or another relaxing essential oil can do wonders to help one sleep, as can soft music or natural sounds like a running creek or the sound of the ocean.

Many herbs and other supplements can also be used, such as kava kava, passionflower, chamomile, skullcap, pulsatilla, St. John's wort, or oats, to name just a few. I sometimes suggest a single herb for sleep and at other times a compound based on the individual's needs. Depending on the herbs used and the individual situation, the dosage can vary from 5 drops to 1 teaspoon (about 120 drops) two to six times daily. Sometimes adding an herbal extract or compound to a cup of hot tea (perhaps a relaxing tea like chamomile) or water can help induce a restful and deep sleep. See a qualified herbalist for specific herbs or compounds for your situation.

DMSO

Dimethyl sulfoxide (DMSO), a by-product from wood processing, has been used for many years as an external treatment for inflammation and pain.

DMSO has been shown to:

- Be a scavenger of hydroxal radicals
- Stimulate the immune system, specifically interferon

- Be antiviral and antibacterial
- Be helpful at softening scar tissue
- Cause differentiation in a number of human cancer-cell lines *in vitro*[170]

DMSO is a potent solvent and a great transdermal agent. This means it can carry molecules of low molecular weight through intact membranes, such as the skin, including the blood-brain barrier. I use DMSO for one purpose—to carry agents, such as herbs and essential oils, through the skin into specific organs and/or the blood.

Hydrazine Sulfate

This anticancer agent has been given a very unjust and biased treatment by the National Cancer Institute. Hydrazine sulfate is not a natural product, but it is worth listing because I do recommend it in certain rare circumstances.

Hydrazine sulfate is a very effective anticachexia agent, capable of improving glucose tolerance, decreasing glucose turnover, increasing caloric intake and weight gain, or at the very least, weight stabilization. This is a very important agent that can save many lives often lost because of the wasting away that is brought on by the cancer, the cancer treatment, or both. I have recommended hydrazine sulfate for several years; it is very inexpensive and free of side effects.

The fact that hydrazine can effectively inhibit cachexia is of immense importance but this is only half the story. Hydrazine possesses antitumor/cytotoxic activity against many types of cancer, including some of the worst and most life-threatening types, for example, glioblastomas. It has also been found to enhance the cytotoxic effects of other cancer drugs.[171]

Table 5.4 **Hydrazine Sulfate Protocol**

Amount	Timing
a) One 60 mg capsule, once daily	With or before breakfast for days 1 to 3
b) One 60 mg capsule, twice daily	Before breakfast and dinner for days 4 to 6
c) One 60 mg capsule, three times daily	Before breakfast, lunch, and dinner, every 8 hours, from day 7 onward

Table 5.4, a hydrazine sulfate protocol, is recommended by Joseph Gold, M.D.

This protocol is intended for people who weigh 100 pounds or more. Those under 100 pounds should start with 30 mg capsules.

Hydrazine sulfate is most effective when daily treatment is maintained for forty-five days followed by an interruption of one to two weeks. The treatment can then be resumed for another forty-five days. This periodic interruption has been reported to prevent peripheral neuritis.

People taking hydrazine sulfate should avoid alcohol, tranquilizers, and barbiturates.

6

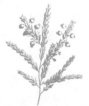

Spiritual Focus

Commune with your hearts and be silent. . . .
—Psalm 4:4, 46:10

T his chapter is written from my heart—a heart that is touched daily by others who are struggling with serious health issues and have come to me for help.

For most people, when an illness such as cancer occurs, its diagnosis has a profoundly negative impact on their emotional well-being. At a moment in time when one needs focus and clarity in order to face the many decisions required to treat an illness, fear and panic are common and usually result in confusion and a deep sense of being lost.

Aside from any herbal or nutritional protocols that I can recommend as a path to wellness, I am acutely aware of another need that in my opinion is equally important—the need for comfort and support. While we can offer comfort and support to one another, it is the nurturing of our inner strength that brings with it the hope of emotional peace so sorely needed at a time of crisis. For me, this inner strength is faith in God. I honor each person's individual path to Spirit; there is no "one way only" formula for faith. I hope that by sharing my beliefs with you, I will inspire you to explore your own deepest feelings about life in general and your own life in particular.

LIVING SPIRITUALITY

I believe that we are first and foremost spirits that exist in physical bodies. To me, spirituality is the pursuit of holiness, and that pursuit is an everyday activity of life in communion with God. I believe that a spiritual life is one that is inspired and guided by the spirit of God and leads us to pursue God's will in our lives. A spiritual connection with God opens one to the power of love in a very real sense. It is possible to see God's infinite love in many ways—by opening your heart to someone else and watching a deep relationship unfold; by breathing in the healing aroma of a flower; by marveling at a night sky full of stars. When infused with a spiritual connection, simple everyday life becomes special—cooking a meal together with someone dear can be as nourishing as the meal itself; loving care for a sick parent or friend who needs help can be healing to both of you.

As I begin to understand death by coming closer to it in others, and as I reflect on life in general and my contact with all people, I begin to understand that physical cancer pales in comparison with the terrible cancer that grows in the hearts of so many all over the world. The violence, hatred, and lack of compassion that exists in our world today is a worse type of cancer, one that can truly hurt us, which we must avoid if we can.

Someday we will all succumb to mortal death and begin a new life. When we open ourselves to the notion that we have come from eternity and will return to eternity, we will begin to experience a tremendous peace, a peace that shatters the division between life and death. Before we reach this peaceful place, we need to learn to forgive; it is in our forgiving that we are forgiven. This is fundamental to our spiritual growth. Many Americans have an obsession with death, fearing it greatly. Our culture over the years has emphasized aggressiveness, competitiveness, aesthetic youthfulness, and overfilling the mind with information. Unfortunately, it has neglected the soul, the inner spirit from which true strength originates.

When you see yourself as a soul, an eternal spirit ever growing in the presence of God, you will be free of fear. This is the point at which you realize that death is a bridge between the now and forever and it can bring you freedom, peace, and everlasting joy. Every day is a preparation for death, or better put, a transition into eternal life. Death is going back home, in a sense. This realization truly helps, because what the dying go through today, I will go through tomorrow. Death is not an end, but a beginning. It is a continuation of life.

To begin the pursuit of holiness and a spiritual life you must first be "poor in spirit" and recognize that all a spirit needs is the grace of God. It will set you free and enable you to be healed. This kind of healing goes deeper than the physical; this is the healing of the soul and spirit, and the soul is eternal. Every religion speaks of eternity, another life. People who fear death believe this life on earth is all there is; when we die it's the end. If you have witnessed the love of God you will not die in fear. We need to make peace with God daily. People die suddenly all the time, so it could happen to any one of us at any moment. Yesterday is gone and tomorrow has not yet come; we must live each day as if it were our last.

PRAYER IN DAILY LIFE

I personally believe that true healing must begin with God and prayer. When you have the emotional peace that comes with prayer, fear is lifted and nothing, not even cancer, can truly hurt you. In my opinion, this tops the list of factors involved in the healing process.

Data is accumulating that supports the theory that prayer makes a difference and can actually aid in physical healing. Studies have already shown that strong religious belief is associated with lower levels of blood pressure.[1] More and more research is under way that supports the mind-body-spirit concept of healing as well as the idea that prayer has a powerful healing effect—on those who are prayed for as well as on those who pray themselves. One provocative study undertaken in the coronary care unit of San Francisco General Hospital showed a dramatic difference in the recovery process between two groups of patients. One group was prayed for regularly by committed church members. The other group did not receive prayers from this source. All patients knew of the study itself but did not know whether or not they were being prayed for; the findings showed that the patients in the unprayed-for control group were twice as likely to suffer complications than were the patients in the prayed-for group.[2] Of course, spiritual communities have always been aware of this connection. A common practice in many monasteries is to sound bells when a member of the community is sick. Other members are reminded of their brother's need, and the ailing monk feels a deep connection to the power of his community's prayers—not to mention the healing sound of the bells themselves.

To bring prayer into your daily life, begin each day by becoming still and lifting your heart to God, praying that all the cobwebs of fear, selfishness, greed, and narrow-heartedness may be cleared from your soul; that the light of the Spirit might descend to give you courage to begin again. Make every effort to keep the presence of God in your daily life, to see God in everyone you meet, and to live your morning meditation throughout the day.

God speaks to us in silence, for those who know how to listen. It is within this silence that faith is built. For me, silent communication with God forms the person—the spirit—that is truly who we are. This is also the place where plants reveal their deep connection to us—a place where scientific and abstract knowledge of plants and medicine is replaced with personal communion with life.

At first, the silence may not feel comfortable, but if you give it a chance it will become familiar and at some point you will welcome it more and more often; then there will be a time when it comes to stay. At that time grace will overcome you and you will be fearless and filled with peace and love. This is where you will go to pray. Praying involves going to meet God; it means to be interactive and to listen. One needs to be still and silent, to listen and hear God speaking. Prayer is having a conversation with God who is all love, non-judgmental, compassionate, and always listening.

Prayer must be in solitude, where the mind and heart unite within the soul; the mind should not wander or roam among the things and affairs of the world. It must stay within, in the heart and soul—the *poustinia*.

The Poustinia

The poustinia is a place (really a state of mind, body, and spirit) where we go to be intimate with God. Literally, poustinia means "to go to the desert," and a *poustinik* is one who is living in a poustinia. The poustinik is an eternal pilgrim exploring the vast spaces of God. This journey is exquisitely beautiful and deeply satisfying to the soul. Within this journey one becomes poor in spirit and begins to realize "the need to have becomes the need not to have." This is when one begins to understand that all we really need is God. This is no easy journey and requires the ability to let go, to detach, and to trust.

As we grow spiritually, it is important to remember that our spirit resides in our physical body. Thus, the body is a temple of the Holy Spirit and we have a responsibility to it. We need to feed it, clothe it, provide rest for it, and take proper care of it with all the resources available to us. We need to love ourselves and all of creation—the animals, the trees, the plants, and all others—in the way that God loves everything.

Many people live out their entire lives eating right, exercising, being successful in the world, but never coming close to developing a poustinia. Yet others I have known are just the opposite; they pay no attention to the physical body but strive to be poustiniks in their daily lives.

At one time in my life, I put all my energies into trying to be a poustinik, a modern-day St. Francis. I cared little about anything of the world. I owned practically nothing, lived trusting in God and caring for others. There is a Franciscan saying that goes like this:

The more you own, the more it owns you.

I believe this is true. At the monastery where I lived, we had a retreat center I helped to run. I cooked, cleaned, made beds, and prayed three times a day. I was fed and given a room for sleeping. I did not make any money, yet my life was full of freedom and joy. After two years I left the monastery to help run a soup kitchen and shelter for the homeless. Two years later, I was ready to return to the field of herbal medicine and nutrition with a whole new light and dedication. Today, I have a successful clinic, a loving and supportive wife, a child, and a vision to create a healing retreat center. My busy life with its added responsibilities has made it more challenging to continue to be a poustinik, but my vision has come from listening to my inner self. I still ask myself these questions daily: Where do I come from? Where am I going? Am I trusting in God? Am I allowing my spirit to emerge and become who I am? If love is the image of God, how well am I loving?

LIFTING FEAR AND "WORRIMENT OF MIND"

Incorporating prayer and a sense of spirituality into daily life is one of the best ways to ease mental stress, an essential part of healing. Worries and anxieties have been shown to be a contributory cause of cancer. In 1889, Eli Jones wrote in *Cancer, Its Causes and Symptoms* that "Worrying weakens the nervous system, lowers the nerve power and thus opens the way for the invasion of cancer." Jones believed the number-one cause of cancer is "worriment of mind." Today, over a hundred years later, clinical studies that link depression with cancer are beginning to be published.[3]

> Dismiss all anxiety from your minds. Present your needs to God in every form of prayer and in petitions full of gratitude. Then God's own peace, which is beyond all understanding, will stand guard over your hearts and minds.
>
> *Letter of Paul to the Philippians 4:6–7*

A positive mental attitude is essential for true healing to occur; in fact, some regard toxic emotions as a major cause of cancer. A long-term emotional state of fear, hopelessness, helplessness, depression, and even anger can all contribute to an impaired immune system and susceptibility to cancer. I believe fear is one of the primary contributing factors to ill health of any kind. On the other hand, a positive mental attitude can contribute to the healing of cancer. Through guided imagery and other psychological techniques, recovery can be enhanced. A new branch of medicine called *psychoneuroimmunology* has documented this.

Many of the cancer patients I see tend to dwell on their past with anger; for example, one patient with lung cancer had a hard time getting past his self-inflicted anger at having once been a smoker. However, what is important is the present; the past must be let go. The past is like a cancelled check, and the future is like a promissory note. Leaving the past with all its anger and pessimism behind is an important step in alleviating fear about the future and allowing hope to emerge.

 We live in a culture where stress is an integral part of our everyday existence. In order to grow in health, happiness, and wisdom, we need to continually create ways to rise above it while discovering and becoming comfortable with the true meaning of life as well as death. I have found the Serenity Prayer extremely comforting both for myself and for the patients who often ask me, "What are my chances?" or "Do you think I'm going to make it?"

> God, grant me the ability to change the things in my life that I can change, the serenity to accept the things that I cannot change, and the wisdom to know the difference.

When a patient is told he has an incurable form of cancer or when all possible forms of therapy have failed, the main focus must be prayer. Clinics in every part of the world claim to have a cure for cancer, from enemas to magnets and everything in between. These claims offer false hope.

What is real is prayer and support by family and friends. We need to believe that God is forgiving and merciful and can offer help, love, and peace to troubled souls. To do God's will involves patience, persistence, and surrender. If one is able to focus on God and not on cancer, guidance and direction will follow. When we pray, we are able to understand and receive grace that inspires the depths of our spirit to allow room for peace and healing. Prayer is to the soul what breathing is to the body.

If the only prayer you say in your whole life is "thank you," that would suffice.

Meister Eckhart

I have seen people dying of cancer, but only in the physical sense. In the greater, overall view of existence, however, they are living because their spirit and soul have emerged. I have helped a great number of people who have come to me for herbs and nutritional counseling in their last months, weeks, and even days. I have helped people leave their physical existence without debilitating pain medication, yet often without any pain at all, possessed of all their cognitive faculties, at home with their family members and most of all, in peace. I have gained a deeper sense of inner peace myself by being involved with so many of these people. I have stacks and stacks of letters written to me by people in their final days; these letters do not depress me, they inspire me. These people have shown me the face of God within their own spirits. They have given me insights into my spiritual life, a sense of my soul, who I am, and where I am going. What I have seen of God in others has brought me to a deeper understanding of God's spirit. Even the immense beauty of nature, which is so deep, wonderful, and dear to me and has so much to reveal and teach me, could not teach or touch me more profoundly than the contacts I have had with other human spirits.

A SPECIAL MESSAGE FOR HEALERS

Anyone who knows me knows that I am not a "preacher," nor do I try to convert anyone to my personal religious beliefs. I am merely trying to share God's love so others may have true joy and peace by learning to pray, thirst for love, and experience the healing power of compassion. This is important not just for those who are ill and seeking to be healed, but for those who are healers. This includes natural healers, such as herbalists, naturopathic physicians, massage therapists, and natural-food chefs, as well as conventional doctors, such as oncologists and surgeons. All healers need to be:

• *Compassionate.* People who are very ill with cancer are afraid and need to be loved and nurtured.

• *Humble.* Nobody has all the answers, particularly when it comes to cancer.

• *Open to a variety of healing modalities.* When people are striving together to bring about a healing of the sick, especially those with cancer, miracles can happen. I can't tell you how happy it makes a person who is following one of my protocols to report back to me that their oncologist has been supportive rather than critical of my approach to cancer.

Those who choose to work with the sick need to understand that this is not a profession but a vocation. The sick do not need pity and sympathy; they need love and compassion. When someone very sick enters my office, the first thing I do is pray in silence. This is private, between me and God, and not a process that anyone else is aware of. I feel, however, that it is crucial to what I do.

Modern medicine today has become a big business, an institution—and also, alas, a formula. The responsibility for healing is often in the hands of a faceless medical establishment, not accountable, caring human beings. Time after time I've had cancer patients tell me they're going to a famous hospital that specializes in treating cancer. Such a hospital may know the latest in treatments for a particular kind of cancer, but what can it offer or teach about healing? What wisdom does it have that can help a person heal?

In traditional healing practices, prayer and medical treatments were applied together to heal the sick. Today, we separate the two. Why the separation? Why can't we use prayer with herbal medicine, with nutrition, and with conventional treatments to heal the sick? Hopefully, this concept is beginning to gain more credibility, and we will see a change before long.

LISTEN TO YOUR HEART

After you have decided on a form of treatment and have incorporated prayer into your daily life, I urge you to try to make every effort to be positive and take charge of your life and your treatment in a proactive way. You may need the help of a therapist or a support group. Commit yourself to living long and well. Seek to understand who you are and why you are here. This will give you a sense of identity as well as peace of mind. Believe that you have a purpose in life and go about seeking that purpose with passion, allowing your heart to guide the way. Learn to forgive and allow room for laughter and joy in your day. Once you have a sense of purpose, let it be guided by your heart and your spirit and pursue it without fear or doubt. Most important, spend time in meditation and prayer, help others, build relationships, show compassion and humility, be a peace-maker, and offer love. Sharing your love is profoundly healing.

Remember that the mind, spirit, and body are inextricably interrelated. The mind affects the brain, and the brain affects all physiological systems of the body.

We are spiritual creatures. I believe that this life is but a beginning to another life, and death is a transformation into that life. I deeply believe that a good herbalist understands that the clinical practice of herbal medicine requires a balance between science and art. I myself try to maintain this balance in my practice. As I am thinking about which remedy or remedies I might suggest and blend for an individual, I look to my spirit for help and discernment. I also add faith into the mix when I explain my personal practice of herbal and nutritional medicine.

I end this chapter with a wonderful text written by St. John of Kronstadt, a Russian Orthodox priest and teacher who was beloved by the people of Russia for his unwavering faith and compassion for the human struggle to attain spirituality. He died in 1908 and was canonized as a saint in 1964. These words of wisdom are especially helpful for those who need healing.

> You are accustomed to look upon your body as upon your own inalienable property, but that is quite wrong, because your body is God's temple. Afflictions are a great teacher . . . [they] cleanse the soul. My brother, bear your illness bravely, and do not be despondent, but on the contrary, rejoice if you can in your illness . . . This sickness of yours may be the opportunity of a lifetime. Listen to God while you are on your back recuperating. Much good can come out of this experience that you might not gain in any other way. We know that for those who love God all things work together for good. Let there come to you out of this illness a blessing instead of a breakdown. Do not let this sickness get your spirit down. While lying on your bed, look up instead of down. Look into yourself and see how helpless you are without God.

Finally, whatever your choices, as this anonymous saying counsels: Do the best you can and don't worry about the rest. Angels do no more.

7

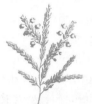

Lifestyle Guidelines

Nature, time, and patience are the three great
physicians.

—Chinese proverb

As the incidence of cancer continues to rise, researchers are pointing
to our environment as a major cause. The truth is, we are one with
our environment because the same life force that flows through our
bodies flows through all other creatures; sustains the planets in their orbits;
moves the oceans, rivers, and streams; and enriches the earth and all that
grows therein.

Just think about it for a moment, and you will understand why we are not
separate from the world around us. We are most clearly connected to the plant
world in a very physical way through the exchange of oxygen, but it goes even
deeper than that. The earth, animal life, and plant life codepend on each other
for existence. We are all part of a vital life force, a creation of God, and in this
perfect plan we are supplied with everything we need to sustain life.

Herbs and foods come from the soil and are just as much a part of creation as we are; thus their healing powers are connected to our life force. This mystery cannot be explained scientifically, but when healers work from this perspective, true healing can take place.

Living in harmony with the environment is a healing exercise, one that is both physical and spiritual. It encompasses all that we do for ourselves as well as all others who touch our lives; the foods we grow, prepare, and eat; the water we drink and bathe in; how we rest and sleep; the care, time, and companionship we give to others; the love we share; the spirituality we acknowledge and live by.

As you read these lifestyle guidelines, be aware of the deep healing connection that exists between us and our world. The guidelines themselves are quite simple and basic. Being mindful of them, eating wholesome organic food, using herbs as food and medicine, and living more simply will enhance your health and your life.

SUNLIGHT AND FRESH AIR

Get fresh air daily and sunshine whenever you can. However, don't expose yourself to direct sunlight for long, especially if you have fair skin. Be sure to get out of the sun if your skin begins to feel hot and starts to redden. Early morning or late afternoon is the best time to enjoy the sun because its rays are less intense. Sunlight provides many of us with countless benefits, not the least of which is its ability to elevate mood. It also helps to modify our endocrine system and is the best source of vitamin D, which has been shown to protect against many forms of cancer, particularly of the colon and breast.[1-3] Sunlight also has a protective benefit against ovarian cancer, according to one research study. A study of mortality rates from ovarian cancer in the one hundred largest counties in the United States between 1979 and 1988 showed that ovarian cancer deaths were inversely proportional to mean daily sunlight. This statistic remained constant after adjusting for variables, suggesting the protective effect of sunlight against ovarian cancer. Not surprisingly, the study also found a higher risk for developing ovarian cancer in northern latitudes, where there is less sunlight, as compared to southern latitudes.[4]

It's best to expose yourself to moderate amounts of sunlight regularly; if you wear glasses, remove them occasionally and, without looking directly at the sun, let the beneficial light pass through the optic nerve to the pineal gland, which regulates several endocrine functions, such as biological rhythm synchronization and the sleep/wake cycle. We now know that melatonin, an immunostimulatory neurohormone and powerful antioxidant, is secreted by the pineal gland.[5,6] Spend time going for walks in the woods or away from traffic, breathing in the fresh, clean air.

Melanoma and Sunscreens

There has been a steep rise in the rates of melanoma since the mid-1970s. Sun avoidance and the use of chemical sunscreens have been the major strategies for risk reduction, yet there has been a steady rise in the incidence of melanoma mortality. There is a good deal of research showing a correlation between skin cancer and the use of sunscreens.[7] Most sunscreens block ultraviolet-B (UVB) radiation but do not block ultraviolet-A (UVA) radiation, which is 90 to 95 percent of the solar spectrum. Sunscreens that block UVB radiation may not only be ineffective in preventing cancers; their use may actually increase the risk. This is because sunscreens protect the skin from redness and sunburn, so people stay out in the sun longer than they should. In fact, in countries that have encouraged the use of sunscreens in recent years (Australia, Britain, France, and Switzerland) there has been a sharp increase in the incidence and mortality from melanoma. Aside from prolonged exposure to ultraviolet radiation, sunscreens also create an imbalance in the skin's accommodation to sunlight, thereby interfering with the cutaneous synthesis of vitamin D_3.

For these reasons, I do not recommend using synthetic sunscreens. As stated in chapter 2, the only commercial sun protection product that I recommend is made by Aubrey (available in health food stores). This is a sunscreen that inhibits or reduces oxidative damage to the skin when exposed to sunlight. Rich in shea butter and African nut butter, which provide natural skin protection because of their high fatty acid content, Aubrey sunscreens are especially helpful for those who must spend lengthy periods of time in the sun.

Slightly more than half the cases of melanoma can be explained solely as sun-caused, but the conventional model does not explain the rest of them. I believe that the predominant theory suggesting that increased exposure to sunlight accounts for more incidences of melanoma is misleading and oversimplified. There is also consistent evidence of higher rates of melanoma among indoor workers and among those of higher socioeconomic status. Some studies are considering these factors as possible causes:

- The increase in consumption of transfatty acids from polyunsaturated oils[8,9]
- Environmental factors, including exposure to artificial light and electromagnetic radiation[10]
- Photosensitizing chemicals that are added to many processed foods
- Intake of a wide range of medical drugs
- Alcohol intake of more than two drinks daily[11]

The most protective nutritive factors against melanoma include carotenoids, lipoic acid, turmeric, green tea, a moderate intake of saturated fat, vitamin E, zinc, and a high intake of fish in the diet.

Full-Spectrum Lights

Too little sun may be more of a problem today than too much sun. Many people work in environments where work continues throughout the night under banks of fluorescent lights. Full-spectrum lights are now commercially available for people who do not get enough sun exposure. Their light spectrum is very close to actual sunlight and they help elevate mood. The light they produce is also less glaring and intense than fluorescent light and therefore is much kinder to the eyes. Another benefit of full-spectrum light is that it enhances the immune system by promoting a synergy between nutrients (such as St. John's wort) that possess photodynamic qualities. Exposure to natural light enhances the nutrients' functioning.

Gardening

A good way to bring the sun into daily life is by gardening, a major healing and stress-reducing activity. So many of my patients who garden have shared with me the wonderful healing effects it has had on them. The planting of flowers, vegetables, and herbs; watching them come alive and grow day by day; smelling their aromatic scents; and harvesting them when ready are all ways to truly bond with nature—the best healing tonic in the world.

EXERCISE

Exercise, from stretching, tai chi, yoga, walking, and running, to swimming and bicycling, can improve circulation and detoxification of the lymph system. It is also extremely beneficial emotionally; the endorphins it releases have a very uplifting effect. Exercise should be relaxing and not a burden—that's the real key to a successful program. Each individual must find the exercise program that is right for him or her. It is best to do a variety of exercises, both aerobic and anaerobic, that work all parts of the body in order to improve both endurance and strength. Many recent studies have shown the correlation of exercise with a reduced rate of cancer.[12,13]

Yoga and Tai Chi

Both yoga and tai chi, commonly practiced in the East, can help strengthen vitality. They not only balance the body but the emotions as well. Remember that the immune system cannot be healthy unless body, mind, and spirit are in harmony.

Yoga, which means union, is not just about stretching. Externally, it strengthens and tones the physical body; internally, it not only expands the spirit but, over time, can loosen and release any destructive emotional patterns that may impair well-being. During yoga, the nervous system is in a parasympathetic (relaxed) mode, while all other forms of exercise require a sympathetic (active) mode. It is therefore able to calm the mind and act as a kind of meditation-in-motion. Quieting the mind through yoga, meditation, or prayer is essential for health and healing. I highly recommend yoga as a daily practice.

PROPER SLEEP AND REST

One of the most important ways to heal cancer is by getting adequate sound sleep. During deep sleep all the detoxifying liver enzymes go to work. This is when the nervous system switches into its parasympathetic mode and the body changes its priorities—from creating energy and digesting food to rebuilding and detoxifying. The liver, which has a complex enzyme system, goes to work breaking down and excreting carcinogens and other waste materials. Without sufficient deep sleep, healing is impeded. Sleeping pills are not the solution.

There are many problems associated with sleeping pills, not the least of which is that over a period of time the body becomes resistant to them. They do not promote delta sleep, the deepest level of sleep from which true rest and healing are derived. What is more, they add stress to the liver for they must be metabolized and then excreted.

We average about one hour less sleep per night than people did just eighty years ago because we tend to go to bed later than people did before the advent of artificial light. This could be a major contributor to the increase in cancer, a factor that has not yet been seriously considered. We now know, for example, that many people with cancer, particularly breast and prostate, have lower levels of melatonin, a neurohormone secreted by the pineal gland, especially in response to darkness. Melatonin has been linked to the regulation of circadian rhythms, such as the wake/sleep cycle, as well as to many other important endocrine functions.

It is important to consider the possibility that you are not getting enough sleep; then consider which solutions are compatible with your lifestyle. One solution might be to go to bed earlier—when you feel tired. It's okay to miss the late news once in a while! Another helpful approach is to take a camping trip. When there are no light switches, life becomes simpler for a time. Become aware of the environment, the darkness, the moon, the stars—this is the natural environment that puts us in touch with our natural rhythms, not the environment where work shifts continue throughout the night in buildings flooded with fluorescent light.

There are many natural ways to enhance sleep:

• Melatonin and 5-hydroxy tryptophane (5HTP) both raise seratonin levels naturally, leading to restful sleep.

• Avoid eating protein before bed. Instead, eat complex carbohydrates, such as oatmeal or a banana, because they help to convert 5HTP to sleep-inducing seratonin.

• Aromatic baths and hot Epsom salt baths are very soothing and can help one to relax before going to bed. See chapter 8 for more information and directions.

• Massage, especially following a relaxing bath, will induce sleep, sometimes when all other therapies, including drugs, have failed.

• Herbs can be especially helpful. Some of the most effective are passionflower, kava kava, oatstraw, skullcap, and, for those with poor cerebral circulation, valerian. It is best to use a fluid extract of the herb, adding 30 to 120 drops (¼ to 1 teaspoon, depending on the herb used) to hot water or a soothing herb tea such as chamomile or lemon balm.

Sleep problems are unique to each individual, therefore, I recommend seeking the advice of a qualified herbalist. Many herbs help in specific ways: for example, pulsatilla is indicated for emotional upset. On the other hand, some herbs can have opposite effects on different people: Valerian can stimulate one person and calm another.

• Soothing sounds can help one fall asleep; again, this is unique to the individual. Environmental sounds such as wind or water are calming to some; others prefer soft music.

THINGS TO AVOID

Chemical Products

Many potential cancer-causing chemicals are in our homes: paints, harsh solvents; commercial deodorants; hair-coloring; the chemicals from air fresheners; oven, carpet, and other household cleaners; building materials; insect repellents; dry-cleaned clothes; deodorizers; and disinfectants.

In the 1930s, benzene was introduced as a cleaning agent. My grandfather, who was an Italian tailor, died from acute leukemia, which he contracted by working with this harmful chemical. Today, we are still at risk for exposure to high levels of benzene, which is found in many cleaning agents as well as in secondhand smoke and fumes from glues, gasoline, and some paints. In addition, carbon monoxide from gas stoves and furnaces is found in high levels inside our homes.

Avoid these chemicals as much as possible; try to protect yourself and the planet in every way you can. For example, don't use toxic pesticides on your lawn or garden. In the United States alone, approximately 886 million pounds of pesticides are used each year to produce food and crops. Four of the top ten heaviest pesticide-using crops are fruits and vegetables, with potatoes, peaches, grapes, citrus fruits, and tomatoes ranking near the top.[14] Become proactive about this poisoning of our food supply; write your congressmen about your concerns. Over a thousand new chemicals, many of them carcinogenic, are developed each year by powerful corporations. We must speak out about the unacceptably high levels of pesticides in our fruits and vegetables, about the lack of pure water and air. I believe that every voice makes a difference. We must go back to basic, simple living in harmony with nature before it is too late.

In the meantime, here are a few tips to make the home environment a safer place:

- Don't use electric blankets. They alter the electromagnetic polarization of the cell membrane; cancer cells are defined by a loss of cell-membrane polarization.

- Use ceramic or glass containers for storing or heating food, since polyvinyl chloride (PVC) plastics emit carcinogens. For this reason, it is important to keep plastic from touching your food, e.g., you can put food in a glass bowl and cover the bowl with plastic wrap, but leave space between the wrap and the food.

- For the same reason, reduce consumption of any foods packaged in plastic and heat-sealed containers.

- Also, never microwave food or drinks in plastic containers. In fact, it is best to avoid microwave cooking entirely.

- Choose pacifiers and children's teething toys that do not contain PVC. Buy toys that are PVC-free, such as those made from wood.[15]

8

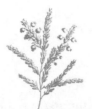

Other Important Modalities for Healing

Go, and wash seven times in the river Jordan, and
thy flesh shall recover health, and thou shall be clean.
                                                    —*Kings V, 10*

HYDROTHERAPY

Hydrotherapy is the therapeutic use of water both internally or externally in any of its three forms (solid, liquid, or vapor) to treat disease or trauma or simply to strengthen one's constitution.

Sebastian Kneipp was a German physician and priest who utilized hydrotherapy more than any other healer. In his book *My Water Cure*, he gives detailed information on the application of water for medicinal purposes. Some of his suggestions include walking barefoot in wet grass, on wet stones, in newly fallen snow, and in cold water; the use of steam baths, hot baths, cold baths, footbaths; wrapping the body with wet sheets; and the use of various compresses.

In 1891, Kneipp wrote, "A frequent disease of the present time is cancer. I have treated several cases of cancer in the early stages, also smaller advanced cancers. They are easily cured. All applications aim solely at purifying the blood." He goes on to discuss a successful treatment of advanced tongue cancer by the use of aloe water mouth rinses along with vapor steams.[1]

Epsom Salt Baths

A very important part of a good cancer-healing program includes an Epsom salt bath three to five times a week before bed. Epsom salt baths neutralize toxins by assisting the body's elimination through the skin, soothing tired nerves in the process. Eli Jones felt that no cancer therapy was complete without these baths.

Drinking diaphoretic teas, which induce the body to perspire—such as elder, yarrow, peppermint, boneset, or ginger—while taking an Epsom salt bath will help eliminate toxins through the skin and mucous membranes. Also, pyrogens (which raise the body's temperature) are released, which enhance resistance, activate the immune system, and stimulate phagocytosis, ridding the body of harmful bacteria. The hot Epsom salt bath also increases heart rate, respiratory rate, metabolism, and circulation.

Epsom salt baths are not recommended for people with low red blood-cell count.

The Aromatic Epsom Salt Bath

I often combine aromatherapy with the Epsom salt bath by adding essential oils to the bath. Lavender oil is my first choice, but tangerine and rosemary, particularly for morning baths, are also recommended. These baths are simple but profoundly healing. Lavender, tangerine, and rosemary all possess anticancer activity, and the Epsom salt bath can be a simple but effective way to employ these aromatic plants.

Directions: Soak in a tub of hot water (106 to 108 degrees Fahrenheit), with 2 cups of Epsom salts and 10 to 20 drops of lavender or other essential oil added, until your body temperature increases to about 101 degrees. Check pulse rate before starting and during treatment; it should be kept under 92 beats per minute. The bath should last from fifteen to twenty minutes.

Cool-Water Bathing

Cool-water bathing is a wonderful and powerful way to strengthen vitality. It is also the least expensive—all you need is access to some cool water and the ability to warm your body after the bath. Begin by dressing warmly (wear a few heavy shirts), and go for a vigorous walk until you are sweating. Then undress and briefly dunk yourself in cool, or cold, water (a river, lake, or your own bathtub). After spending just a few seconds in the cool water, immediately get out, put your clothes back on, and resume walking until you feel warm again.

This may sound a little eccentric, but once you try it and feel the enhanced vitality that this simple practice can produce, you'll be convinced of its value. The cool water bath is not for someone with advanced cancer or for the very weak. Before attempting this on your own, seek a professional in the field of hydrotherapy to see if you are a good candidate for cool-water bathing and also for proper guidelines.

HYPERTHERMIA

Hyperthermia uses heated water, such as hot tubs, hot fomentations, or hot footbaths. By applying heat (up to 109 degrees Fahrenheit), cancer cells begin to die, and the immune system becomes active to fight the cancer. The high temperature slows down the growth of malignant cells and their oxygen respiration. Some scientists believe that hyperthermia works because of a defect in the tumor's blood supply. Heat also makes cells more sensitive to radiation by preventing them from repairing radiation damage. In addition, it seems to enhance the effects of some chemotherapeutic drugs, such as cisplatin, cyclophosphamide, and malphalan.[2]

Hippocrates was the first to offer anecdotal evidence that cancer was susceptible to high temperatures. Centuries later, in 1856, a German physician reported that a patient in whom a fever was induced had been completely cured of a soft-tissue sarcoma. Recently, in the 1970s, it was shown that chemotherapy and radiation therapy, augmented with hyperthermia, controlled more tumors than either treatment when administered alone. Many clinical studies have proven that whole-body hyperthermia (WBH) enhances radiation and chemotherapy. WBH has been shown to induce elevated levels of granulocyte-colony stimulating factor, interleukin-1 beta, interleukin-6, interleukin-8, interleukin-10, and tumor necrosis factor-alpha within hours after administration.[3,4]

Results from nonrandomized Phase I and Phase II trials showed that the combination of hyperthermia and radiation produced a twofold increase in the response rate over standard radiation alone. A Phase III trial is currently under way.[5]

Multi-institutional clinical studies on hyperthermia of many deep-seated and highly resistant tumors of the lung, liver, pancreas, stomach, bladder, and rectum were undertaken using 8Mhz radio-frequency capacity heating devices at seven different institutions. A total of 177 people were used in the trial; 81 (46 percent) received hyperthemia with chemotherapy. Complete responses and partial responses were obtained in 80 percent of the cases with lung cancer, 39 percent with stomach cancer, 56 percent with liver cancer, 35 percent with pancreatic cancer, 71 percent with bladder cancer, 100 percent with primary rectal cancer, and 47 percent with recurrent rectal cancer.[6]

Compelling evidence exists that hyperthermia therapy as part of a multimodal treatment approach is a viable tool that should be used more often in cancer therapies, either systemically, which involves the whole body, or locally, just around the area of a tumor.[7] Hyperthermia can be carried out in saunas, steam rooms, or sweat lodges, but should always be supervised by a trained professional. It is important to drink copious amounts of fluid during hyperthermia treatments.

CASTOR OIL PACKS

Castor oil packs are used to augment detoxification, stimulate the immune system, and improve circulation to the area over which they are placed. Castor oil acts as a counterirritant that stimulates the tissues under the pack and attracts immune-enhancing cells to the area where it is applied, the liver being the most common. Castor oil packs are best applied on three consecutive days.

Materials needed:
- 4 to 6 ounces castor oil
- Wool flannel cloth (use cotton, if allergic)
- Plastic wrap
- Hot water bottle
- Bath towel

Directions: Fold two to four thicknesses of flannel to 12 by 14 inches to cover the abdomen. Dampen the cloth and soak it with castor oil so that it is wet, but not dripping. Heat in a low oven on a cookie sheet until the cloth is as hot as possible but not hot enough to burn your skin or to ignite while in the oven. Place a bath towel over the surface on which you will be lying. Place the pack over your abdomen and cover it with plastic. Bring the ends of the towel up and wrap it around your abdomen, placing a hot water bottle on top. The pack should remain in place a minimum of one hour.

ENEMAS

Enemas can be very useful therapeutically as a way to thoroughly cleanse the entire colon and stimulate the liver. They are most useful when there are tumors in the bile duct causing partial or total obstruction. This can lead to constipation, bile backup, and toxemia. Also, many pain medications and some chemotherapies cause bowel sluggishness or constipation. A simple coffee enema can alleviate this condition. It can also alleviate the pain caused by cancer, particularly when there are tumors in the lower abdomen or pelvic area.

Here are some general guidelines:

- Take an enema three mornings in a row followed by a rest for four days.
- Use 2 to 4 quarts of filtered or distilled water.
- Use a plain water enema, an herbal enema, an acidophilus enema, or a coffee enema. Consult an experienced health care practitioner for which type, if any, would be appropriate for your condition.

Herbal Enema

Make a tea using 2 heaping tablespoons of herbs to 1 quart of filtered/distilled water. A qualified herbalist will prescribe appropriate herbs for specific conditions (for example, bowel inflammation is helped by soothing herbs such as slippery elm and marshmallow root). When using roots and barks, be sure to simmer for at least twenty minutes. If using leaves or flowers, steep for ten minutes. After the tea is ready, strain and dilute with 1 to 3 quarts of plain water. Let cool to body temperature and then proceed to fill the enema bag.

Lie on a towel on your left side with your knees drawn up to your chest and place the bag at doorknob height. Gently insert the lubricated tip and slowly let the solution enter the bowel over the next five to fifteen minutes. Roll onto your back and massage the periphery of your abdomen counterclockwise, beginning in the left corner of the lower bowel.

Roll onto your right side and continue gently massaging. Sometimes the contents are expelled right away, and at other times it is important to retain the contents for five to fifteen minutes. Your health practitioner will give you the appropriate instructions.

Coffee Enema

Coffee enemas are a major part of the Gerson anticancer program. The actions of coffee enemas are multiple. The caffeine in the coffee is carried to the portal vein from the rectum, where it stimulates the liver, the major organ of detoxification. Since it is crucial that people with cancer avoid constipation, enemas, particularly coffee enemas, are a safe and effective way to have a bowel movement without the use of laxatives.

Directions: Prepare 1 pint of strong organic coffee, using 3 tablespoons of coffee per pint of water. Dilute with 1 to 2 quarts of filtered/distilled water. Fill the enema bag, gently insert the lubricated tube, and retain as much of the contents as you can for fifteen minutes, if possible.

MUSIC THERAPY

Since cells vibrate dynamically and may transmit information via harmonic wave motions, it is possible that certain types of music may possess healing properties.

A 1996 study reported in *Alternative Therapies in Clinical Practice* demonstrated the effect of different sounds on the growth of human cancer-cell lines *in vitro*. Five tumor-cell lines (lung, colon, brain, breast, and skin) all showed decreased growth when exposed to the primordial sounds of *sama veda* (traditional Indian) music as compared to increased growth when exposed to hard rock music.[8]

Music is also a wonderful tool to alleviate the anxiety and pain surrounding surgery and other medical procedures. Studies are beginning to appear showing the positive results of soothing music on the healing process.[9,10]

Although I do not currently use music therapy in my practice, if I were diagnosed with cancer, one of the first things I would turn to would be music—specifically jazz. There aren't too many things that would make me feel better than listening to Bill Evans, John Coltrane, or a group like Weather Report. Music is an important part of my life.

As both an herbalist and a bass player, I see a beautiful congruence between music and herbs. Each is unique to the moment—no two musical performances are ever exactly alike, and so it is with the world of herbs and their unique ability to heal when blended in accordance with the needs of the patient. Second to jazz, some type of spiritual music would be my choice—music for the soul. Spiritual music can help one center on prayer and has a profound effect on healing.

Combining soothing sounds with the uplifting smells of aromatherapy creates a wonderful synergistic effect. Imagine combining the morning sounds of birds chirping with the fragrance of your favorite flower essence—ylang-ylang, rose, lavender, or perhaps tangerine if you are suffering from nausea.

My vision for a natural healing center would offer not only the best botanical and nutritional medicine, acupuncture, massage, organically grown food, and hydrotherapy, but music and sound therapy, aromatherapy, and most of all, love and compassion.

MASSAGE

Massage therapists are among our most effective healers. Just touching a person can have a tremendous healing effect. As tense muscles begin to relax during a massage, a great deal of the emotional stress that caused the physical tightness in the first place can be released, at least temporarily. Cancer patients frequently feel isolated and alone; the healing touch of a massage therapist does more than soothe aching muscles, it provides much-needed emotional comfort as well. I consider massage an important part of any natural healing protocol.

ACUPUNCTURE AND QIGONG

Acupuncture and qigong are Chinese therapies used to enhance one's overall vitality and for treating all illnesses, including cancer. Both methods increase the flow of life energy, *chi*, and rebalance the body's energy channels or meridians. Acupuncture, by stimulating certain points on the body with extremely fine needles or massage, unblocks energy pathways and allows the *chi* to flow freely.

Acupuncture can also relieve pain. In China, it is often used during surgery, making it possible to reduce the amount of anesthesia needed or even eliminate it entirely.

Qigong also cultivates *chi*. Its movement techniques have been the foundation of Traditional Chinese Medicine for over five thousand years. There is nothing like it in Western medicine.

Research has shown that acupuncture and qigong have the ability to boost the immune system in cancer patients by increasing overall white blood-cell counts, B-cells, elevating natural killer-cell activity, and stimulating production of red blood cells.[11]

9

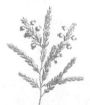

Current Mainstream
Cancer Therapies

As I did the green herb, I have given you all things.
—*Genesis 9:3*

S urgery, radiation, chemotherapy, hormone therapy, and immunotherapy
are the main tools used by doctors today at conventional cancer treatment centers. The kind of therapy used is selected on the basis of many
factors, such as the type and location of the cancer and its sensitivity to particular chemicals; whether or not the cancer is *in situ* (is localized, has not
invaded neighboring tissue, and has not metastasized); the aggressiveness of
the cancer; the considered treatment's cure, morbidity, and mortality rates;
and the age and general health of the patient.

The standard conventional medical treatments for cancer are aimed at
eliminating cancer cells. Progress is measured by the degree of selectivity a
treatment exhibits—how well it kills off malignant cells without destroying

too many healthy cells. Unfortunately, attacking cancer cells in this way also brings with it the risk of attacking the entire body. Because most conventional treatments damage healthy cells and tissues while they destroy cancerous cells, they can cause numerous unpleasant or life-disrupting side effects, the worst of which is the growth many years later of additional cancers.

Many of these side effects, however, can be successfully treated with proper nutritional intervention. Common problems that are responsive to herbs or nutrition include dry mouth, mouth sores, hemorrhaging, cachexia, nausea, diarrhea, bone marrow suppression, and pain. (See chapter 11.)

Can conventional cancer therapies work together with natural medicine? Not only can they work together, but when used appropriately, they actually complement one another and greatly enhance success by increasing cure rates and improving both longevity and quality of life.

The majority of the cancer patients I have worked with are also undergoing some form of conventional cancer treatment. Thus I can say with complete confidence based on my own observations that natural therapies, particularly herbal medicine, can not only greatly improve the effectiveness of conventional therapies while reducing the side effects but can affect the "spirit" of the disease, the underlying causes. The multiple causative factors of cancer development can be addressed by targeted natural medicine because, as described in chapters 4 and 5, nutrients and herbs can inhibit some of the cellular mutations that allowed the cancer to begin in the first place, as well as control many promotional agents involved in cancer growth. Therefore, once conventional therapy has ended, these natural remedies can greatly diminish recurrences. For example, the regenerative and liver-protective effects of a botanical formula that includes turmeric, schizandra, milk thistle, and artichoke leaf can help reduce the toxicity of conventional therapies while allowing the body its best chance of attaining a vital state when such therapies are completed.

SURGERY

Surgery is the oldest and still considered the most effective mainstream treatment choice for solid tumors. It is often curative for localized cancer (particularly small tumors) in which all or nearly all cancerous tissue can be removed. Radical surgery is performed and a tumor is removed along with the nearby lymph glands, tissues, and even organs when the surgeon has evidence that the cancer has spread locally or regionally. Sometimes surgery is used palliatively in advanced stages of cancer when a tumor may be interfering with a healthy organ. In other cases, surgery may be performed preventively to remove growths that are considered precancerous.

Advances in surgery include a move toward less radical operations for some cancers. For example, in early-stage breast cancer, a lumpectomy is now done more frequently than a mastectomy. Studies have shown that, at least in the case of early-stage breast cancer, the long-term survival rate is just as good.

Types of Cancer Surgery

Specific surgery removes the discrete visible tumor plus some of the adjacent normal-appearing tissue—to ensure removal of any cancer cells that might have made their way from the tumor and could cause recurrence.

Radical surgery removes the cancer, adjacent tissues, and also nearby organs or lymph nodes that might have been invaded by cancer cells.

Palliative surgery treats the complications of the cancer to help relieve pain or pressure and also to remove hormone-secreting glands, such as the ovaries or prostate.

Less common surgical techniques used to treat cancer include electrosurgery (which uses electric current), cryosurgery (which uses applications of liquid nitrogen), and laser surgery (which uses laser beams).

Herbal and nutritional protocols for maximizing the effectiveness of surgery are discussed in chapter 11.

RADIATION THERAPY

Radiation therapy, or radiotherapy, is a local treatment that uses high-energy rays to damage cancer cells and destroy their ability to grow and divide. It is administered either externally (by machine) or internally (either by implanting small containers of radioactive material near or directly into the cancer or by giving radioactive material orally or by injection). Radiotherapy is used in the following ways:

1. As an adjunct to surgery or chemotherapy in order to eliminate cancer cells that might remain in the area where the tumor once was.

2. To shrink tumors so they can be removed.

3. As a palliative treatment for advanced cancer to reduce the pain of bone metastases and to shrink tumors in particular parts of the body, such as the spinal cord, where tumors may be pressing on a sensitive area.

Radiation is commonly used as a standard form of adjunct therapy for cancers of the colon and rectum, one of the most common types of cancer in the United States, even though research suggests that it offers little or no survival advantage beyond the benefits of surgery, which is the primary treatment.[1]

Depending on the dose and the part of the body that is treated, radiation therapy has various side effects of different intensity that may or may not be permanent. They include skin reactions (dryness, itchiness, rashes, redness, darkening, irritation, blistering, cracking), hair loss, pneumonia and other respiratory infections, permanent hoarseness, cataracts, earaches, dry mouth, sore mouth and throat, difficulty swallowing, tooth problems, loss of appetite, nausea or vomiting, diarrhea or constipation, abdominal cramps, sterility, impotence or decreased sexual desire, cystitis, menopausal symptoms, fatigue or weakness, decrease in the number of white blood cells, nerve damage, and other tissue and organ damage.

In addition, the radiation absorbed by the body can cause cancer later in the patient's life because it induces free-radical damage and cell mutation and disturbs the functioning of solar photon energy electrons, which allow for normal cellular functions and reactions.

Radiation reacts with all of the body's cells but particularly with lipids, which in turn leads to an acceleration of oxidative processes, mutations, and perhaps the spread of cancer. Radiation therapy is also a known cause of second cancers, particularly leukemia.

Chapter 11 presents protocols that are helpful and offer protection for those undergoing radiation therapy.

CHEMOTHERAPY

Chemotherapy involves the administration of various chemical compounds and drugs for the treatment of cancer. It is used as a primary treatment for some cancers, including leukemias and lymphomas. It can also be used in addition to surgery for solid tumors that have advanced beyond their original location, both regionally and distantly.

Cancer cells that are fast-growing are most susceptible to chemotherapy, which kills them by various mechanisms that usually act at different stages of the mitotic (cell-division) cycle. The potent chemicals that chemotherapy uses to kill cancer cells are given by mouth or injected into a vein or muscle, beneath the skin, into an artery, into the spinal cord, or into the lung or abdominal cavities.

Alkaloids, which are natural compounds derived from plants, such as the periwinkle, are made into chemotherapeutic agents. Alkylating agents work differently, in that they bind nonspecifically to DNA and protein to inhibit cell growth. Some antibiotics from molds, such as actinomycin-D, are also used as chemotherapeutic drugs.

General guidelines for administering cancer chemotherapy recommend that the highest tolerated dose be used and that several drugs be used in combination. The use of high doses, the systemic administration, and the toxic properties of many anticancer drugs account for the often severe side effects of chemotherapy. Some cancers are resistant or become resistant to the effects of some of the drugs. The emergence of resistant clones and the regrowth of drug-resistant cancers is a particular problem during and after treatment.

Efforts to improve the effectiveness of chemotherapy include:

1. Developing ways to specifically target the tumor.

2. Linking cell-killing agents to monoclonal antibodies that are attracted to specific proteins on the surface of the cancer cells.

3. Further developing photodynamic therapy (PDT), which beams light into a tumor that has been injected with hematoporphyrin, a chemical that causes oxygen to become toxic to the cells it touches. The use of this localized cancer treatment is still quite limited. PDT capitalizes on the greater attraction of hematoporphyrin molecules to tumor tissue rather than to normal tissue.

Major Types of Chemotherapy

Alkylating Agents

These agents block reproduction of the chain of cancer cell DNA during cell division.

Examples: Carboplatin, cisplatin, cyclophosphamide, decarbazine, etoposide IV, etoposide oral, ifosfamide, lomustine, mitomycin, thiotepa.

Uses: Ovarian, breast, and lung cancers and some leukemias and lymphomas.

Antimetabolites

These drugs cause cancer cells to die by preventing the production of proteins and nucleic acids that are required by cancer cells to form DNA. They trick cancer cells into accepting them, leading to the formation of defective DNA, which breaks the normal growth cycle of cancer.

Examples: Fluorouracil, gemcitabine, hydroxyurea, methotrexate, docetaxel (Taxotere), and paclitaxel (taxol).

Uses: Leukemias and ovarian, breast, colon, and pancreatic cancers.

Tumoricidal Antibiotics

These antibiotics interfere with cancer-cell functioning and can inhibit DNA, RNA, or protein synthesis. Because they are so toxic, they are not normally used against bacterial infections like other antibiotics. They are derived from substances that occur in nature, such as fungi in the soil.

Examples: Doxorubicin (Adriamycin) and bleomycin.

Uses: Hodgkin's disease and cervical, testicular, breast, bladder, thyroid, and some other cancers.

Mitotic Inhibitors

These natural substances, derived from the periwinkle plant, stop cancer cells from dividing normally.

Examples: Vinblastine and vincristine.

Uses: Hodgkin's disease, choriocarcinoma, neuroblastoma, acute lymphocytic leukemia, and breast, lung, and testicular cancers.

Biological Modifiers

Another group of chemotherapeutic drugs modify the growth and reproduction of cancer cells.

Examples: Bacillus (BCG), interferon, interleukin-2, irinotecan (CPT-11), topotecan, and vinorelbine tartrate.

Uses: Kaposi's sarcoma, leukemias, melanoma, and bladder, kidney, colon, and ovarian cancers.

Protecting Agents

In addition, there are protecting agents that are used with other chemotherapeutic drugs to either enhance or minimize their side effects.

Examples: Leucovorin (folate) is used as an antidote to the anticancer drug methotrexate, and as a synergist with the drug fluorouracil.[2] Steroids are also used to diminish allergic reactions to chemotherapy, but sometimes their side effects can be as serious as those of the chemotherapy itself.

Side Effects of Chemotherapy

The powerful drugs used in chemotherapy destroy constantly dividing cancer cells, but unfortunately, they also affect healthy dividing cells, causing many side effects, such as nausea and vomiting; loss of appetite; weakness; mouth ulcers; fatigue; hair loss; menstrual changes; a weakened immune system, which lowers resistance to infections; anemia; heart problems; kidney and/or liver toxicity; and even more cancer. Although most of these side effects are temporary and will gradually go away once treatment is stopped, some of them can be permanent. For example, the drug Adriamycin can injure the heart. However, the appropriate nutritional supplements can be protective. The most effective nutritional supplements known to be protective against the harmful effects of Adriamycin (along with their divided daily doses) are:

- Vitamin E succinate, 400 IU
- Selenium, 200 mcg
- Vitamin C ascorbate, 1,000 to 2,000 mg
- Quercetin, 600 to 1,000 mg
- Bromelain, 500 to 1,000 mg
- CoQ10, 100 to 400 mg
- Lipoic acid, 100 to 600 mg
- N-acetyl cysteine, 1,000 to 2,000 mg
- PCOs or flavonoid-rich plant extracts such as hawthorn, 200 to 300 mg

These supplements should be taken with meals, except for quercetin, brome-lain, and vitamin C, which should be taken thirty minutes before meals.

The widespread use of chemotherapy with patients unlikely to benefit either because the negative side effects outweigh the expected benefits, or because specific benefits have not yet been demonstrated at all, has drawn criticism from respected researchers. The cancer research community needs to reexamine the value of long-accepted chemotherapy for certain types of cancer.

I have been working for many years with people who have cancer, and I've seen many circumstances where chemotherapy has done more harm than good—situations where no therapy at all may have given a longer life or certainly a higher quality of life. On the other hand, I have seen chemotherapy, used along with natural therapies, save lives. There are several questions doctors must consider before deciding whether chemotherapy should be used, and if so, what type. Some of these include:

1. *The overall health of the person.* This includes physical as well as mental health. Is the person's health strong enough to survive this therapy and are they emotionally healthy enough to go through it with a good attitude? Do they want to undergo chemotherapy? I often see elderly people with late-stage cancers who would prefer to be at home in comfortable surroundings rather than in a hospital setting where the treatments they receive will not add to the quality or length of their lives.

2. *How sensitive is the chemotherapy to this particular cancer-cell line?* Normally, the first cycle of chemotherapy will demonstrate some effectiveness if it is the correct agent. However, I have seen patients undergo four or five cycles of chemotherapy only to discover that there has been no success at all. It is important to realize that when chemotherapy is not working, it is doing harm by causing damage to healthy cells and vital organs, suppressing the immune system, and reducing the patient's vitality.

Herbal and nutritional therapies can make chemotherapy more sensitive to the particular cancer being treated. For example, bromelain and quercetin are especially compatible with most chemotherapies used in cases of breast, ovarian, and colon cancers, as well as leukemia and most melanomas, while reishi, coriolus, astragalus, and Siberian ginseng work well with all chemotherapies for all types of cancers.

Using herbal support produces a more effective attack upon the cancer, reduces the overall toxicity of the chemotherapy, and lowers the chance of eventual cancer-cell mutation. Cancer-cell mutation occurs when chemotherapy that was once effective is no longer working because the cancer-cell line has become immune to it. When this happens, and this is not an uncommon situation, the protocol needs to change.

HORMONE THERAPY

Hormone therapy has been somewhat successful in treating types of cancer that are hormone-dependent, notably breast cancer and prostate cancer. In these two types of cancer, sometimes the ovaries or the testicles are removed so that the hormones that were supporting the cancer will no longer be produced.

Androgens (male hormones) are sometimes given to patients to treat breast cancer, and estrogens, which are female hormones, such as DES-flutamide (Eulexin), are given to treat prostate cancer. Hormone-blocking drugs, such as tamoxifen, which is used to treat and prevent recurrence of breast cancer, are very often used. Because of the estrogenlike effects of tamoxifen, bone density increases and cholesterol is sometimes lowered in postmenopausal women who take this drug. Another drug, raloxifene, has recently been developed and has similar effects. However, it has a much broader application as preventive maintenance therapy for breast cancer as well as osteoporosis. Both tamoxifen and raloxifene work by binding to specific estrogen receptors on the surface of tumor cells where the hormones would normally bind, and they inhibit the cell from growing and reproducing. These drugs are generally taken following surgery and/or chemotherapy to prevent a local recurrence or metastasis of cancers that are hormone dependent.

Some of the possible side effects of hormone therapy are:

1. Nausea, vomiting, loss of fertility.
2. In women—deepening of the voice, increased sexual desire, increased growth of body hair, menopausal symptoms in premenopausal women, bleeding in postmenopausal women.
3. In men—raising of the voice, decreased sexual desire, impotence, enlarged breasts.

These changes are temporary for some and permanent for others. One of the major problems with the use of hormone therapies is that after a while the cancer can become not only resistant to the hormone antagonist, but it can actually become more aggressive and can feed on that drug. An estrogen-positive tumor, for example, may grow in response to estradiol and/or tamoxifen, and because of mutant receptor, the tamoxifen can actually stimulate rather than inhibit cancer.

For this reason, I would only endorse the use of tamoxifen and/or raloxifene for those female cancer patients who have chosen a conventional therapy course. I do not recommend using either of these drugs as preventive therapy, particularly in postmenopausal women.

IMMUNOTHERAPY

Immunotherapy, also called biological therapy or cell-transfer therapy, is relatively new in the field of conventional cancer treatments. Immunotherapy works through the use of certain drugs designed to artificially mimic specific immune system substances called biological response modifiers, such as interferon, interleukin-2, lymphokine-activated killer-cells, and monoclonal antibodies. Another approach is to give the patient pathogenic organisms that stimulate the immune system while simultaneously attacking tumor cells.

Vaccines are being developed to prevent and treat certain cancers. At this time, there is also research being done that focuses on cancer vaccines that are unique to each individual. This research is seeking ways to isolate each tumor's genetic codes so that cellular aberrations may be treated through the use of personalized vaccines that will call up and utilize each body's own immune arsenal.[3,4]

The following side effects of immunotherapy vary according to the different types of treatment and are generally temporary: loss of appetite, nausea, vomiting, diarrhea, chills, fever, muscle aches, weakness, rashes, bruising, immune suppression, and easy bleeding.

When alpha-interferon was first discovered it was thought to be a major breakthrough in treating both cancer and HIV disease. When the body produces its own interferon, it does so through a complex process involving communication and harmony. We have only just begun to understand that process, although for me it is just another example of the innate wisdom our bodies possess.

TUMOR MARKERS

It has long been known that malignant tumors are associated with abnormal production of proteins, enzymes, and circulating hormones, but only recently has it been found that some of these substances can act as tumor markers. A tumor marker is basically a substance that is synthesized by the tumor and released into the circulation of patients with cancer. It's important to know if a cancer is excreting specific tumor markers so that the patient and doctor can assess treatment options and values. Following are a few of the more common tumor markers (see table 9.1).

Table 9.1 **Some Tumor Markers and Their Clinical Use**

Marker	Type of Tumor Identified
Carcinoembryonic antigen (CEA)	Various carcinomas: colorectal, breast, thyroid, prostate cancer; the most commonly used tumor marker
CA-125	Nonmucinous ovarian carcinomas, various other carcinomas
CA19-9	Gastrointestinal and colorectal carcinomas
CA15-3	Metastatic breast cancer, ovarian cancer
Prostatic acid phosphatase (PAP)	Prostate carcinomas
Prostate-specific antigen (PSA)	Prostate carcinomas
Ovarian cancer antigen (OCA)	Ovarian carcinomas
Human chorionic gonadotropin (HCG)	Trophoblastic tumors, ovarian, breast, liver, lung carcinomas
Plasminogen activators (PA)	Prostate cancer
Alkaline phosphatase	Bone tumors and bone metastases
Ferritin	Liver tumors

(Continued)

Table 9.1 **Continued**

Marker	Type of Tumor Identified
Antimalignin antibody (AMA)	New test that can help with early detection
CA 27-29	A tumor marker similar to CA15-3 antigen, used primarily to help with detection of a recurrence of breast cancer
Fibroblastic growth factor (FGF)	A simple blood or urine test to detect early cancer activity; fibroblastic growth factor (FGF) is a protein that is released from some cells and stimulates new blood vessels, an action necessary to feed tumors; scientists have now detected elevated levels of FGF in the urine of cancer patients; in general, the more FGF released, the bigger the tumor's blood supply and the greater the risk of metastasis[5,6]

10

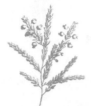

Making Decisions

I believe there is a subtle magnetism in nature, which, if we unconsciously yield to it, will direct us aright.
—*Henry David Thoreau*

CONVENTIONAL THERAPIES—PROS AND CONS

Should I use conventional therapies, like chemotherapy and radiation therapy? If so, what questions should I ask? If not, what should I do?

Odds are, one out of every three or four people will face a cancer diagnosis at some point. When that happens, the most likely medical protocol will be surgery, chemotherapy, and/or radiation therapy. These treatments are intended to help cure the disease, slow its progress, or to relieve pain or other symptoms. Decisions about whether or not to use these therapies and/or other conventional therapies can be fraught with fear and anxiety, not only for the patients themselves but for close family members and friends.

A multitude of choices will come from many directions. There may be a variety of health care providers involved—a surgeon or two, an oncologist, a radiologist, an internist, an OB-GYN or urologist, perhaps a nutritionist, and, in a few cases, maybe even an herbalist. Everyone will have an opinion. The surgeon will usually recommend surgery, sometimes invasive surgery, with the promise that the cancer will be removed along with an extra layer of tissue in order to get "clean margins." Next, the oncologist will step in with a recommendation of chemotherapy; this may be one chemo drug or a combination of drugs. And then, just to make sure the cancer is eliminated, local radiation therapy will probably also be suggested. After all this, breast cancer patients will likely be advised to undergo hormone or tamoxifen therapy. This complicated barrage of surgery, chemo, radiation, and perhaps hormone therapy is all directed against the return of one single cancer cell. How can you decide what's best for you? For openers, at least one other opinion is definitely advisable.

Although I believe that chemotherapy, radiation therapy, and surgery may be necessary in certain circumstances, I deeply believe that they are not the best choices all the time. The more experience I gain in working with people who have cancer, the more confidence I have that the natural approach I recommend can be successful in combination with the conventional medical approach or even all by itself in many cases. At this time, I am not ready to make this claim for every person with every type of cancer, but maybe some day I will be able to do that, too. I feel very confident using my approach alone for certain cancers—for example, prostate cancer, postmenopausal breast cancer, cervical cancer, and many low-grade lymphomas. With other aggressive cancers, such as pancreatic cancer, acute leukemias, and childhood brain tumors, the challenge remains difficult, but I continue to seek and find more effective ways to deal with these forms of cancer in natural ways. Many of the people I see do not come to me until all else has failed and it is hard to know what the outcome would have been had seen them when they were first diagnosed, before surgery and chemotherapy treatments. This is when cancer is what I call "virgin" cancer: It has not yet mutated or become resistant, which leads to "super" cancer. Cancer is easier to prevent than to cure.

Surgery will remove the primary tumor or the cancerous growth but not the causative factors; in many cases it can and will cause aggressive spreading of the cancerous growth. Radiation may inhibit a local recurrence, but neither surgery nor radiation addresses cancer as a systemic disease.

Surgery

Eli Jones, the famous Eclectic physician, stated, "I have never seen a cancerous tumor cut out by the knife that has not returned." Surgery can only "cure" the local tumor by removing it; it does not reduce the risk for the spread of cancer, and may even increase the chance of metastases.

Let's take a closer look at surgery. According to conventional wisdom, when a cancerous tumor is removed, the cancer is gone (or so we think). I tell breast cancer patients that it is not the breast they need to worry about but the liver, bones, brain, and the lungs; this is where the cancer is really life-threatening. So the question becomes: does having this operation inhibit or increase the chance of the cancer spreading to one of these sites? Sometimes, surgery may increase the chance, especially if the cancer has moved outside of the local area. Surgery causes trauma and inflammation, both of which weaken the patient. It also overtaxes the immune system's ability to fight the cancer, perhaps enabling the cancer to move at a more aggressive rate.

One problem that occurs frequently after surgery is that certain metastatic gene-inhibiting proteins diminish, thereby allowing aggressive cancer cells to invade and migrate. This can lead to the formation of life-threatening, organ-invading tumors at a much faster rate than if the primary tumor had not been removed. The nm (nonmetastatic) 23 gene is one such gene that has been identified.

I believe we need to look at this process and question the removal of all primary tumors as standard procedure if we are to maximize healing potential, inhibit recurrences, and prevent metastatic, life-threatening cancers. One possible solution is an aggressive cancer-inhibiting protocol to be used before and after surgery. This would help to prevent and/or reduce the risk of systemic cancer-cell activity. (See chapter 11.)

A recent report published in the *Lancet* questions the use, or misuse, of surgery. It states that surgery can kickstart cancer to spread and that cancer may work faster on injured tissue when the body's immune system is suppressed and in an inflammatory state. One breast cancer study showed an increase in damage, relapse, or death within three years after surgery.[1]

However, surgery alone can be the treatment of choice for certain early cancers of the cervix, breast, stomach, rectum, thyroid, colon, skin, and testis.

It can and does save lives in many cases. When conservative surgery alone is done, the survival rate is no less than surgery combined with radiation. Further, in some cases, such as certain cases of postmenopausal breast cancer, surgery without either chemotherapy or radiation is a valid option.

As I have stated earlier, I support each person's choice, whatever that might be. I will help, regardless of whether or not I agree with the treatments that have been chosen. Frankly, I myself do not always know for sure what is best.

Radiation

From what I have seen and from what I now know, I can say with confidence that prophylactic radiation therapy for many types of cancer not only spreads the cancer rather than eradicating it, but in some cases it actually causes cancer in healthy tissue. For instance, breast cancer patients may be at risk of developing lung cancer or leukemia after radiation. In one study of thirty-one patients who received radiation therapy for breast cancer, nineteen went on to develop lung cancer an average of seventeen years later (usually in the lung on the same side as the breast that had been irradiated).[2]

However, used correctly in certain types of cancer, and in certain circumstances, radiation therapy can be a useful tool. It can, for instance, be used to reduce the size of some tumors before an operation, to kill microscopic cancer cells following an operation, and, in advanced cancer, to reduce pain.

Radiation therapy can work in some cancers, although I personally question its effectiveness, and it is certainly no wonder-cure treatment. I offer patients undergoing radiation some adjunctive support, including herbs, nutritional supplements, and specific dietary suggestions, to diminish the systemic damage radiation does and to inhibit recurrence of the cancer and reduce the chance of developing a second type of cancer.

Radiation can help eradicate the following types of cancer:

- Cancers of the oral cavity, tongue, and lip
- Cancers of the larynx and nasal cavity
- Skin cancers and other melanomas
- Small-cell lung cancer
- Early Hodgkin's disease and some other early non-Hodgkin's forms of lymphoma

Types of cancers that are not generally responsive to radiation therapy include:

- Breast cancer
- Uterine cancer
- Lung cancers other than small-cell
- Bladder and prostate cancer
- Thyroid cancer
- Connective tissue sarcomas

Some of the most common short-term side effects of radiation therapy include:

- Fatigue
- Sunburnlike redness to the skin
- Hair loss in the treated area
- Damage to the salivary glands causing dry mouth and dry eyes, sometimes doing permanent damage
- Nausea and vomiting
- Diarrhea
- Scar tissue damage
- Bone marrow suppression and immune weakness
- Osteoporosis, following prolonged use

Chemotherapy

Toxic chemotherapy as well as other conventional therapies can compromise quality of life or even lead to life-threatening complications. I see this every day as I work with people who have cancer. Because I approach each cancer patient and the cancer itself as unique entities, it is difficult for me to generalize about treatment decisions. However, there are two general rules I can offer when making decisions about chemotherapy.

1. Generally, if you have an aggressive cancer that responds well to a particular cytotoxic drug, chemotherapy supported by a natural protocol to reduce side effects might be the best option. On the other hand, in the case of slow-growing cancers, natural therapies alone might be preferable.

2. Age is a factor to be considered. Older people tend to do better with natural therapies alone; chemotherapy seems to work better for younger cancer patients.

The faster the cancer cells grow, the more they tend to differ from normal cells; therefore, cytotoxic agents can recognize and destroy such cells more effectively. If the same cytotoxic agents are used to destroy slow-growing cells that are less differentiated, many healthy cells are destroyed in the process. The reason many people lose their hair during chemotherapy is because hair cells divide more rapidly than many other cells and therefore are more affected by cytotoxic agents.

Slow-growing cancer cells respond better to herbal and natural therapies because these therapies tend to induce the cancer cell to die through apoptosis (natural cell death) as opposed to necrosis (the explosive bomblike death produced by chemotherapy). Some natural agents that have been shown to induce apoptosis include quercetin, baicalein, genistein, catechins, and podophyllotoxin.

Some cancer-cell lines in which chemotherapy has been either curative or very helpful include Hodgkin's disease, childhood leukemias and other childhood cancers, testicular cancer, some lymphomas and, to a certain degree, ovarian cancer, nonsmall-cell lung cancer, and certain types of breast cancer.

When faced with a decision about whether or not to undergo chemotherapy or radiation, you should always get a second opinion. A new study has shown that second opinions frequently change treatment options for a significant number of patients.[3] It is essential to gather all the information available when faced with a radiation, chemotherapy, or other toxic therapy decision. Asking the right questions can help you understand goals and possible tradeoffs to the therapy, and that information can help you make a decision with confidence—which is valuable in and of itself. Some important questions to ask include:

- *What is the goal of the treatment?* If I undergo this treatment, am I taking a realistic shot at a cure, will it assure me a few extra years or months, or is this treatment simply to offer pain relief?
- *What is the success rate?* How effective has this treatment been for others with a similar condition who have undergone it in the past?
- *How is success measured?* Is it measured only by tumor shrinkage? Unfortunately, tumor shrinkage doesn't always correlate with significant

improvement in survival rate. If the treatment is not a cure but may extend your life, understand that it can also reduce the quality of your life.

• *What are the short-term and long-term side effects of this treatment?* Will I lose my hair? Can I still work? Will I lose weight? Many people who undergo certain chemotherapy protocols, particularly ones that include steroids, gain weight. Will I be able to have children in the future?

• *What can be done about the side effects?* Hopefully, after reading this book, you will have many answers to this question, but you should still ask your doctor.

• *Do you know anyone I can talk to who has undergone this treatment?* Many times physicians will be happy to put you in touch with someone who has undergone the therapy or therapies you are about to experience.

• *Is this the best place to be treated?* If you have a rare cancer or are thinking about an experimental therapy, you may want to go to a hospital that specializes in that therapy.

Always remember—this is *your* decision. No one person has all the definitive answers. A surgeon will most likely recommend surgery; a radiologist will recommend radiation treatments; and an oncologist will more often than not recommend chemotherapy. Many men with prostate cancer who consult me have been told that surgery is the only way to assure a cure. Anyone who is up-to-date on prostate cancer knows that removing the prostate gland does not guarantee anything other than the fact that the prostate gland is no longer there. I personally believe that this can increase one's chances of the cancer becoming invasive.

CONVENTIONAL THERAPIES AND NATURAL MEDICINE

Can conventional cancer therapies, including chemotherapy and radiation, work with natural medicine?

If we could come to a place of harmony and use the best of conventional medicine and the best of complementary medicine, I believe we could make an enormous difference in the lives of many people. I believe natural medicine, in particular herbal medicine, has the potential to cure most cancers, as well as many other diseases that plague our world today; still, I am willing to work with any other discipline or therapy that might be useful to someone who is ill. Most oncologists will agree that even chemotherapy has many limitations and they would welcome better options, particularly an intelligent holistic protocol that would complement their toxic therapies.

The protocols I recommend have been part of the cure for many people with cancer—patients who have used every existing conventional therapy. Many of these cures would not have occurred without my adjunctive protocols. Every day I learn more about what herb or supplement can enhance a particular therapy, reduce its toxic effects, and prolong its ability to be effective.

There are many questions that need to be answered before recommending the correct herbal or nutritional supplement.

- How does this supplement or herb interact with the type of chemotherapy being used?
- How much is needed and when should the supplements be started?
- Should administration of supplements occur during chemotherapy or should it wait until a few days or weeks after?

I am constantly finding more and more answers to these sometimes complicated questions, and hope this book can help the health care professional as well as the cancer patient.

I believe there is a general metabolic imbalance in at least 90 percent of all cancer patients. If this is true, how is it possible to completely eradicate cancer by simply removing the cancer through surgery, chemotherapy, and/or radiation? Do any of these therapies address the cause of the cancer in the first place? No, they do not. Does conventional medicine do anything at all to address the environment that has enabled the cancer to form in the first place? No, again. So what has been done to prevent a recurrence or to aid in a cure other than to destroy the visible tumor?

On the other hand, might surgery, chemotherapy, or radiation enable the cancer to become more aggressive and come back stronger? If an impairment in cellular health precedes cancer, then what happens to that impaired system after it has been through an operation, six months of chemotherapy, and one month of radiation therapy? I believe that the vitality of a person treated in this way must be several levels below what it was when the cancer first materialized, even if many or all of the cancer cells have been destroyed. Cancer, by itself, puts an enormous stress on the system and contributes to a loss of health and emotional well-being. Studies are beginning to appear that demonstrate how the stress of a cancer diagnosis negatively affects an individual's overall vitality.[4] If nothing is done to address this, the individual may be at high risk for cancer recurrence or even for developing a new type of cancer.

Everything we do affects our vitality index: the fried potato chips or piece of cake we eat; the lack of sunlight, clean water, and fresh air; mental stress, anger, and worry—all add up to a decline in vitality. Suppose a person becomes unable to sustain normal cellular health. This individual develops cancer and has a vitality index of only 5 on a scale of 1 to 10. If it is successful, conventional therapy may eliminate all traces of abnormal cells, but it is likely to bring the vitality index down still further. With vitality even more impaired than before treatment, this individual is now at risk for cancer to recur, perhaps even a metastatic life-threatening cancer that is resistant to the chemotherapy that worked before.

Wouldn't it be wonderful if there were a different scenario! What if, during and after the elimination of abnormal cells, the patient's vitality could be built up to 8 or 9. Cancer therapies would be more effective and health would be enhanced, giving the patient the greatest chance for a cure.

RESOURCES TO HELP MAKE THE NECESSARY CHOICES

The following resources can help you make the choices that are best for you regarding treatment for cancer.

Onotech

Onotech is a lab located in Irvine, California, that tests chemotherapeutic drugs for their efficacy in killing particular cancer cells (phone: 1-800-662-6832). Most physicians do not think its testing is reliable, but for those who are not sure which drug to use, it might be helpful. Test results are returned with a chart showing the various drugs and their sensitivity to your particular cancer. Although this test is controversial, I recommend using it to assist in the decision-making process.

BOOKS

An Alternative Medicine Definitive Guide to Cancer by John Diamond, M.D., and Lee Cowden, M.D. (Puyallup, Wash.: Future Medicine Publishing Co., 1997.)

Biology of Female Cancers by S. Langdon. (Boca Raton, Fla.: CRC Press, l997.)

Breast Cancer? Breast Health! The Wise Woman Way by Susun S. Weed. (Woodstock, N.Y.: Ash Tree Publishing, 1996.)

Cancer: Prevention, Detection, Causes, Treatment by Clifford T. Stewart. (Wallingford, Penn.: Hampton Court Press, 1988.)

Cancer & Natural Medicine by John Boik. (Princeton, Minn.: Oregon Medical Press, 1995.)

The Cancer Reference Book by Paul M. Levitt and Elissa S. Guralnick. (New York: Facts on File, Inc., 1983.)

Choices: Realistic Alternatives in Cancer Treatment by Marion Morra and Eve Potts. (New York: Avon Books, 1987.)

Herbs Against Cancer by Ralph W. Moss, Ph.D. (Brooklyn, N.Y.: Equinox Press, 1998.)

Making the Chemotherapy Decision by David Drum. (Los Angeles: Lowell House, 1996.)

My Healing from Breast Cancer by Barbara Joseph. (Los Angeles: Keats Publishing, 1997.)

Nutrition and Women's Cancers by Barbara C. Pence and Dale M. Dunn. (Boca Raton, Fla.: CRC Press, 1998.)

Prostate Cancer: A Survivor's Guide by Don Kaltenbach. (New Port Richey, Fla.: Seneca House Press, 1995.)

Questioning Chemotherapy by Ralph W. Moss, Ph.D. (Brooklyn, N.Y.: Equinox Press, 1995.)

Total Breast Health by Robin Keuneke. (New York: Kensington Books, 1998.)

Understanding Cancer by John Laszlo, M.D. (New York: Harper & Row, 1987.)

What You Really Need to Know About Cancer by Dr. Robert Buckman. (Toronto: Key Porter Books, 1996.)

11

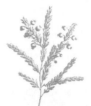

Natural Ways to Relieve Common Side Effects of Cancer and Cancer Therapies

And the fruit thereof shall be for meat, and the leaf thereof for medicine.

—*Ezekiel 47:12*

There are many serious and debilitating side effects of cancer and conventional cancer therapies, including body wasting, loss of appetite, loss of the sense of taste, nausea, diarrhea, constipation, dry mouth, mouth sores, pain, neuropathy, hemorrhaging, and anemia. Herbal protocols and nutritional supplements can offer relief from these conditions and provide the body and its immune system with much-needed support while undergoing conventional therapies. This chapter provides many herbal and holistic strategies that can be used to great advantage by cancer patients. Remember that in herbal medicine, each individual's protocol is unique; therefore, these remedies are offered as broad guidelines with general and conservative doses. Seek the advice of a qualified health professional for specific protocols. Unfamiliar supplements (those not available in most health food stores) are listed in the Resources.

LOSS OF APPETITE, WEIGHT LOSS, BODY WASTING

Weight loss is one of the most important factors in dealing with cancer and the effects of conventional cancer therapies. It is caused by altered metabolism due to cytokine activity (an increased level of tumor necrosis factor), malabsorption (which always involves diarrhea), and reduction of energy intake. One of the major causes of reduced energy intake is loss of appetite. Pancreatic cancer, in particular, is characterized by progressive weight loss and nutritional deterioration. A recent study has shown that increasing calorie intake can prolong survival for patients with advanced pancreatic cancer.[1] For recipes utilizing many of the nutrients listed in this section, see the section on nutritional smoothies in chapter 14.

• Essential fatty acids, in particular, omega-3 fatty acids, such as fish oils and flaxseed oil, have been shown to prevent body wasting (cachexia) in both animal and human studies. Medium-chain triglycerides (derived from coconut oil), another form of fatty acid, are very helpful for those who are suffering from malabsorption.

Dose: 1 to 4 tablespoons daily.

• Low-temperature whey protein will decrease diarrhea, improve amino acid uptake, slow catabolic breakdown, promote muscle growth, enhance glutathione, and aid in the growth of healthy intestinal flora.

Dose: 1 to 4 tablespoons daily, blended with juice or yogurt.

• Digestive herbal bitters, such as boldo, gentian, goldenseal, collinsonia, quassia, dandelion, wormwood, boneset, kola, and alfalfa, can be taken in extract form mixed with water or tea prior to eating. Herbs such as these with bitter properties can aid in the stimulation of various digestive enzymes.

Dose: 10 to 60 drops before each meal (depending on the specific herbs used and the individual's constitution). Seek professional guidance for specific herbal compounds.

• Nux vomica extract is especially suited for people who are very weak and have low vitality and a poor appetite. This extract can only be obtained through a doctor. It is an excellent way to build up the nervous and digestive systems and restore vitality.

Dose: 1 to 5 drops diluted in water and taken before meals. An herbalist might also mix nux vomica extract with other appropriate herbs into a compound.

• Digestive enzymes, such as papin-rich papaya (I use Biogestin [see Resources]), hydrochloric acid (critical for digesting meat protein and mineral absorption), lipase (to aid in fat absorption), pancreatin, and plant enzymes, should be taken just before eating or in one of the nutritional smoothies (see chapter 14) to increase the absorption of many nutrients and reduce diarrhea.

Dose: Papaya or full-spectrum plant enzymes—2 to 4 tablets before eating; hydrochloric acid—1 to 4 tablets before eating. Although I recommend the use of these enzymes in some cases, it is better, when possible, to use herbal bitters to stimulate the body's production of hydrochloric acid.

• Hydrazine sulfate cuts off a tumor's supply of new glucose, which stops the preferential depletion of the body's energy pool. It also increases caloric intake and weight gain, which puts an end to cachexia.

Dose: Generally, 1 to 3 tablets (50 to 100 mg each) between meals. Should be taken only under professional supervision.

• L-glutamine U.S.P., which has been shown to prevent muscle wasting, is best taken between meals, under the tongue.

Dose: 2 to 6 teaspoons of powder, blended with water. It can also be blended into a shake.

• Coconut milk can be very helpful for weight gain. Fresh is best, but you can buy the canned variety in most health food stores. It helps with intestinal absorption of food, is rich in lauric acid and medium-chain triglycerides, and is an excellent antimicrobial fatty acid. Many cancer patients suffering from malabsorption are at great risk for infection, and coconut helps to resist numerous bacterial assaults.

Dose: Use coconut milk in shakes and take with meals, or use coconut meat shredded, as a garnish, on food.

• Deer antler extract. Improves appetite and sleep, decreases muscular fatigue, promotes lymphocyte transformation, and increases white blood count. In China, antler extract is clinically used for anemia, platelet disorders, lassitude, malnutrition, and protein metabolic disorders.

Dose: 10 to 30 drops diluted in water or tea and taken before meals.

DIARRHEA

As a result of radiation therapy, chemotherapy, and the regular use of antibiotics (which are often given to cancer patients with suppressed immune systems to inhibit bacterial infections), bowel health is seriously disrupted and very often can lead to chronic diarrhea and malabsorption. A few supplements can really help. The first thing to do is to normalize the gut flora. I recommend the following three supplements:

1. *Saccharomyces boulardii (SB)* is a nonpathogenic yeast originally isolated from the surface of lichee nuts. It has recently been getting attention as a treatment for AIDS-related diarrhea. In my experience, I have found this to be one of the best supplements available not only for AIDS-related diarrhea, but for all drug-induced gastric conditions, particularly diarrhea caused by antibiotics that disrupt the gut's flora. SB is very effective against yeast infections as well as bacterial infections. Because it enhances the immunological system of the gut's barrier function, SB is widely used in Western Europe to prevent diarrhea and other gastrointestinal diseases associated with antibiotic use. Unlike other probiotic supplements, such as lactobacillus, SB works in a full pH range; it resists gastric acid and is not killed off by antibiotics.

Dose: 2 to 3 capsules three to four times daily.

2. *Whey protein.* The benefits of low-temperature whey protein, as discussed in the previous section include its ability to promote muscle growth, inhibit wasting syndrome, enhance glutathione, and enhance many immune-modulating functions.

Dose: 1 to 4 tablespoons daily, mixed into juice or yogurt. I recommend Probioplex (see Resources).

3. *Lactobacillus acidophilus* and other live, active cultures help to restore healthy bacteria.

Dose: 2 to 3 capsules of PB8 acidophilus daily (see Resources).

Other Helpful Supplements

• Berberine-containing plants, such as goldenseal, are not only excellent for their antidiarrheal activity, but they also inhibit many bacterial, viral, and fungal pathogens.

Dose: 2 to 3 capsules three to four times daily.

• Tanabit is a tannin-rich plant-extract product that has remarkable antidiarrheal, antifungal, and cancer-inhibiting properties.

Dose: 2 to 4 capsules three times daily.

• Bentonite clay water. Bentonite is a volcanic clay that is very useful in absorbing toxins and stopping diarrhea. It acts like a sponge, picking up toxins in the gut. In a fluid medium, it has been shown to absorb the toxins of cholera, typhoid, dysentery, and proteolytic bacteria.[2] Be careful, however, not to use too much because over a considerable period of time its strong absorptive powers could render vitamin A and other necessary nutrients unavailable by absorbing them from the alimentary canal. Studies have shown no ill effects when the intake of bentonite did not exceed 25 percent of the total diet.[3]

Dose: ½ to 2 teaspoons added to water or a water/juice mix; stir and let stand for a while or overnight, and drink once a day until diarrhea stops. Sometimes it is helpful to add some mucilaginous bulking agent to the mixture, such as freshly ground flaxseeds, just before drinking.

• Citrucidal (grapefruit seed extract) is an excellent antibacterial, antifungal, and antiviral nutrient that offers protection against a wide range of organisms. It is especially helpful for diarrhea that is caused by infection.

Dose: Liquid extract—10 drops in water three to four times daily. Tablets (100 mg each)—1 to 2 tablets three to four times daily.

• Belladonna is particularly helpful in cases of diarrhea that are accompanied by spasms and cramping.

Dose: 5 to 10 drops, used only under the care of a qualified health care professional.

Recipes for Treating Diarrhea

Herbal Extracts

Herbal extracts that help resolve diarrhea include wild geranium, collinsonia, atractylodes, uno de gato, red root, sundew, hawthorn, blueberry leaf, and panax ginseng. Belladonna, as mentioned above, is particularly helpful in cases of diarrhea accompanied by spasms and cramping but should only be used under the care of a qualified health care professional. An example of an herbal formula for this condition follows.

Antidiarrhea Herbal Formula

Wild geranium	40 ml	Blueberry leaf	10 ml
Sundew	15 ml	Atractylodes	10 ml
Collinsonia	15 ml	Cinnamon	2 ml
Red root	15 ml	Ginger	3 ml
Bayberry	10 ml		

Dose: 30 to 60 drops four to six times daily, taken in cold water or blackberry or red currant juice. Note: If you cannot find all these herbs, use wild geranium alone, 40 to 60 drops four to six times daily.

Antidiarrhea Drink

4	ounces water	1 teaspoon bentonite clay
2 to 4	ounces juice (use an astringent fruit, such as black currant)	1 tablespoon Probioplex

Optional: 1 tablespoon freshly ground flaxseed powder and 1 to 2 teaspoons slippery elm powder, added right before drinking. Put all ingredients in a blender or shaker jar and blend well.

Antidiarrhea Tea

1 papaya leaf	1 slippery elm or marshmallow root
1 uno de gato (cat's claw)	Pinch of peppermint and/or cinnamon
1 white oak bark	

Add 1 level tablespoon of this mixture to a pint of water. Let herbs sit overnight in water. Bring to a boil the next morning; turn heat to low and simmer fifteen to twenty minutes. Strain and drink during the day.

Revitalizing Broth

Take five or six non-gas-forming vegetables, such as carrots, celery, squash, parsley, beets, potatoes, or parsnips, and cut into small pieces. Cook in 1 to 2 pints of water until soft. Cool. Put in blender and liquefy. This will break down the fiber in the vegetables and make them easier to digest. Return to pot and simmer. Add 1 to 2 teaspoons of granulated seaweed.

Add to 1 cup cooked barley or basmati rice. Drink throughout the day. This broth nourishes the very sick and it is easy to assimilate.

If these remedies and recipes don't work, ask your doctor to prescribe tincture of opium. Start with a very low dose and slowly increase until the desired effects are reached.

YEAST INFECTIONS

Vaginal, intestinal, or throat (thrush) yeast infections commonly occur while people are undergoing chemotherapy and radiation therapy because antibiotics destroy most of the good bacterial flora that resist infections. Many of the supplements recommended for diarrhea, such as SB, lactobacillus acidophilus, tanabit, and berberine-containing plants, such as goldenseal or bayberry, are also excellent treatments for yeast infections. Specific herbs to consider for fungal infections include usnea, spylanthes, and propolis.

Dose: 10 to 30 drops three to six times daily (use a single herb or a combination of all three).

Vaginal Infections

For vaginal infections, there are a number of herbal suppositories sold in health food stores. I often recommend Earth's Harvest products (see Resources) because they offer a variety of suppositories for this condition, including those that contain essential oils, goldenseal, and soothing and astringent plant extract. Boric acid suppositories also work well for some.

CONSTIPATION

Just imagine the increased load of toxins the body confronts when dealing with cancer and conventional cancer therapies. The importance of elimination in the healing process is obvious. And yet, constipation is a common problem with cancer patients. Many pain medications and some chemotherapies cause sluggishness and constipation. The entire digestive system, the key to restoring vitality, suffers. Diet can play a major role in restoring proper bowel function.

First of all, be sure to drink plenty of fluids (hot fluids or herbal teas are best) and eat high-fiber foods such as fruits, vegetables, and whole grains. Avoid cheese and refined carbohydrates, such as white rice, flour, and sugar. Also include soaked dried fruit, ground flaxseeds, and flaxseed oil in your diet. Do not take laxatives. Helpful nutritional supplements include:

• Magnesium, nature's natural laxative, or trace-mineral tablets rich in magnesium.

Dose: Magnesium—200 to 1,000 mg daily in divided doses. Trace mineral tablets—2 to 6 tablets daily in divided doses.

• Liver-detoxifying formula containing choline, inositol, and taurine, along with herbs such as dandelion and fringe tree. Stronger herbs, such as cascara sagrada and/or mayapple, can be used along with soothing herbs such as marshmallow or slippery elm bark, and with a stimulating herb like ginger or prickly ash bark. This type of combination can be very helpful. Formulas such as these can be compounded by an herbalist and are usually taken in the form of teas throughout the day.

Enemas

Enemas are useful to cleanse the colon and stimulate the liver. Herbal, acidophilus, or coffee enemas are all helpful for constipation. Coffee enemas, in particular, are a safe and effective way to avoid the use of laxatives. See chapter 8 for formulas and instructions for taking enemas.

It is important to remember that when treating cancer, both diarrhea and constipation should be treated immediately.

NAUSEA AND VOMITING

Although there is a drug called Zofran (ondansetron HCL) that works very well in combating the nausea from chemotherapy, I am not convinced that this is beneficial. Chemotherapy is very toxic to both cancerous and noncancerous or healthy cells. When so much destruction is going on inside the body, nausea occurs as a way for the body to rid itself of the dead cells killed off by chemo. Perhaps trying to live with some nausea might be better in the long run. I do think it is useful to be able to minimize severe nausea but not to eliminate it totally. I recommend eating frequent, small meals of nutritious, organic food throughout the day. During this time, the last thing one should do is to eat heavy meals, which will only create more stress on the detoxifying systems of the body.

Citrus, in the form of oranges or tangerines, can be very helpful in combating chemotherapy-induced nausea. In addition to peeling an orange and eating it, you can also add the essential oil of orange or tangerine to a diffuser and let the aroma of the essential oil fill your room.

Real, 100 percent ginger ale, such as Premium Blend Ginger Brew, works well for nausea as do certain herbal teas, such as peppermint, alfalfa, slippery elm, fennel, chamomile, and ginger. At the same time, they also aid digestion.

PAIN

All of the following herbal and nutritional remedies offer pain relief and are far better for the body than morphine. Frequently prescribed for cancer pain, morphine actually causes constipation, depletes the vital force, and reduces body temperature and circulation. It is best for the patient if pain can be relieved without the use of morphine.

SPES is a Chinese herbal preparation that is the most effective natural treatment for controlling pain associated with cancer. It is effective, quick-acting, without side effects, and can inhibit cancer growth and metastasis. I know of no other product that equals this one for cancer pain. See chapter 5 for more information on SPES. (Also see Resources.)

• Vitamin K_1 (nontoxic form) has demonstrated an analgesic effect nearly as effective as that of morphine in patients with inoperable carcinomas. Vitamin K_1 has also shown antitumor action.

Dose: 5 to 10 drops two to four times daily.

• Butterbur has shown both cytostatic action and marked analgesic properties in patients with tumors.

Dose: 10 to 30 drops three to six times daily.

• Belladonna is not sold over the counter. Consult a health care practitioner for use.

General dose: 5 drops three to four times daily. If dry mouth develops, take less.

• Corydalis is one of the best plants to use for the pain associated with cancer, particularly abdominal pain. Corydalis is one of the primary ingredients in the Chinese herbal pain formula, SPES.

Dose: 30 to 60 drops three to four times daily.

• Kava kava, the popular herb used for anxiety, stress, and insomia, is also a very effective pain reliever and muscle relaxant. A powdered extract with about 30 percent kavalactones or a good fluid extract are the best forms to use. I have found the fluid extract to be more effective overall than the standardized herbal preparations on the market. The extract has another advantage in that it can be combined with other pain-relieving herbs or herbal sedatives, such as passionflower and valerian, to help induce a restful sleep.

Dose: 30 to 60 drops in hot water or a tea made of chamomile and lemon balm, twenty to thirty minutes before bed.

• Lapacho is an analgesic that also possesses antibacterial, antiparasitic, and antifungal properties. It is completely safe as a whole herb and is usually taken as a tea, using 1 teaspoon per cup. Up to 1 quart can be taken daily.

• Meadowsweet and white willow contain natural aspirinlike compounds that will relieve pain and inflammation without any side effects. Meadowsweet is particularly helpful for gastric pain.

White willow dose: 2 to 4 capsules of extract, three to four times daily (Willowprin by Nature's Herbs).

Meadowsweet dose: 30 to 60 drops three to four times daily.

• Echinacea, a popular herb used for boosting immunity, is also very effective in advanced cases of cancer for its help in relieving pain. As long ago as the late 1800s, Eli Jones wrote about echinacea's pain-relieving qualities in his book on cancer.

Dose: 60 to 120 drops (½ to 1 teaspoon) of extract three to six times daily.

• Condurango, a South American herb, has repeatedly been found to be beneficial in cancer treatment. It increases the appetite, reduces pain, and restores weight.

Dose: 20 to 60 drops three to six times daily.

• Cannabis, popularly known as marijuana, alleviates nausea and vomiting caused by chemotherapy, is a great appetite stimulant, and is an effective pain reliever. It has also been found to have anticancer effects. As reported in the *Journal of the National Cancer Institute* in 1975, A.E. Munson and his colleagues found that cannabis retarded the growth of lung cancer. Marijuana is certainly safer than morphine, which is often the drug of choice for people with late-stage cancer. It is very sad to watch a patient struggle to die after having been pumped up on morphine. Fortunately, many states are now passing laws that allow legal access to this medicinal plant for those who need it.

• Coffee enemas, among other benefits, can relieve pain, particularly when there are bowel or bile duct obstructions and/or constipation that must be corrected before healing can begin. See chapter 8 for more information and instructions.

• Lipoic acid reduces the production of lactic and peruvic acids that are generated by cancer cells, thereby causing severe muscular pain.

Dose: 300 to 600 mg daily in divided doses, taken with meals.

NEUROPATHY

Neuropathy is nerve damage that has occurred causing pain and numbness, particularly in the extremities. See table 11.1 for nutritional supplements that can inhibit and/or treat chemotherapy-induced neuropathy.

Table 11.1 **Nutritional Supplements for Chemotherapy**

Nutritional Supplement	Daily Dose
Lipoic acid	200–600 mg
Fat-soluble vitamin B_1	50–200 mg
Coenzyme B_6	50–200 mg
Liquid vitamin B_{12} and folic acid (Hydroxy Folate)	2–4 mg each taken under the tongue
Vitamin B complex or multivitamin with each B vitamin	20–50 mg
PCO phytosome (grape seed or pycnogenol)	200–400 mg
Hypericum (St. John's wort)	3–6 capsules daily (use 0.3 hypericum standardized 300 mg capsules); or use 30–60 drops of extract 3 times daily

DRY MOUTH

The radiation therapy used to treat throat cancer inhibits salivary secretions. Sometimes the effects are short-term, but at other times the damage may become permanent. The herbal extract of pilocarpine jaborandi and/or prickly ash may ease this condition. Pure oral pilocarpine is now used by conventional medical doctors as a treatment to reduce dry mouth (xerostomia) caused by radiation to the neck and head.

Dose: Pilocarpine—2 to 3 drops three to six times daily. Prickly ash—10 to 20 drops in 1 ounce of water three to six times daily.

Evening primrose oil or other GLA-rich oils can also be effective in treating this condition.

It is also helpful to drink several cups of slippery elm tea throughout the day and to take 4 to 6 ounces of aloe vera leaf juice.

The following is a formula I often recommend for this condition:

Dry Mouth Formula

Pilocarpine jaborandi	20 ml	Kava kava	15 ml
Prickly ash	15 ml	Aloe leaf extract	50 ml
Echinacea	15 ml	Herbaswee	5 ml

(5 ml is equal to 1 teaspoon. These quantities will produce ½ cup of formula.)

Dose: Place 30 to 40 drops (1 dropperful) directly in the mouth three to six times daily before meals.

MOUTH SORES

Mouth sores are often caused by chemotherapy or radiation and can be very painful. Because of the severe discomfort they cause, eating can be difficult. There are a number of natural remedies that can be used to inhibit or treat this condition. One remedy I frequently recommend is a tincture of 50 percent propolis applied directly to sores several times daily. Other herbal extracts that are very effective include collinsonia, chamomile, licorice, echinacea, poke, and thuja.

Mouth Sore Formula

Aloe leaf concentrate	30 ml	Collinsonia	10 ml
Glycerin or Throat	30 ml	Echinacea	10 ml
Care (by Nutritional		Chamomile	5 ml
Therapeutics)		Thuja	5 ml
Licorice	15 ml	Essential oil of clove	5–10 drops
Propolis	15 ml		

Dose: Use 60 drops of this formula (about ½ teaspoon) per tablespoon or two of warm saltwater and rinse mouth every two hours, while awake.

Tooth and Gum Tonic (see Resources) is an herbal mouth rinse that is also effective at inhibiting mouth sores. You will not find this product in any health food store or pharmacy, but it can be ordered by a dentist or health care professional.

Other suggestions for relieving mouth sores:

• Rinse mouth with a decoction of white oak bark, sage, licorice, and slippery elm; use four to six times daily.

• Take acidophilus tablets internally and also rinse mouth with ½ to 1 teaspoon of acidophilus in 1 ounce of warm water before bed.

• DGL, a licorice-derived powder, is available in tablet form. Dissolve 2 tablets in mouth four to five times daily.

• L-glutamine powder. Take 2 to 3 teaspoons daily, directly in the mouth. Wash down with water.

If these natural remedies don't solve the problem, ask your doctor to prescribe an allopurinol mouth rinse.

HEMORRHAGING

There are many herbs that can relieve hemorrhaging caused by cancer without any risk of side effects. Some of the most common herbs include wild geranium, red root, thuja, goldenseal, yarrow, shepherd's purse, and cinnamon. A sample formula that an herbal practitioner might compound for this condition would include:

Wild geranium	110 ml	Goldenseal	10 ml
Red root	40 ml	Cinnamon	10 ml
Yarrow	30 ml	Cotton root	10 ml
Shepherd's purse	30 ml		

Dose: ½ to 1 teaspoon three to six times daily.

Supplements that help this condition include vitamin K_1 (5 to 10 drops three times daily) because of its blood-clotting properties and fat-soluble chlorophyll (2 to 3 capsules, three times daily). Chlorophyll, the substance that gives plants their green color, has the same molecular structure as hemoglobin.

LOW PLATELETS

Low platelet count (thrombocytopenia) is a problem facing most cancer patients and can be worsened by some chemotherapies. Idiopathic thrombocytopenia is now thought to be a causative factor in some cases of chronic lymphocytic leukemia, in which hepatitis-C virus is found even though there is no clinical or biochemical sign of hepatitis. (See table 11.2.)

ANEMIA

There are many types of anemia, some of which are not caused by iron deficiency, yet most doctors indiscriminately treat all anemias the same by giving

Table 11.2 Supplements for Low Platelet Count

Supplement	Daily dose
Red root	60–120 drops (½–1 teaspoon) 3 times daily (It is truly amazing how well this works)
Marrow Plus *or* Composition-A	4 tablets, 3 times daily or 4–5 tablets, 3 times daily
SP500 (Spleen Extract)	2–6 tablets daily with meals
Melatonin	1–10 mg taken before bed
Shark oil	1,000 mg, 3–6 times daily

Table 11.3 Herbal Formulas and Supplements for Anemia

Supplement	Daily Dose
Hydroxy Folate (B_{12} and folic acid)	10–20 drops (200 mcg per drop), taken sublingually
Aqueous Liver Extract	2 capsules, 3 times daily
Laktoferrin	4 capsules, before bed
Marrow Plus or Composition-A	3–5 tablets, 3–4 times daily

iron supplementation. Iron reacts in the body with oxygen to release hydroxal radical, one of the most deadly free radicals. (See table 11.3.)

Other herbs and nutrients specific for anemia include:

• Nettles leaf (1:1 extract), 1 to 5 ml, one to three times daily.
• Yellow dock, 1 to 2 ml, one to three times daily.
• An herbal bitter taken before meals. This will not only improve the appetite but will also improve the assimilation of blood-building nutrients.
• Beet-root juice mixed with carrot juice.
• Organic liver and small amounts of organic meat (be sure to take an herbal bitter before eating).
• Bone marrow soup with plenty of dark leafy greens.
Note: 1 dropperful = 1 ml.

LYMPHEDEMA

When cancer invades the lymph system or when lymph glands are removed (as is the case with breast cancer), it may cause edema, particularly in the arms and legs. Tumors, because they attract sodium and repel potassium, can also contribute to this problem.

Helpful herbs and supplements include the following.

• Horse chestnut. I recommend a supplement by Phyto Pharmica called Varicosin, which contains extracts of horse chestnut, butcher's broom, and gotu kola.

Dose: 3 to 6 tablets daily. Or use 3 to 6 capsules of standardized horse chestnut alone.

- OPCs. *Dose:* 100 to 400 mg caps. Use 2 to 4 caps, 3 times daily.
- Bromelain. *Dose:* Use 500 to 750 mg tablets and take 1 tablet with turmeric (and possibly horse chestnut extract) three to four times daily, thirty minutes before meals or two hours after meals.

Herbal Lymphatic Formula

Echinacea	30 ml	Blue flag	10 ml
Red root	20 ml	Bladderwrack	10 ml
Poke	10 ml	Stillingia	5 ml
Figwort	15 ml	Corydalis	5 ml
Baptisia	15 ml		

Dose: 60 to 120 drops (½ to 1 teaspoons) three times daily in a small amount of water.

Another very good way to stimulate the lymph system and remove waste material is a saltwater glow massage. Use either a washcloth or loofah sponge to rub the entire body with saltwater.

MENOPAUSAL SYMPTOMS

Frequently, women who have had breast or ovarian cancer develop menopausal symptoms. Menopause can be brought on prematurely because of chemotherapy or certain drugs. For example, tamoxifen, although a weak estrogen itself, diminishes a woman's own estrogen production, which can lead to menopausal symptoms. Hormone replacement therapy is usually out of the question in this case because of the risk of cancer recurrence. The supplements, herbs, and foods that inhibit breast cancer, however, will also alleviate menopausal symptoms. Freshly ground flaxseed (1 to 2 tablespoons) added to cereal, yogurt, juice, or salad is an excellent food to include in your diet. Spending time outdoors and making time for regular exercise are both important to support the endocrine system and pave the way for a smooth transition. I recommend a supplement called Every Woman II (see Resources). It is a food-grown, low-potency multivitamin with herbal extracts and superfoods made to support a woman during and after menopause.

Natural supplements for menopausal symptoms include:

- Breast Basics (see Resources).

  Dose: 2 to 4 tablets daily. This supplement contains vitamins C and E, selenium, folic acid, beta-carotene, and potency assured herbal extracts of astragalus, rosemary, orange peel, turmeric, red clover, lavender, ginger, burdock, dandelion, Siberian ginseng, vitex, plus reishi, maitake, and shiitake mushrooms.

- Harmonizer (see Resources).

  Dose: 1 to 2 tablets two to three times daily. This supplement contains vitamins C, E, B$_6$, folic acid, selenium, alpha-lipoic acid, boron, tocotrienols, black cohosh, chaste berry, dong quai, gamma-oryzanol, green tea extract, garlic, lactoferrin, and low-temperature isoflavone extracts and phosphoglycolipids from soy.

- Gamma-oryzanol, a growth-promoting substance found in most grains, has been isolated from rice bran oil and is used to treat various health conditions, including many menopausal symptoms, particularly in Japan. Due to its ability to reduce leutinizing hormone by the pituitary and promote endorphin release by the hypothalamus, gamma-oryzanol is very effective for treating hot flashes, insomnia, mild depression, and minor anxiety in addition to lowering high cholesterol and triglyceride levels.

  Other important factors that make gamma-oryzanol so impressive are its antioxidant properties, its anticancer effects in animal studies, and its ability to protect against the damages of radiation and chemotherapy.

  Dose: 50 to 100 mg, two to three times daily. Best results are usually found with a total of 300 mg daily.

- Hesperidin. This lesser-known bioflavonoid is seldom used by most health care practioners, yet it is very effective at relieving hot flashes. Other flavonoids, such as those in grape seed extracts, can also help relieve many of the symptoms of menopause.

  Dose: 4 to 6 capsules (500 ml each), three to four times daily.

  Other key supplements helpful for menopausal symptoms include evening primrose oil and the trace mineral boron, as well as calcium and magnesium.

The following herbal compounds may also be helpful (see Resources):

- Women's Transition (Pioneer Nutritional Formulas)
- FemTone (Phyto Pharmica)
- Two Immortals (Health Concerns)
- Black Cohosh Extract (Source Naturals), yielding 2 mg of triterpene glycosides. Some of the specific indications for black cohosh include night sweats, hot flashes, hypertension, heart disturbances, flulike symptoms, minor anxiety, insomnia, and nervousness.

Vaginal Dryness

Another common problem of menopause is vaginal dryness. Earth's Harvest makes a great suppository out of vitamin E and black cohosh. Simply insert one before going to bed, as needed. Vitamin E oil can also be used by piercing a capsule and inserting it one to three times weekly, or as needed. Make sure your diet is adequate in essential fatty acids. This is very important in the treatment and prevention of vaginal dryness.

HEALING FROM SURGERY AND RADIATION

There are two important reasons to assist your body before and after an operation for removal of a cancerous growth, and before and after receiving radiation therapy. The first is to maximize healing, reduce inflammation, reduce oxidative systemic stress, and prevent scar tissue buildup (a particular concern in any gastrointestinal tract or for surgery in the peritoneal area). The second is to prevent systemic cancer cells from escaping or becoming more aggressive, thereby reducing the risk of recurrence. During and after an operation, your defenses are down because the body systems are working primarily to heal, thereby reducing the body's systemic immune surveillance, which inhibits cancer growth.

Some healing aids to use before and after surgery include:

- Bromelain. *Dose:* 500 to 750 mg *and* turmeric (made of 95 to 97 percent curcumin). *Dose:* 300 to 500 mg, taken together on an empty stomach, three to four times daily.
- OPCs. *Dose:* 1 to 2 tablets (100 mg each), taken three times daily.

• Beta-glucan. *Dose:* 2 to 4 capsules daily *or* Reishi 5. *Dose:* 4 to 6 capsules daily.

• Glucosamine sulfate (Phyto Pharmica). *Dose:* 2 capsules (500 mg each) two times daily.

• Varicosin (Phyto Pharmica). Contains extracts of horse chestnut, butcher's broom, and gotu kola.

Dose: 3 to 6 tablets daily between meals.

• Colloidal silver. *Dose:* Internally—60 to 120 drops three to four times daily. Externally, applied to a wound or burn—two to three times daily.

• Arnica-Ginger Gel (New Chapter) is a good healing salve when applied locally after surgery or radiation.

• Full-spectrum supplement containing 500 mg vitamin C ascorbate; 200 IU vitamin E succinate; 25,000 IU carotenoid complex; 10 mcg selenium; and 10 mg zinc. (Extra zinc, 30 to 50 mg, may be used to enhance healing for a short period of time.)

Two supplements that I recommend are Cyto-Redoxin (Tyler Encapsulations) and Clinical Nutrients Antioxidant (Phyto Pharmica). These are high-quality multicell protective complexes that contain plant extracts as well as vitamins and minerals. Cyto-Redoxin contains balanced amounts of lipoic acid; dry-form vitamin E; vitamin C ascorbate, carotene complex, selenium, zinc, grape seed extract, green tea extract, and CoQ10.

Dose: 2 to 4 capsules daily.

• Herbal extract compounded by an herbalist, using such herbs as panax ginseng, echinacea, baptisia, thuja, gotu kola, Chinese skullcap, hawthorn, arnica, and horsetail. Use as directed.

• Nutritional smoothie, particularly one using Greens Plus, whey protein, and flaxseed oil, can be used as a drink during the day. (See chapter 14.)

If you are undergoing radiation therapy, the following will be helpful:

• Substitute Wobenzym (Marlyn Healthcare Group) for bromelain and turmeric.

Dose: 3 to 5 tablets three times daily.

• Add 2 to 3 teaspoons L-glutamine powder to the daily intake of nutrients.

• Drink 4 ounces cold-pressed aloe leaf juice mixed with another juice daily.

- Take 1 to 6 teaspoons Chlorella or Greens Plus in powdered form daily.
- Other helpful herbs include Siberian ginseng, astragalus, ginkgo, ashwaganda, schizandra, licorice, green tea, uno de gato, and reishi. I usually make an 8-ounce mixture of herbal extracts for postradiation patients, and recommend that they take 1 teaspoon in 1 ounce of aloe leaf juice three to four times daily.

Postradiation Tea

Make a mucilaginous tea with slippery elm bark, marshmallow, plantain, mullein, horsetail, and comfrey. Add 2 heaping tablespoons of herbs to 3 pints of cool water. Let sit several hours or overnight. Then gently heat herbs, being careful not to boil. Strain and drink throughout the day. This tea is very soothing and healing to the mucous membranes of all tissues in the body, particularly the linings of the respiratory, urinary, and digestive tracts.

GOUT

Gout, a painful arthritic condition brought about by excess uric acid, afflicts many people undergoing chemotherapy because of the negative effect cytotoxic drugs have on the kidneys. For gout I usually recommend the following herbal compound.

Gout Formula

Celery seed	60 ml	Juniper	10 ml
Nettles (leaf, root, seed)	60 ml	Avena	20 ml
Burdock seed	30 ml	Colchicum	15 ml
Devil's claw	30 ml	Pipsissewa	15 ml

Dose: 1 teaspoon three to six times daily, taken in black cherry concentrate or a cup of watermelon seed tea.

I also recommend taking 10 drops of Hydroxy Folate (B_{12} and folic acid) along with 500 mg each of bromelain and quercetin, three times daily between meals. It is very important to avoid meat, shellfish, and all alcohol while treating this condition.

12

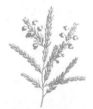

Breast Cancer

*. . . and now faith, hope, and love abide, these three;
and the greatest is love.*

—Corinthians 13:1–3, 13

B reast cancer, like other cancers, is the end result of a multistage process of carcinogenesis. This process involves a series of genetic changes resulting in an altered cell and, ultimately, in the clinical appearance of breast cancer. This complex process includes inherited and acquired susceptibility factors as well as endogenous and exogenous exposures; they lead to genetic or other biological changes that alter cell function and growth, causing increased cell proliferation. Eventually, these mutations can lead to invasive cancer. (See table 12.1.)

That's the bad news. The good news is that while there are many initiating and promoting factors for breast cancer, there are just as many protective factors that can inhibit or even reverse these stages.

Let's take a look at breast cancer statistics and demographics.

Table 12.1 **Stages of Breast Disease Leading to Breast Cancer**

1. Normal breast epithelial cell	Normal and healthy tissue.
2. Intermediate or mutant cell	Exposure to a carcinogen, such as radiation, or the result of acquired genetic alterations.
3. Atypia	Atypical appearance of cells. Various promoting factors, such as hormones and/or dietary influences can cause atypia. Hyperplasia, a condition in which there are too many cells in the tissue, precedes atypia.
4. Carcinoma *in situ*	Cancer is confined to a particular site and has not formed a tumor mass that can be detected by examination. These cancers are usually detected by mammography.
5. Invasive or infiltrating cancer	Cancer cells have penetrated the membranes that surround the duct or lobule. They will eventually form a lump that can be felt.
6. Angiogenesis/dissemination	The cancer has spread out of its primary tumor site.
7. Axillary lymph node metastases	There is lymph node involvement.
8. Distant micrometastases	The cancer has spread outside the lymph nodes and has invaded an organ.
9. Overt metastatic disease	The cancer has spread to more than one site.

DEMOGRAPHICS AND STATISTICS

• Breast cancer is the most common cancer among women worldwide and accounts for about 30 percent of all newly diagnosed cancers in women in the United States.[1] A much smaller percentage of men also get breast cancer.

• Ninety-nine percent of all malignant breast neoplasms are carcinomas, of which nearly all are adenocarcinomas (malignant tumors originating in glandular epithelium).[2]

• The lifetime risk of breast cancer for women is now one person in eight.[3]

• There has been a sharp increase in breast cancer rates: a 25 percent rise overall between 1973 and 1993,[4] a 45 percent rise in Portland, Oregon,[5] and a 31 percent increase in Seattle, Washington.[6]

• The incidence of *in situ* breast cancer has increased roughly fivefold since the 1970s, somewhat attributable to the widespread use of mammography screening, and also to the increased use of hormone replacement therapy.[7]

A recent study points to the urgent need for women to better understand the difference between mammographically detected ductal carcinoma *in situ* (DCIS) and invasive and potentially life-threatening breast cancer. Few cases of DCIS are clinically significant, but almost all will be treated surgically.[8]

• Even with increased diagnostic capabilities and awareness, mortality rates have not changed in the last fifty years. Breast cancer still accounts for 17 percent of cancer deaths in females.[9]

• The latest U.S. statistics estimated about 180,300 cases of breast cancer in 1998; that 14 percent of women will be diagnosed with this disease in their lifetime; and that the potential reduction of risk through diet and lifestyle ranges from 33 to 50 percent. In addition, global statistics show that two to five out of every 100,000 women in Thailand and Sri Lanka die of breast cancers compared to the United States' rate of thirty to forty out of 100,000.[10]

SYMPTOMS AND DETECTION

Breast cancer is most often discovered by the patient and presents itself as a painless lump with no cyclical variations. There is usually no bilateral lumpiness, as with cystic breasts, and the lump is normally rock hard and not always apparent. Nipple discharge, unless bloody, is not likely to be an indicator of cancer.

Routine mammography may pick up and be of benefit in postmenopausal women, but it does not seem to help premenopausal women. False negatives are twice as likely to occur in premenopousal mammograms because of their denser breast tissue. The risk of death from breast cancer appears to be higher in premenopausal women who undergo annual mammography compared with those who undergo a simple annual physical examination and complete a health questionnaire.[11,12]

STAGES OF BREAST CANCER

Once breast cancer has been diagnosed, the stage of the cancer and the course of treatment will be determined by a number of factors, including the size of the tumor, its location, specific characteristics of the cancer cells, and the patient's age, menopausal status, and general state of health. (See table 2.2.)

The following system of clinical staging has been adopted by most U.S. cancer centers.

Table 12.2 **Stages of Breast Cancer**

In situ	About 5 to 10 percent of breast cancers are discovered very early. They are sometimes called carcinoma *in situ* (found only in the local area, not invading nearby tissues). Other terms for this type of cancer are intraductal carcinoma, ductal carcinoma *in situ*, and lobular carcinoma *in situ*.
Stage I	The cancer that is no larger than 2 centimeters (just under 1 inch), has no nodal involvement, and has not spread beyond the breast. Statistics show an 80 percent five-year survival rate at this stage.
Stage II	Any of the following may be true: • The cancer has spread to the axillary lymph nodes (under the arm) but is no bigger than 2 centimeters. • The cancer is between 2 and 5 centimeters and may or may not have spread to the lymph nodes. • The cancer is larger than 5 centimeters but has not spread to the lymph nodes under the arms. Statistics show a 65 percent five-year survival rate at this stage.
Stage III	*Stage IIIA* is defined by either of the following: • The cancer is smaller than 5 centimeters, has spread under the arm to the lymph nodes, and has cells that have grown together and become attached to the lymph nodes. • The cancer is larger than 5 centimeters and has spread to the lymph nodes. *Stage IIIB* is defined by either of the following: • The cancer has attached to tissues near the breast-chest wall, including muscles and ribs. • Cancer that has spread to lymph nodes near the collarbone but without disseminated metastases. Statistics show a 40 percent five-year survival rate at this stage.
Stage IV	The cancer has metastasized and spread to other organs of the body. Statistics show a 10 percent five-year survival rate at this stage.[13]

RISK FACTORS

Genetics

Although it is estimated that 85 percent of breast cancers occur in women without a strong genetic predisposition, 15 percent of all breast cancers can be directly attributed to genetic causes such as the BRCA 1 and BRCA 2 genes.

The genetic risk for premenopausal breast cancer is much greater.[14,15] Studies have shown that Jewish Ashkenazi women are at high risk for mutations in the BRCA 2 gene.[16]

Dietary Factors

Dietary fat intake. In some studies, overall fat intake has shown a modest increase in risk, but fried food and refined fat (hydrogenated and transfatty acids) continues to demonstrate a much stronger and more conculsive risk factor. Obesity, particularly in women with upper-body fat, is a significant risk factor.[17,18]

    Vegetable intake. Studies have demonstrated a strong inverse relationship between vegetable consumption and breast cancer,[19] i.e., the fewer the vegetables in the diet, the higher the breast cancer risk.

    Cooked meat mutagens. Heterocyclic amines (HCAs), a food derived mutagen found in "blackened" or overcooked meat, has long been shown to induce breast cancer in rodents. Recent studies, however, have demonstrated a strong association between eating overcooked meats and breast cancer in human subjects.[20,21]

    Alcohol. Studies have demonstrated an increased risk factor for breast cancer, even at moderate levels of consumption.[22,23]

Exogenous Hormones

Hormone replacement therapy. Current findings support a causal relationship between use of estrogens and progestins and breast cancer incidence in postmenopausal women. Further, these hormones may actually promote the late stages of carcinogenesis among postmenopausal women and facilitate the proliferation of malignant cells.[24]

    Oral contraceptive use. Oral contraceptives affect the proportions of estrogen and proliferating cells that occur during natural menstrual cycles. These changes are interrupted by oral contraceptives and result in a greater suppression of estrogen and a longer period of high proliferation during the menstrual cycle, both factors linked to increased risk of breast cancer.[25]

Reproductive Factors

Early menarche. Women with an early menarche (before age twelve) compared to woman whose menarche occurred after age thirteen have a fourfold increase in breast cancer risk. A longer menstrual cycle seems to give an overall reduced risk.[26]

Not breast-feeding. This risk factor is attributed to the fact that lactation delays ovulation, which causes a woman to have a lower estrogen exposure over her lifetime. Having a first child before the age of twenty lowers this risk by half.[27,28]

Late menopause. The body is exposed to estrogen for a longer period of time.

No pregnancies. Pregnancy brings with it an increase in estriol, an anti-cancer fraction of estrogen.

Environmental Factors

Electromagnetic fields. Exposure to electromagnetic fields can decrease production of melatonin by the pineal gland. Melatonin has been shown to suppress mammary tumorigenesis in experimental animals.[29]

Environmental toxins. Exposure to environmental toxins, such as pesticides, hydrocarbons, PCBs, and DDT, are risk factors for breast cancer. I believe environmental chemical contamination is an important etiological factor in breast cancer that has been greatly understated. Studies have shown that exposure to PCBs and DDE, the major metabolite of DDT, are associated with breast cancer risk in women. In one study, a fourfold increase in the risk of breast cancer was demonstrated when serum DDE levels increased from 2.0 ng/ml to 191 ng/ml.[30,31] Environmental chemical compounds that accumulate and remain in human adipose tissue reach levels two to three hundred times higher than those observed in serum. In breast cancer cells, DDT causes proliferation by itself and also enhances proliferation in collaboration with estradiol. Other examples of estrogen-mimicking (xenoestrogenic) chemicals that tend to accumulate in the body include kepone, dieldrin, methoxychlor, alkyl phenols, and bisphenol-A.[32,33]

Fission products. Low doses of radiation that are released from nuclear power plants result in the appearance of fission products in our food supply.[34] Radiation causes genetic damage, which increases the overall risk for breast cancer. It is now known that radiation causes mutation of the important p53 suppressor gene. For this reason, I do not recommend postlumpectomy radiation. Even though it may decrease the risk of a local recurrence of cancer, it does not help to inhibit metastatic cancer.

Mammograms

Recent findings show that women receiving mammograms should be cautious of overexposure to radiation emitted by equipment that is not professionally and regularly monitored. Such equipment can deliver doses of radiation far above what are assumed today to be safe levels.[35] For women under age fifty, the benefit-to-risk ratio of mammograms is controversial.[36]

Increased mammographic density is associated with a fourfold to sixfold risk factor for breast cancer.[37,38]

Lack of Sunlight

There is an inverse epidemiologic correlation between sunlight availability and the risk of breast cancer in the United States, Canada, and the former USSR.[39,40] Sunlight is a source of vitamin D, which may be the reason for its protective effects.

Lack of Exercise

Physical activity can reduce breast cancer risk, as demonstrated by many recent studies that concluded that 36 percent of breast cancer cases could be prevented by increasing physical activity.[41,42]

Fibrocystic Breast Disease

The pooled estimate from all studies to date shows that the ratio for the association between atypical hyperplasia and breast cancer is 3:67.[43]

Hypothyroidism

At least two-thirds of my breast cancer patients also have an underactive thyroid or an underactive endocrine system that is manifesting as hypothyroidism, frequently undetected.[44,45]

MAINSTREAM TREATMENTS

Surgery

Surgery remains the most frequent choice when breast cancer has been diagnosed. There are, however, a few important questions that should be answered before proceeding with this option.

1. *When should a mastectomy be performed as opposed to a lumpectomy?* When there are multiple tumors or when the size of the tumor is too large and lumpectomy will cause significant deformity.

2. *What about axillary lymph node dissection. Is it necessary?* Axillary lymph node dissection, the removal of lymph nodes for analysis, is often recommended by conventional oncologists. The theory is that axillary nodes can provide information about the probability of cancer recurrence and can therefore be used to help make decisions about the need for radiation and chemotherapy.

Recent studies have investigated the possibility of avoiding axillary dissection by relying on clinical information and primary tumor characteristics instead of nodal status for the staging of breast cancer. Better identification can be attained at the primary tumor than by axillary dissection, including tumor size, grading, and overexpression of certain genes (such as c-erbB-2 and p53).[46] In addition, use of a relatively new procedure called *sentinel lymph node evaluation*, a much less invasive procedure, is rising. In this procedure, also called *lymphoscintography*, dye and radioisotope tracers are used to identify one node that may signal the spread of cancer without disturbing the rest of the nodes. Use of this procedure helps to prevent complete axillary dissection in 80 to 90 percent of patients with early-stage breast cancer and avoids several complications, including chronic arm swelling (lymphedema).

My View

I am not in favor of axillary dissection because it can seriously compromise the immune system. In my opinion, the more surgical procedures (and accompanying disruptions to the immune system), the greater the risk of cancer spreading and manifesting in another location. I feel that enough data for creating a specific natural protocol can be provided by clinical information, primary tumor characteristics, and the patient herself.

Breast-Conserving Surgery

The use of lumpectomy for breast cancer increased from 16 percent in 1983 to 37 percent in 1991, while use of modified radical mastectomy declined from 75 percent to 58 percent in the same period. Lumpectomy was used more frequently for early-stage breast cancer than for later stages of the disease. By 1991, more than 50 percent of *in situ* cases and slightly fewer than 50 percent of Stage I cases were treated with lumpectomy.[47]

Reasons not to use breast-conserving surgery include:

- Large tumor size
- Multifocal breast carcinoma
- Lobula carcinoma
- Tumor necrosis
- High S-phase (stage during which DNA is synthesized)
- Low estrogen-receptor content
- Vessel invasion and lymph node metastases
- Certain mammographic patterns
- Premenopausal
- Overexpression of the mutant p53 protein and/or erbB-2
- Overexpression of glutathione S-transferase[48]
- Low levels of alpha-linolenic acid (ALA) and high levels of prostaglandin E2.[49]

My View

I believe that surgery can actually enhance the growth of systemic cancer because the removal of a tumor creates a tremendous amount of damage to healthy tissue and causes significant inflammation. Inflammation and the breakdown of tissue create an environment of very high free-radical activity in which cells are actively dividing in order to replace damaged cells, thus making it possible for an increase in the growth of the cancer itself. Postsurgical healing causes tremendous stress to the immune system, leading to systemic immune suppression that renders one vulnerable to a host of infections and/or more aggressive systemic cancer growth.

I believe we need to look at and question the mainstream practice of removing all primary tumors as standard procedure if we are to maximize healing potential, inhibit recurrences, and prevent metastatic life-threatening cancers. A solution that I often prescribe for my clients who have chosen surgery is an aggressive cancer-inhibiting protocol to be used before, during, and after surgery. This helps to prevent and/or reduce the risk of systemic cancer-cell activity. (See chapter 11 for more information.)

The timing of surgery. Immediate primary tumor removal is usually reconsidered for women in their fifties taking hormone replacement therapy (HRT) who have developed an estrogen-driven tumor. Rather than rushing into surgery, I would recommend stopping the estrogen and allowing the body to clear itself of these hormones. At the same time, I would recommend a specific nutritional protocol and dietary modifications that would reduce any and all tumor-promoting activities throughout the body. (See chapters 3, 4, and 5.) After this has been accomplished (allow at least one to two months) and the tumor has been brought into a less aggressive status or even "put to sleep," the surgical removal of the tumor (which has probably gotten smaller once the exogenous estrogen has been halted and positive measures taken) can be most effectively carried out.

Studies have also shown positive benefits for the scheduling of breast cancer surgery at certain points in the menstrual cycle of premenopausal women. In a retrospective study of 283 women who had undergone mastectomies for primary breast cancer, the recurrence rate was twice as high for those women who underwent a mastectomy during the first part of the cycle (follicular phase) than for those whose surgery took place in the later part of the cycle (luteal phase).[50]

Radiation

Although some studies show a slightly higher disease-free survival rate after radiation,[51] other studies find no difference in overall survival rates. For instance, one recent clinical trial of breast cancer radiation following lumpectomy of node-negative breast cancer found that the radiation reduced the recurrence of the cancer returning to the breast, but neither reduced the risk of metastatic cancer, nor produced a reduction in mortality.[52]

Aside from this, there are significant negative side effects of radiation to be considered. They include:

- Suppression of sweat glands and dry mouth (xerostomia)
- Weakening of the immune system that can cause respiratory illnesses like pneumonia
- Electrocardiogram changes
- An increased risk of developing sarcomas, leukemias, and additional breast cancer

My View

Although radiation is commonly used today after a lumpectomy, particularly to inhibit local recurrence, I do not believe it adds any benefit to either life expectancy or quality of life. Aside from the many negative side effects described in chapter 11, it may actually cause other cancers to form at a later date. See chapter 10 for more information on radiation.

Chemotherapy

Chemotherapy, treatment with cytotoxic drugs designed to attack cancer cells, is virtually standard protocol following surgery, but studies have shown that if a tumor is 1 cm or smaller, chemotherapy is not needed[53] and further, that if lymph nodes test negative, chemotherapy may not be beneficial at all.[54]

My View

It's important to seriously weigh the decision to have chemotherapy because of the intense nature of its side effects, which include:

- Early menopause
- Immune suppression
- Suppressed appetite, nausea, and vomiting

- Hair loss
- Decreased libido
- Atopic vaginitis
- Chronic health problems associated with specific cytotoxic drugs, for example, heart damage caused by Adriamycin

See chapter 10 for a more detailed review of chemotherapeutic drugs.

Hormone Treatment

Hormone therapy has been somewhat successful in treating cancers that are hormone dependent, notably breast and prostate cancers. In order to stop production of the hormones that fed the cancer in the first place, the testicles or ovaries are occasionally removed when dealing with these two types of cancer. Androgens (male hormones) are sometimes given to patients to treat breast cancer, and estrogens (female hormones) may be given to treat prostate cancer. Hormone-blocking drugs, such as tamoxifen, are also used to treat and prevent recurrences of breast cancer. Estrogen stimulates cancer growth because it binds to a nuclear receptor that contains a heat-shock protein (HSP) molecule. Upon binding, the HSP disassociates itself and allows changes in the receptors to occur. This leads to activation of DNA transcription. Hormone-blocking drugs work by binding to specific estrogen receptors on the surface of tumor cells where hormones would normally bind, inhibiting the cell from growing and reproducing. These drugs are generally taken following surgery and/or chemotherapy to prevent a local recurrence or metastasis of cancers that are hormone-dependent.

Tamoxifen

Tamoxifen is a hormone antagonist that works by competing with the estrogen receptors, thus inhibiting the effects of estrogen on target cells. It is usually given to women with estrogen-positive breast cancer, the theory being that breast cancer is suppressed by inhibiting estrogen production. Although tamoxifen therapy has been found to be beneficial, it does have some unpleasant side effects, which include:

- Early menopause, with hot flashes and other menopausal side effects, depression being perhaps the most common.

- Increased risk of liver and endometrial cancer.[55]
- Ocular toxicity[56] including decreased visual acuity, macular edema, and other abnormalities that are often reversible after tamoxifen withdrawal.
- Increased levels of estradiol, the damaging form of estrogen.
- Increased level of thrombocytes, which can lead to phlebitis, stroke, or blood-clotting disorders.
- While tamoxifen may show some positive effects on bone mineral density,[57] it has also been shown to depress thyroid function.[58]
- Tamoxifen resistance may allow the proliferation of a more aggressive form of cancer that can be difficult to treat. This resistance can develop to the extent that tamoxifen itself actually stimulates cancer growth. It should be noted that tamoxifen is not effective in all estrogen-receptor-positive tumors because it is only a partial antagonist to estrogen.[59]

Megace

Primarily used as hormonal therapy for advanced breast cancer, Megace is also used as a primary treatment for endometrial cancer. It is a synthetic form of the hormone progesterone, which is sometimes used as an estrogen antagonist, particularly when tamoxifen and Arimidex therapies are no longer effective at inhibiting the growth of cancer. It is also used to prevent excessive weight loss or wasting.

Danazol

Another synthetic steroid used in the treatment of endometriosis and benign breast disease, danazol has recently been found to be useful in metastatic breast cancer, specifically in postmenopausal women. It has four mechanisms of action:

- Inhibition of pituitary gonadotropin secretion
- Inhibition of adrenal and gonadal steroidogenesis
- Binding to androgen, estrogen, and progesterone receptors
- Binding to sex-hormone-binding globulin and corticosteroid-binding globulin[60]

Arimidex and Femara

These drugs are aromatase inhibitors that reduce circulating estrogen. Aromatase is an enzyme complex involving cytochrome P450, which mediates the conversion of androgens to estrogens. Following menopause, aromatization increases in extragonadal sites, such as fat and muscle, and becomes the main source of estrogens. Breast cancer that is driven by estrogen expresses aromatase activity. This is particularly true once tamoxifen resistance has occurred and the cancer that was previously driven by estrogen is now able to convert androgens into estrogens to aid in further proliferation of the cancer. This is more often the case in postmenopausal women. It is this unique ability to inhibit estrogen circulation that makes Arimidex and Femara so different from tamoxifen. Both of these relatively new drugs are being used as a second line of defense against estrogen-receptor-positive breast cancer, particularly after tamoxifen has stopped working. Based on my experience with women who have used these drugs, Femara appears to be a better choice.

Raloxifene

Another new drug that is currently being promoted as a breast cancer and osteoporosis preventative, raloxifene, is too new for me to comment on at this time. Like tamoxifen, it works by binding to specific estrogen receptors on the surface of tumor cells where hormones would normally bind, thereby inhibiting tumor-cell growth and reproduction. It seems to produce fewer side effects than tamoxifen, although tamoxifen is still regarded as the standard treatment for breast cancer.

In general, chemotherapy is thought to work best in premenopausal women, while hormone therapy works best in postmenopausal women, particularly those whose tumors are hormone-positive.

Side Effects of Hormone Therapy

The possible side effects of hormone therapy include:

- Nausea, vomiting, loss of fertility.
- In women: deepening of the voice, increased libido, increased growth of body hair, menopausal symptoms in premenopausal women, bleeding in postmenopausal women.

- In men: raising of the voice, decreased libido, impotence, enlarged breasts.

These changes are temporary for some and permanent for others. One of the major problems with the use of hormone therapies is that cancer can become not only resistant to the hormone antagonist, it can actually become more aggressive and feed on the drug itself.

My View

Chemotherapy and hormone therapy use drugs that circulate throughout the bloodstream and are, theoretically, systemic therapies. Eventually, however, the cancer cells mutate with both of these treatments and can become more aggressive. Refractive hormonal cancers tend to be more aggressive and harder to treat in both conventional and nonconventional methods. When a cancer is very aggressive to begin with, chemotherapy makes more sense as long as the drugs being used are sensitive to an individual's particular cancer-cell line. If that is not the case, it may do more harm than good.

Personally, I do not recommend prophylactic tamoxifen, that is, prescribing it as a preventive medicine for inhibiting breast cancer following other therapies. Currently, in my practice I see approximately three hundred women with breast cancer. Of this number, two hundred have been instructed to take tamoxifen as a five-year posttreatment cancer-prevention therapy. I would say that about 50 percent of that group take the drug as directed, 25 percent begin to take it but stop because they are uncomfortable with the side effects, and the remaining 25 percent never start. Recently, tamoxifen is also being recommended by some doctors as preventive treatment for all disease-free women at high risk for breast cancer.

While I maintain my commitment to work with each patient's own treatment choices, my personal opinion is that tamoxifen should be used only as a treatment for active breast cancer and not as preventive therapy. I believe that if a patient takes tamoxifen prophylactically to prevent recurrence, she will never know whether she is truly in remission or if the tamoxifen is acting as a hormone to suppress cancer growth temporarily. I prefer to see multiple natural modalities used to inhibit the cancer from returning, saving tamoxifen as a possible treatment if it is ever needed in the future. There are so many natural ways to inhibit cancer growth by hormonal modulation, for example, with flaxseeds, soy foods, calcium D-glucarate, and the many herbs mentioned throughout this book.

Bone Marrow Transplant

Bone marrow transplantation is a relatively new type of treatment that is sometimes used when breast cancer is first diagnosed at an advanced stage or it has become resistant to treatment with standard chemotherapy. Normally, very high doses of chemotherapy are used in this process, doses so high they can destroy bone marrow. Therefore, marrow is removed from the bones and frozen before treatment begins. High doses of chemotherapy, usually alkylating agents, with or without radiation therapy, are then given to treat the cancer. After this treatment, the patient has no residual bone marrow necessary to produce the white blood cells that protect against infection or the platelets that prevent bleeding. The marrow that was removed is then thawed and injected into a vein to replace the marrow that was destroyed. Autologous bone marrow transplant (use of the patient's own bone marrow) is the usual procedure in cases of breast cancer.

Bone marrow transplants, which have not yet been proven to have curative effects, are very costly; moreover, we do not yet know the long-term effects of this form of therapy. Based on my experience with patients in my practice who have undergone bone marrow transplants, I have serious questions about this procedure. This drastic attempt to put the cancer into remission rarely works for more than a year or two. Many times, the person is never the same again after it is done because of the weakened systemic vitality that often results. In evaluating over 19,000 patients who received transplants between 1964 and 1992, studies have shown that those undergoing bone marrow transplantation had an increase of other solid tumors following the transplant.[61]

My View

In general, conventional medicine tends to overtreat when not really sure what to do next. Hundreds of hospitals throughout the country have spent small fortunes to add bone marrow facilities to their institutions, without knowing the long-term results of such a procedure. As of this writing, there is no conclusive study that shows that bone marrow transplants are any more effective than any other breast cancer therapies in extending a patient's life or enhancing the quality of life. Even so, bone marrow transplants continue to be a mainstream treatment that is very costly to the patient but generates a significant amount of income for the medical establishment.

I am also dubious about vaccines or gene therapy for cancer, which are currently the focus of research for possible cures for cancer. Once again, we need to remember to look at the whole person, not just the tumor, when treating cancer.

AFTER THE DIAGNOSIS: WHAT TO DO FIRST

A diagnosis of breast cancer brings with it an enormous cargo of decision-making. I try to help my clients find sources for information and advice so that they can confront their condition as warriors, with strength and positive feelings of control. I believe that the act of being proactive and making one's own decisions about one's health is healing in and of itself. Remember, cancer does not happen overnight. Very often it has taken years to develop. You have time to read, ask questions, and make the decisions that are right for you. Take as much time as you need to be comfortable with the healing path you have chosen.

After a breast cancer diagnosis, every woman should take these steps:

• Ask your physician to explain the current stage and type of cancer you have. Ask for the pathology report, even if you don't understand it at first. Ask if there is anything unusual about your case and, if so, where (and who) are the best people suited to deal with your particular situation.

• Call the Cancer Information Service at 1-800-4-CANCER for current information about your particular form of cancer and current research and treatment options. It is essential to do plenty of research before deciding which treatment is best. See page 294 of chapter 10 for a list of recommended reading material.

• Find a good holistic health care professional (herbalist or naturopathic physician) who can provide guidance about all the natural and complementary therapies that can help you. Be sure that this person is experienced in the area of cancer. Be comfortable with the person you choose.

• Start a file of your medical records and keep all information current.

• Consider joining a support group. Although this is not for everyone, it can bring you in touch with others who are going through similar situations.

• Seek a second opinion if you have any doubts at all about the advice you receive; this goes for holistic practitioners as well as conventional doctors.

• If you have a mastectomy and decide to have breast reconstruction, be sure to explore all options currently available; choose an experienced doctor and ask how many surgeries will be required to complete the process.

• Be sure to have your husband/partner involved as an integral part of your healing process. Even though you must make all the final decisions about treatment yourself, it is important to have someone who is close to share in the many experiences you will encounter along the way. Know that love is the greatest healer.

• Most important, use your heart, mind, and spirit to direct and guide you in your choices—and never look back.

Once a woman has done her homework and made her decisions, she must feel comfortable with the course of action to be taken. If she opts for allopathic (conventional) therapies, there are still many choices to be made. Whatever a patient's decision, if she decides on the allopathic mode, I try to complement and enhance the therapies that have been chosen.

FIBROCYSTIC BREAST DISEASE AND CANCER

Proliferative benign breast disease, also referred to as fibrocystic breast disease (FBD), particularly when associated with atypia, places women at increased risk of developing breast cancer. However, not all women diagnosed with fibrocystic breast disease will develop breast cancer. FBD is characterized by the formation of benign breast cysts that are enlarged during the luteal phase of the menstrual cycle.

Fibrocystic breast disease may be caused by:

• Excess estrogen or too little progesterone during the luteal phase of the menstrual cycle.

• Caffeine, theophylline, and theobromine, found in coffee, tea, and chocolate.

• Hypothyroid/iodine deficiency.

• Reduced or impaired liver function. The liver is the primary site for estrogen clearance, and factors that interfere with proper liver function can lead to estrogen excess. From an herbalist's perspective, in order to understand the progression from PMS, swollen breasts, and fibrocystic breast disease to breast cancer, one must address the possibility of liver stagnation. There is a strong association between the detoxifying mechanisms that take place in the liver and protection against breast cancer.

• Colon function. Constipation, bowel dysfunction, and a poor diet can cause an imbalance of bacterial flora in the large intestine. This can be improved by proper diet and by acidophilus supplementation. Women who have fewer than three bowel movements per week have a risk of fibrocystic breast disease that is four-and-a-half times greater than women who have at least one bowel movement a day.

Treatment of Fibrocystic Breast Disease

Dietary Changes

It is best to eat a primarily organic vegetarian diet rich in vegetables and fruits. Eliminate red meat and chicken and completely avoid caffeine and the trans fatty acids found in commercially processed foods. Eat plenty of complex carbohydrates and fiber-rich foods, particularly flaxseeds, which are rich in lignans. Consume fish and soy products, such as tofu and tempeh, for protein. Add bitter greens, such as arugula and chicory, to salads to help the liver excrete excess hormones.

Herbal Strategies

Consult with an herbalist for specific protocols. The following classes of herbs are extremely helpful in treating fibrocystic breast disease.

1. Liver-detoxifying herbs, such as dandelion, fringe tree, agrimony, and bupleurum, improve liver function and increase bile flow.

2. Alterative and lymphatic herbs, such as red root, poke, tiger lily, and blue flag, improve the function of the lymph system and can actually help absorb and dissolve cysts.

Table 12.3 **Supplements to Prevent or Help Fibrocystic Breast Disease**

Supplement	General Daily Dose
Lipotrophic supplement containing choline, methionine, and taurine	2–3 capsules, 1–3 times daily
Vitamin E succinate, dry form	600–1200 IU
Vitamin B$_6$	50–200 mg
Bromelain	500 mg, 3 times daily
Acidophilus	1–2 capsules, 1–3 times daily
Sea herbs	1–3 grams daily
Potassium iodide	2–8 drops
Evening primrose oil	3–6 500 mg capsules daily
Beta-Plex	2–6 drops
Herbal tonic	Individually prescribed

3. Herbs that can regulate hormone function, such as alfalfa, black cohosh, and red clover, decrease excessive estrogen and adhere to estrogen-receptor-binding sites. Other herbs, such as chaste tree, pulsatilla, wild yam, and evening primrose, increase luteinizing hormone production and inhibit the release of FSH (follicle-stimulating hormone), thus causing a shift in the ratio of estrogen to progesterone. Additionally, herbs such as bladderwrack, kelp, and Oregon grape balance the endocrine system and improve thyroid function. (See also table 12.3 for supplements for fibrocystic breast disease.)

External herbal treatments

Poke oil. Poke Oil Plus is available from WellSprings Center for Natural Healing (see Resources) and is also sold over the counter in natural food stores. *Directions:* Apply to the breast twice daily.

Flaxseed/slippery elm/fenugreek poultice. A poultice of ground flax-seeds, slippery elm bark, and fenugreek is also helpful. Use 1 to 3 ounces of flax, fenugreek, and slippery elm bark ground to a powder. Slowly add boiling water to create a paste. *Directions:* As a poultice, spread the wrap mixture on a cloth and apply to the breast. As a compress, soak a cloth in the mixture and apply to the breast. Another option is to cover the poultice or compress with plastic wrap and apply low heat for fifteen to twenty minutes. As a plaster, apply mixture directly on breast (this can be messier, but it's more effective).

Clay poultice. See chapter 4 for ingredients and directions.

Castor oil pack. See chapter 8 for ingredients and directions.

A SAMPLE PROTOCOL TO PREVENT
THE RECURRENCE OF BREAST CANCER

As you read this sample protocol, please remember that I look at each person as an individual, a human spirit with a complex set of symptoms, characteristics, and constitutional strengths and weaknesses. I do not treat or look at cancer itself as a separate entity, and therefore have no set protocol for treating cancer. What I do is treat a person who is exhibiting symptoms of imbalance in the body. I change the protocol for that individual whenever necessary, according to the body's reactions.

The sample protocol that follows is based upon many of the more common characteristics of a woman with breast cancer. I'll call my subject Mary.

Mary is a postmenopausal woman in her midfifties. She is slightly pear-shaped and large-breasted, and has a history of lumpy and cystic breasts. She has dry hair and skin, receding gums, varicose veins, and a subnormal body temperature that indicates a slightly low thyroid function. Mary always puts others first and is mildly depressed on a deep level. She tends to worry and is often sad, although most people around her, including her husband and children, are not aware of this. Mary works in an office, does little exercise, and does not get much sunlight or fresh air. Her sleep is never deep, and she often wakes up at night, thinking too much or worrying. She often diets, trying to reduce her fat intake and lose weight. Mary shops in large commercial supermarkets and does not buy organic food. Her daily diet is something like this:

Breakfast: Bagel or muffin with coffee and a glass of processed orange juice.

Lunch: Salad bar platter with low-fat dressing; diet soft drink (Mary usually consumes two or three of these drinks throughout the day).

Midday: Chocolate, candy, or a cookie to help ward off the drop in blood sugar and the accompanying fatigue that occur every afternoon.

Dinner: After a long hard day at work, Mary does not feel much like cooking, so she picks up a prepared chicken and some frozen vegetables and cooks some refined pasta. After dinner, she often has a cup of low-fat ice cream.

During an annual gynecological checkup and mammogram, Mary is diagnosed with breast cancer; the next week she has a lumpectomy. Because her cancer was found early, it appears to be a less aggressive form, and there is no lymph node involvement. It is therefore recommended that she undergo six treatments of a mild chemotherapy (CMF) and three weeks of radiation. Following this treatment, tamoxifen is prescribed. Before long, Mary becomes very depressed, stops taking the drug, and comes in to see me because she is looking for ways to improve her health and prevent the cancer from coming back. (See table 12.4 for sample protocol.)

Mary's Herbal Tonic*

American ginseng	40 ml	Horse chestnut	15 ml
Gotu kola	30 ml	Bladderwrack	15 ml
Licorice	25 ml	Poke	10 ml
Reishi	20 ml	Pulsatilla	10 ml
Red root	20 ml	Foxglove	5 ml
Echinacea	20 ml	Ginger	5 ml
Thuja	15 ml		

*Formulated for Mary's specific constitution and needs as presented at the time of her visit. *Dose:* Take 1 teaspoon in a little water two times daily.

Dietary Recommendations for Mary

• Morning smoothie for weekday breakfasts when time is short. See chapter 14. Otherwise enjoy organic eggs or whole grain breads or cereals.

• Eat more of the superfoods listed in chapter 3, such as soy foods, fresh vegetables and fruits, garlic and onions, nuts and seeds; sprout broccoli, buckwheat, and sunflower seeds and add to salad.

• Include sea vegetables in soups, salads, and grain dishes.

Table 12.4 Mary's Herb and Supplement Protocol

Supplement	Dose
Breast Basics	3 capsules daily (2 in the morning; 1 in the evening)
Ocean Herbs	3 capsules daily (2 in the morning; 1 in the evening)
Cyto-Redoxin	3 capsules daily (2 in the morning; 1 in the evening)
Calcium D-glucarate	2–3 capsules twice daily
CoQ10 (100 mg capsules)	1 capsule daily taken with an omega-3 fatty acid such as flaxseed oil or Eskimo Oil
Activated quercetin	2 tablets twice daily, 30 minutes before meals
Maitake D-fraction	30 drops twice daily
Super-Tonic	3 capsules daily (2 in the morning; 1 in the evening)
Minor bupleurum	3 capsules twice daily
Cellular Forte (IP6)	2 capsules twice daily
Lipoic acid (100 mg)	1 capsule twice daily
Specific Herbal Tonic (recipe on page 336)	1 teaspoon twice daily
Herbal tea mixture of red clover blossoms, green tea, roasted dandelion, nettles, and pinch of orange peel	1–3 cups daily

See Resources for specific supplements.

- Replace refined flour products with organic sprouted grain breads.
- Eat more legumes and fish and less chicken. Whatever chicken is eaten should be organic or at least hormone-free.
- Switch to organic foods.
- Prepare and cook meals at home, unless you have access to an organic whole foods restaurant.

Lifestyle Recommendations for Mary

- Spend some time in prayer or meditation every day, connecting with your inner spirit.
- Take a yoga class twice a week.
- Exercise outdoors (when possible) three times a week.
- Have a massage once a month.
- Take up some form of art that allows for creative expression.
- Spend about twenty minutes each day outdoors in the sun.
- Get full-spectrum lights for your office desk.

These changes in lifestyle and diet, along with the herbal and supplemental protocol, are enough changes for Mary to deal with right now. Changes like these should come from love and the desire to nurture oneself on many levels. Trying to implement changes in one's life from a perspective of fear can be counterproductive.

13

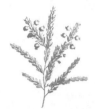

Prostate Cancer

Praise be you, my Lord, with all Your creatures, especially Sir Brother Sun, who is the day through whom
you give us light.

—*St. Francis of Assisi*

rostate cancer is a growing health problem throughout the Western
world. In America, it is now the most common cancer in men and the
second most common cause of cancer-related deaths. The number of
diagnosed cases of prostate cancer has more than tripled in the last decade.
Current statistics show that the disease now accounts for one-third of all U.S.
male cancers, with an estimated 179,300 cases and 37,000 deaths in 1999.[1]

Current estimates indicate that one in nine men will be diagnosed with this
disease during his lifetime (a statistic very similar to female breast cancer estimates). Only one out of three men diagnosed with prostate cancer will die of the
disease, and in at least 25 percent of all cases, no treatment is required because of
the advanced age of the patients and the fact that their cancer is so slow-growing
it will not ever become harmful before they die of other age-related causes.

Many men are past the age of eighty before prostate cancer is found, but recently an alarming number of younger men have been diagnosed with this disease—and in younger men it is usually a more serious condition.

I see many men with prostate cancer and have had a great deal of success in treating this disease (even in advanced stages) using herbs, nutritional supplements, and diet. Many of these men did not use any conventional treatments.

Because natural and holistic protocols for treating prostate cancer work by restoring and detoxifying the body, a significant additional benefit of their use is their ability to inhibit many age-related chronic diseases, such as heart disease. Many of the herbs and nutritional supplements used to treat prostate cancer are especially restorative to the heart as well, as are my dietary and lifestyle guidelines.

RISK FACTORS

Risk factors associated with prostate cancer include:

- *Age.* Incidence increases with age.
- *Race.* African-American men have the highest mortality from prostate cancer in the world, although the disease is uncommon among Africans in African countries. A similar statistic applies to Japanese men—those living in Japan have only one-tenth the risk of dying from prostate cancer compared to those who live in America.[2]
- *Family history and genetic predisposition.* Epidemiologic studies have shown that if a man has a first-degree relative with prostate cancer, his prostate cancer risk is approximately twice that of the general population; when both first- and second-degree relatives are affected, the risk increases about nine times.[3]
- *Reproductive factors.* Several studies have shown a higher incidence of prostate cancer in men who have undergone vasectomies,[4,5] and other research has indicated that prostate cancer risk may be increased by frequent sexual activity begun early in life, multiple sexual partners, or a history of sexually transmitted diseases.[6]
- *Dietary factors.* Epidemiologic studies have shown a connection between a high-fat diet and prostate cancer risk[7] while other research has begun to show significant protection from risk by increasing intake of fruits, vegetables, and vitamin supplements.[8,9] One study demonstrated a 45 percent risk reduction when subjects ate at least ten servings per week of tomato-based foods

rich in lycopene.[10] Other studies have focused on the preventive value of supplements, with promising results:

- Vitamin E has shown an ability to inhibit prostate cancer growth in human cells[11] as well as cell-culture studies.[12]
- In a study involving 29,000 male smokers, researchers found that those who took modest doses of vitamin E supplements over a period of six years were 32 percent less likely to develop prostate cancer and 41 percent less likely to die from the disease.[13]
- Intake of modified citrus pectin (MCP), a compound derived from citrus fruits, has been shown in animal tests to prevent the spread of prostate cancer. MCP appears to inhibit the binding abilities of cancer cells.[14]

SCREENING PROCEDURES

There is much controversy about the value of prostate cancer screening, appropriate staging evaluation, and the optimal treatment for each stage of the disease. The prostate-specific antigen test has become a common diagnostic measure recommended to all men past the age of forty and, as a result, more early-stage cancers have been detected. This has not, however, resulted in a lower mortality rate. The chances of dying from prostate cancer remain the same for those who are screened and those who are not.[15] A multicenter trial sponsored by the National Cancer Institute is currently under way to determine the value of routine PSA screening for reducing mortality.[16] Current screening procedures include:

- *PSA (Prostate-Specific Antigen)*. PSA is a protein that is only produced by cells located within the prostate gland. Both benign and malignant cells produce this protein, and the larger the prostate gland the higher the PSA. Since the PSA count can be high in cases of benign prostate growth, a common occurrence in men as they age, it is not always an accurate marker by itself. A relatively new development that promises more accurate PSA testing is the discovery of the existence of two types of PSA—free and protein-bound. A low ratio of free PSA to protein-bound PSA indicates the presence of prostate cancer with 95 percent accuracy; a high ratio indicates a benign condition.
- *DRE (Digital Rectal Examination)*. Because the prostate gland is located adjacent to the rectum, a physician is able to feel the gland during

an examination to determine if there are any palpable abnormalities in size or shape. While abnormalities of this kind do not necessarily indicate cancer, they indicate the need for further testing. Approximately one-third of all DRE abnormalities are eventually diagnosed as prostate cancer.

• *TRUS (Transrectal Untrasonography)*. In this procedure, a rectal probe is used to pass sound waves from the probe to the prostate gland. Since cancer cells differ from normal cells in the way they absorb sound waves, the distinct patterns of cancer cells indicate the presence of prostate cancer.

• *Biopsy*. If there are abnormalities in both the PSA and DRE, a biopsy will most likely be recommended. Biopsies are usually performed using ultrasound-guiding techniques. Occasionally a number of random biopsies will be done to sample the entire prostate gland.

I am not in favor of biopsies, because they may disturb the cancer, causing it to grow more rapidly and/or to spread to other areas. I would prefer to see research focus on finding new noninvasive procedures rather than on developing surgical or other invasive practices for detecting and treating this disease. Although MRI (magnetic resonance imaging) is sometimes recommended, studies have shown that it is not a reliable diagnostic procedure for prostate cancer.[17]

GRADING AND STAGING

After the presence of prostate cancer has been positively identified, conventional treatment options will depend largely on the appearance of the cancer cells under the microscope, a process known as tumor grading. Once the tumor's characteristics have been assessed in this way, the next step is to determine the stage, or extent, of the cancer.

Grading

The most common way to grade prostate cancer is the Gleason scoring system. This system defines five glandular patterns of cancer cells under low magnification, ranging from 1 (well-differentiated cells) to 5 (completely undifferentiated cells). Some tumors possess more than one cellular pattern; in that case, both patterns are graded and the grades are combined to get a Gleason score ranging from 2 (1+1) to 10 (5+5). Those tumors graded in the low range are significantly less likely to grow rapidly and spread; those with a high score indicate that the cancer is aggressive and is likely to metastasize without treatment.

Staging

One of the most important factors to consider in the management of prostate cancer is the stage. The most commonly used staging system is the Whitmore-Jewett system, which defines four stages with accompanying substages:

Stage A

Undetectable tumor confined to the prostate gland; usually an incidental finding during prostate gland biopsy.

- A1. Tumor presents a low Gleason score and is well differentiated.
- A2. Tumor presents a higher Gleason score, is moderately or poorly differentiated, and possesses a capacity for metastatic activity.

Stage B

Palpable tumor (or nonpalpable but indicated by high PSA count) confined to the prostate gland.

- B1. Focalized palpable tumor confined to one lobe of the prostate gland.
- B2. Palpable tumor involving both lobes of the prostate gland.

Stage C

A tumor localized to the periprostatic area but extending through the prostatic capsule; seminal vesicles may be involved.

- C1. Clinical evidence of extracapsular extension.
- C2. Extracapsular tumor producing bladder or urethral obstruction.

Stage D

Metastatic prostate cancer.

- D1. Regional lymph node involvement.
- D2. Distant metastatic involvement.[18]

CONVENTIONAL TREATMENTS

Current conventional treatment options for prostate cancer are considered either curative (for cases within Stages A and B) or palliative (for cases within Stages C and D) and include the following.

Radical Prostatectomy

This procedure involves removal of the prostate gland, seminal vesicles, and a certain amount of surrounding tissue. It is usually performed on men under the age of sixty-five when the disease is local to the prostate gland. The risks are considerable; there is a 1 to 2 percent mortality rate and complications may include:

- Loss of sexual function
- Loss of bladder control
- Scarring of the urethral channel
- Blood clot formation
- Bowel injury

I have concerns about the true curative effects of a prostatecomy, even when disease is totally confined to the prostate gland. Although physicians consider this procedure curative and able to reduce the risk of metastases, many men who do not elect surgery will have no further spread of cancer, while others who do elect this procedure may still experience spread of the disease at a later date. Although I support the treatment decisions made by my patients and offer them complementary natural protocols to help them heal, I believe that surgery is not the answer to preventing the spread of cancer.

Radiation

External beam radiation, an alternative to radical prostatectomy, is used in cases where the cancer is confined to the prostate gland and surrounding tissues (Stages A, B, and C). Usually recommended to older men (over sixty-five years of age), side effects are fewer and less serious. They may include bladder inflammation, diarrhea, and bloody stools. While most men retain potency after treatment, as many as 50 percent eventually develop erectile dysfunction. While there is controversy about the effectiveness of radiation therapy versus radical prostatectomy, statistics have shown that the results of the two treatments are comparable in outcome up to ten years after treatment.[19]

Brachytherapy

This procedure involves the implantation of radioactive seeds directly into the prostate, using hollow needles guided by real-time imaging—usually transrectal ultrasound, CT scanning, or fluoroscopy—to ensure proper placement of the seeds. Since radioactive seeds implanted in this way deliver radiation directly to the prostate without affecting surrounding tissue and organs, higher doses of radiation can be used. The seeds remain permanently in place within the prostate and become inert and inactive within six to twelve months. Complications accompanying this treatment are minimal—usually urinary problems involving frequency, urgency, or difficulty with urination—and tend to diminish by the time the seeds have lost their radioactivity. Nearly 90 percent of the men receiving this treatment retain sexual function, a very high percentage in relation to all other available curative treatments for prostate cancer.

While this treatment appears to be a good alternative for older patients or those who wish to avoid surgical procedures, it is still too soon to know its long-term effectiveness.

Cryotherapy

This procedure freezes prostate tissue by inserting probes containing liquid nitrogen through the perineum and into the prostate gland. Ultrasound imaging is used to guide the placement of the probes and to control the amount of tissue to be frozen. Although the treatment is performed easily (outpatient basis under general anesthesia) and recovery time is brief, the procedure can have many complications, including a 75 percent risk of impotence. In addition, long-term effectiveness of this treatment has not yet been established.[20]

Hormone Therapy

A standard form of therapy to treat prostate cancer that has gone beyond the prostate gland, hormone therapy is used to inhibit the production of the male hormone, testosterone, thereby inhibiting the growth of the cancer as well. Hormonal drugs currently in use include:

- *Lupron (Zoladex in oral form).* A leutinizing hormone-releasing antagonist that lowers the amount of testosterone available.
- *Flutamine.* An agent that blocks the action of androgen hormones, such as testosterone.
- *Estrogens (such as DES).* Agents that inhibit the binding of testosterone to a cell's hormone receptors.

Common side effects of hormone therapy include mild diarrhea, breast tenderness and enlargement, diminished sex drive, hot flashes, and diminished muscle tone.

Hormone therapy is usually suggested as a primary therapy for older men or for men who have relapsed after surgery or radiation therapy. The potential disadvantage of hormone therapy is that resistant cells may develop and grow more rapidly, causing a more aggressive disease pattern.

Another method used to lower testosterone production is a procedure called bilateral orchiectomy, or surgical removal of the testicles. This is a palliative rather than curative treatment, usually recommended for those with late-stage prostate cancer (Stages C or D). In many cases, the benefits of orchiectomy are temporary, and the cancer reappears. For this reason, an androgen blocker, such as flutamine, is normally recommended to help minimize this risk. The side effects of orchiectomy are similar to those of hormone therapy listed above.

Chemotherapy

Although chemotherapy is sometimes used in advanced stages of prostate cancer, it has not been found to be very effective in treating this disease. Chemotherapeutic agents commonly used include vinblastine, etoposide, mitoxantrone, and taxol.[21]

Of all the forms of cancer I have worked with, prostate cancer is the form of cancer for which most of my patients rely on natural healing protocols as primary healing strategies. More than 50 percent of the men I see with prostate cancer choose natural modalities right from the beginning of their diagnosis; 25 percent have already chosen conventional treatments such as surgery or radiation and come to me after a recurrence, when they choose natural modalities as their primary treatment; another 25 percent choose to use my protocol in combination with one of the conventional therapies.

It is wonderful to have the opportunity to help men with prostate cancer by using herbs, supplements, and dietary and lifestyle guidelines as their primary treatment strategy; to see them get well, thrive, and show no apparent signs of cancer is even better. I have found that many prostate cancers, even some of the more aggressive forms (high PSA, high Gleason score, even a palpable tumor or evidence of metastasis) respond beautifully to natural healing modalities.

A SAMPLE PROTOCOL FOR PROSTATE CANCER

Tom is fifty-five years old and has recently been diagnosed with prostate cancer. He has a PSA count of 12 (normal is 0–5). He has had a biopsy that confirmed the presence of prostate cancer. His Gleason score was 5 (the range being 2–10, the higher the number the more aggressive the cancer).

Tom's personality is passive-aggressive—he's very hardworking and intelligent. In fact, he's a perfectionist. I have found that the majority of men I see with prostate cancer tend to be very detail-oriented and extreme perfectionists. He has a medium build and is about 10 pounds overweight. He works indoors, mostly at a desk, and exercises only on the weekends. Tom is always in a hurry, but not really sure why, and has a family predisposition to heart disease.

Tom is generally a worrier, and now that he finds himself with prostate cancer, he is very concerned about what to do. He doesn't like the choices of surgery or radiation, yet his doctors are telling him he is relatively young and needs to get rid of the cancer before it spreads. They tell him that the cancer is confined to the prostate gland and that he has a good chance of being "cured." Tom is undecided. If Tom had his mind set on surgery, I would not question his decision but would honor it and help him with a natural and complementary protocol designed to help him live a healthy and fulfilling life. But because Tom is not sure what to do, actually does not want surgery or radiation, and would rather deal with his cancer holistically, I suggest we work together for three months.

We agree that since a holistic program is a systemic approach to healing, even if Tom decides to have surgery at a later date, his entire body (including his immune system) will be in better shape than it is now. Tom also realizes that since his prostate cancer was many years in the making, three months would not add any significant risk to his situation. His doctor agrees. Meanwhile, the three-month period can be time for calmness, rational thinking, and prayer (something Tom is not accustomed to but would like to explore).

Tom decides to undertake the program with me, hoping to avoid surgery and/or radiation forever. His PSA count will be monitored during this time.

Tom's Dietary Program

I advised Tom to eat a primarily vegetarian diet, with the exception of fish three times weekly, emphasizing fresh vegetables, fruits, soy foods (like tempeh), and whole grains. Some foods that specifically inhibit prostate cancer include green peas, soy foods, and other legumes, flaxseeds, garlic, foods rich in carotene and lycopene (including tomatoes, pink grapefruit, melons, and mangoes), sprouts of all kinds (such as sunflower seeds, broccoli seeds, and buckwheat seeds), sea herbs, and dark greens, both raw and cooked. I suggest that he diversify his vegetable intake by eating watercress, arugula, bok choy, and dandelion greens, not just the usual broccoli and green leaf lettuce. I also talked with Tom about eating out of love, not fear. One cannot try to eat well (as so many people do) for fear that certain foods will contribute to disease progression. One must eat well because it is natural, normal, and satisfying to one's entire being.

Tom's Lifestyle Changes

In addition to diet and supplements (see table 13.1), another important aspect of Tom's healing protocol included spending more time outdoors engaging in exercise of all kinds, such as hiking in the woods with twenty to thirty minutes a day of exposure to sunlight. I also recommended that he slow down, smell the roses, and find a way to get in touch with his inner self. For the latter, I asked Tom to ask himself several questions every day:

- Where am I going in life?
- Am I fulfilling my heart's desires?
- What is my soul's mission?

I counseled Tom about quieting his mind, focusing on the important things in his life, and living accordingly. We spoke of the blessings his prostate cancer brought to him, such as allowing him to change in ways that would otherwise not have occurred to him, and also by simultaneously addressing and minimizing his risk for heart disease.

Table 13.1 Tom's Herb and Supplement Protocol

Supplement	Dose
CoQ10 (100 mg)	2 capsules with meals, once daily
Lipoic acid (100 mg)	2 capsules with meals, once daily (taken with CoQ10)
Vitamin E (dry form, 400 IU)	1 capsule with meals, once daily
Aged garlic	2 capsules with meals, twice daily
Vitamin D (400 IU)	1 capsule daily during winter only
Zinc (Whole Food Complex by New Chapter*) (30 mg)	1 tablet, once daily
Harmonizer (Nutritional Therapuetics*)	2 tablets with meals, twice daily
PC SPES*	3 capsules just before bedtime
Activated quercetin	2 tablets, three times daily, 30 minutes before meals
Andrographis extract	1 tablet, three times daily, taken with activated quercetin, 30 minutes before meals
Beta-Plex*	5 drops, once daily
All-purpose multivitamin (Every Man II by New Chapter*)	1 tablet, twice daily with meals
Modified citrus pectin*	2–3 teaspoons daily
Eskimo-3 (Eskimo Oil*)	1 teaspoon, once daily, taken with CoQ10 and lipoic acid
Tom's Herbal Tonic	Recipe follows

*See Resources.

Tom's Herbal Tonic*

Nettles root seed	30 ml	Hawthorn leaf and flower	10 ml
Boswellan	20 ml	Reishi	10 ml
Red clover	20 ml	Burdock seed	5 ml
Thuja	10 ml	Licorice	5 ml
Turmeric	10 ml	Ginger	5 ml

*Formulated for Tom's specific needs. *Dose:* Take 60 drops in a little water three times daily.

Notes on the Herb and Supplement Protocol

PC SPES. After three months, depending on Tom's PSA count at that time, the dosage of PC SPES might be reduced. This herbal formula is very concentrated and powerful. My goal for Tom is not just to reduce the dosage over time but eventually to eliminate it altogether. Because both Tom and his doctor want to see a quick drop in the PSA, PC SPES is likely to have the most profound effect, since studies have demonstrated its ability to decrease testosterone levels and serum concentrations of PSA.[22] Everything in Tom's protocol will ultimately contribute to inhibiting prostate cancer and enhancing his total well-being.

Quercetin. Among other things, quercetin inhibits the mutation of the p53 suppressor gene. This is a known malfunction that leads to prostate cancer. I advised Tom to stop taking his usual vitamin C supplement, because the form of quercetin he will take contains vitamin C in the form of magnesium ascorbate as well as bromelain.

Beta-Plex. Regular beta-carotene is not as effective as Beta-Plex, a full-spectrum carotene supplement taken from natural food sources. It contains high amounts of lycopene in synergy with other natural carotenoids. Tom's instructions were to mix 1 tablespoon freshly ground flaxseeds with 1 to 6 ounces organic yogurt and 5 drops of Beta-Plex.

Three months later, Tom had made many positive changes in his life; he was more relaxed and feeling very good. His PSA had dropped into the normal range, and he decided not to have surgery or radiation—at least for the moment. He was intent on continuing my protocol, which remained the same for another three months.

After six months, I made the following changes in Tom's protocol:

- Reduction of PC SPES to 2 capsules daily.
- Replacement of garlic with green tea extract caps, 1 capsule three times daily. (Tom is not particularly fond of tea, or he could have simply drunk three cups of green tea each day.)
- Replacement of andrographis with Cellular Forte (IP6), 2 capsules three times daily.
- Replacement of boswellan and turmeric with American ginseng and milk thistle in the herbal tonic.

It has now been two years since Tom's diagnosis of prostate cancer. He is disease-free, living well, and happy (with his prostate gland intact). He is no longer taking PC SPES, and his PSA count remains normal.

14

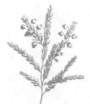

The Healing Kitchen

All praise be yours, my Lord, through Sister Earth, our
mother, who feeds us in her sovereignty and produces
various fruits with colored flowers and herbs.
           —*St. Francis of Assisi*, The Canticle of Brother Sun

This sampling of recipes is intended to illustrate the ease with which good nutrition can be incorporated into your daily life. It's important to understand, however, that food itself is only one part of nourishment. Planning, shopping, cooking, and eating with those loved ones who share your life can bring a wonderful sense of joy to mealtimes. Eating "on the run" or rigidly structuring a diet to fit a current health food trend prevents one from ever truly understanding the deep connection that exists between ourselves and nature—the world of plants and animals that was intended by God to sustain human life.

Nutritious food and herbs are healing; I consider them as much a part of a healing protocol as the herbal remedies themselves. The recipes that follow are recipes for wellness and are intended for all family members—those in excellent health as well as those who are ill or recovering from illness. It has been my experience that many people with cancer become confused about diet and frequently embark on special or extremely restricted diets, hoping for a cure. I don't believe that any one diet will cure or heal cancer in and of itself. If anything, it is love and a passion for life that can enhance the healing process in amazing ways.

Be aware that the organic whole foods you eat have a spirit of their own, one that will blend with your spirit and strengthen and empower your vital force. Learn how the body works and the role that food and herbs play in keeping it running smoothly (see chapter 3), and then commit yourself to cooking with enthusiasm and eating nutritious meals in a spirit of gratefulness and joy.

SHOPPING GUIDE

There are many small companies that make good-quality organic products. Also, check to see if your town has a farmer's market, a great place to find affordable fresh organic foods. Here are some reliable major brand names (ones you can trust). Look for them in your natural foods store.

Pasta:	Eden, Westbrae, DeBoles, Mendocino Pasta Company.
Cereal:	Nature's Path, Health Valley, Arrowhead Mills, Familia Muesli, Walnut Acres 14-Grain Cereal, Erewhon.
Jams:	Cascadian Farms.
Juices:	Santa Cruz, Knudsen, Heinke's, Mountain Sun, Tree of Life.
Nut butters:	Maranatha, Arrowhead Mills, Westbrae, Once Again Nut Butter (tahini).
Cheese:	Organic Valley, Alta Dena, Horizon, Cascadian Farms, Natural by Nature (cream cheese).
Flour:	Shiloh Farms, Arrowhead Mills.
Seaweeds:	Maine Coast Seaweeds, bulk seaweed from Ryan Drum (see Resources).
Tempeh:	Brands vary locally; look for organic. Tempeh Works is good.
Tofu:	Nasoya.
Oils:	Flora, Spectrum, Barlean's.
Bread:	Alvarado, Shiloh Farms, Breads for Life, Garden of Eatin', Food for Life (Ezekiel bread), French Meadow.

Tomatoes (canned):	Muir Glen, Millina's Finest, Green Valley, Tree of Life, GardenValley.
Vegetables (frozen and canned):	Cascadian Farms, Walnut Acres.
Miso:	Westbrae (also a good source of other macrobiotic foods).
Soy sauce:	San-J (shoyu), Arrowhead Mills.
Seeds:	Sow Organic Seeds, Seeds of Change.
Mustard:	Eden.
Salsa:	Parrot.

COOKING EQUIPMENT

Use high-grade stainless-steel cookware. Teflon can scratch, chip and flake, leaving users exposed to aluminum. Teflon can also cause a condition called "polymer-fume fever" (characterized by flulike symptoms) when used to cook at high temperatures. Vegetables cooked in aluminum can produce a hydrooxide poison that neutralizes the digestive juices, leading to intestinal troubles. One can absorb toxic levels of iron from cast-iron pots, if used frequently.

Use glass bowls and wooden spoons; avoid plastics of any kind in the process of preparing and cooking food.

And, once again, avoid microwave cooking; it weakens the vitality of food.

MENU SUGGESTIONS

The following menu options are intended to inspire interest in planning meals that are nutritious, diverse, and seasonal. Use organic products, fresh organic produce, and fish from unpolluted waters. The recipes marked with an asterisk (*) are given in this chapter.

Breakfast

- Morning smoothie.*
- Yogurt (preferably made from goat or sheep's milk) with raisins, chopped dates, figs, or apricots. Garnish with sunflower seeds, almonds, or coconut. Top with grated citrus peel.

- Oatmeal or multigrain cereal with soy milk. Add a tablespoon of ground flaxseeds and top with a little pure maple syrup and grated citrus peel.
- Poached egg with steamed asparagus and a slice of toasted whole-grain bread.
- Seasonal fruit salad. For example, a winter salad might include pomegranate, apples, pears, and citrus; a summer salad might include watermelon, grapes, peaches, plums, and berries.

Lunch

- Black bean and rice burrito* with arugula salad.
- Lentil soup* with mixed green salad.
- Sprouted hummus spread* on whole-grain bread with tomatoes and onions.
- Baked marinated tofu on sprouted whole-wheat bread with greens and mustard.
- Leftovers. Any vegetables, fish, tofu, or tempeh left over from the previous evening's meal can make an excellent cold lunch when combined with fresh greens as a salad or used as a sandwich filler.

Dinner

- Lemon-broiled tempeh,* basmati and wild rice, steamed broccoli, and a salad of mixed fresh greens.
- Roasted salmon with greens,* new potatoes with parsley, stewed tomatoes, and spring fiddlehead fern salad.*
- Vegetable lasagna,* arugula salad, and garlic bread.
- Asian tofu and bok choy,* brown rice, steamed carrots, and a green salad.
- Skillet fish,* millet with scallions, sautéed rutabagas,* and wilted spinach salad.*

Beverages

The best beverage to drink with meals is pure water. It should be sipped for refreshment, not gulped with food. Herbal teas are best for after-dinner drinks. They can be blended according to taste. A combination of red clover, ginger, nettles, and cracked fennel seed topped with a sprinkling of orange peel is delicious and healing.

Desserts

A selection of seasonal fruits is best. Depending on appetite and food preferences, a piece of freshly baked (sugar-free, of course) cake or pie is a wonderful special-occasion treat. See pages 377 to 380.

Vegetables

All vegetables should be organic. Most areas now have at least one local organic source, whether it's a food co-op, a health food store, or a farmer's market. Organic vegetables may cost a little more than grocery store produce, but it's money well spent. With the current escalation in the use of pesticides and chemicals to preserve foods, buying organic is actually much less expensive in the long run. Allergies and other health-related problems can be costly.

Organic food also tends to be seasonal, and eating seasonal produce is very favorable to the digestive process. As your body systems fluctuate with seasonal changes in order to achieve homeostasis, you are connected to your outer environment.

Consider growing some of your own vegetables. There are many positive aspects to having a garden, no matter how simple. Aside from creating your own source of organic produce, it is emotionally healing and very gratifying to put your hands into the earth and create sustenance for yourself.

Vegetables are the major component in a healing diet. Cooking vegetables can be a very creative pursuit. A few basic recipes follow. From simple steaming to more complicated casseroles or stews, vegetables should be a mainstay of every diet.

Surround yourself with vegetables—in the garden, on the counter in baskets, in the refrigerator, and, most of all, on your lunch and dinner plates.

Zucchini and Potatoes

1 onion, chopped	2 small potatoes, peeled and thinly sliced
3 to 6 cloves garlic, finely chopped	Salt and pepper, to taste
2 tablespoons parsley, minced	Parmesan cheese
2 to 4 tablespoons olive oil	2 fresh tomatoes (or 2 cups canned)
3 medium zucchini, thinly sliced	

Quickly sauté the onion, garlic, and parsley in olive oil.

Add zucchini and potatoes and cook over medium heat, stirring occasionally, for about 15 minutes. Season lightly with salt and pepper. Add tomatoes, cover, and simmer slowly for about 15 minutes longer. The potatoes and zucchini will be soft, browned, and infused with flavor.

Serve with a grating of Parmesan cheese.

Serves 4 as a side dish.

Optional: For added protein, add 6 ounces of diced, cooked tofu before serving.

Sautéed Greens

1 pound greens (chard, bok choy, kale, broccoli rabe)	2 to 4 cloves garlic, crushed
	2 to 4 tablespoons olive oil
1 onion, sliced	Salt and pepper, to taste

Wash greens well. Steam until tender (about 5 minutes) and set aside.

In frying pan, sauté onion and garlic in olive oil until golden. Remove from heat.

Add greens to the oil mixture and toss with salt and pepper. Cover and let sit until ready to serve. This is a good hot vegetable, but it also makes a wonderful sandwich filling, so make more than you need and store the leftovers in the refrigerator.

Serves 4 as a side dish.

Portobello Mushrooms

4 tablespoons olive oil	2 pounds portobello mushrooms, sliced
2 tablespoons red wine or balsamic vinegar	Pinch freshly ground fennel seeds
4 cloves garlic, crushed	Salt and pepper, to taste

Mix all ingredients and marinate for one hour. Arrange on a baking sheet and bake at 400 degrees Fahrenheit for 20 minutes, turning once.

Serves 6 as a side dish.

Vegetable Stir-Fry

Oil (toasted sesame oil or olive oil)	¼ head broccoli florets, broken apart
1 onion, chopped	1 cup peas
2 cloves garlic, chopped	½ pound mushrooms, sliced
2 medium zucchini, chopped	Mung beans
2 carrots, chopped	Soy sauce or tamari, to taste

Drizzle a little oil into a wok and sauté the onion and garlic until soft and clear.

Add the rest of the vegetables and the soy sauce or tamari and stir occasionally until done (about 20 minutes).

Serve over rice as a main dish (serves 2), use as a vegetable side dish (serves 4), or use as a sandwich filling.

Note: Just about any vegetables you like and/or have on hand can be substituted for the above ingredients.

Steamed Vegetables

Steaming vegetables is really simple. Put some water in the bottom of a saucepan, drop in the steamer, and arrange upon it the cleaned vegetable of your choice. Most vegetables take only minutes to steam—you'll have to check them at first until you get used to the process.

If you just use your imagination—a really wonderful thing to do in the kitchen—you will find yourself creating surprising combinations of your own favorite veggies.

When combining vegetables of different textures, begin with the hard vegetables first (carrots, yams), then add the softer ones (broccoli, zucchini).

Once they're steamed, you can really get creative with herbs and dressings to add delicious flavors.

Some examples:

- Steamed broccoli with fresh lemon juice and pepper
- Steamed asparagus with oil, balsamic vinegar, and Parmesan cheese
- Steamed carrots with honey and cinnamon
- Steamed sweet potatoes with maple syrup
- Steamed green beans with oil, salt, and pepper

Roasted Mixed Vegetables

Cut into bite-size pieces enough zucchini, yellow squash, carrots, red or white onions, eggplant, and red and/or green peppers to meet your serving requirements.

Toss with olive oil, salt, and pepper plus fresh or dried basil or rosemary.

Roast in oven at 375 degrees Fahrenheit for 35 to 40 minutes, removing from the oven once or twice to stir.

Winter Blend Roasted Vegetables

Use winter root vegetables such as potatoes, yams, rutabagas, turnips, carrots, and daikon and follow above directions. Instead of rosemary, try adding a pinch of garam masala (Indian spice mix).

Roasted Potatoes

White potatoes, sweet potatoes, or yams all work well in this recipe but should be roasted separately. Quantity depends on the number of people you are serving. For a side-dish portion, you should allow one potato per person.

Cut potatoes into uniform bite-size pieces and toss with olive oil, salt, pepper, and rosemary.

Roast in a 375 degree Fahrenheit oven for 35 to 40 minutes, removing once or twice to stir.

Onions that have been roasted separately may be added later.

Spicy version: Substitute a natural Cajun spice mix for the rosemary.

Rutabaga Sauté

1 onion, finely chopped
2 cloves garlic, minced
2 tablespoons olive oil

2 to 3 rutabagas, peeled and
    diced into 1-inch squares
Water
Salt and freshly ground pepper

Sauté garlic and onion in olive oil until lightly golden, about 2 to 3 minutes.

Add rutabagas and continue to cook until soft, about 15 minutes, adding water as necessary.

Add a dash of unrefined salt and freshly ground black pepper to taste.
Serves 4.

Brussels Sprouts and Tomatoes

1 small onion, chopped
2 cloves garlic, diced
2 tablespoons olive oil
1 small package (8 ounces) brussels
    sprouts, washed, dried, and cut in half

1 cup chopped tomatoes
1 tablespoon tamari

Sauté onion and garlic in olive oil.

Add brussels sprouts and sauté slowly for about 5 minutes.

Add tomatoes and tamari and simmer gently for 10 minutes.
Serves 4.

Spring Fiddlehead Fern Salad

1	pound fiddlehead ferns	2 to 3	tablespoons olive oil
⅓	cup dry coconut	½	onion, sliced
1	tablespoon sesame seeds		Salt and pepper, to taste
⅓	cup balsamic vinegar		

Boil 3 quarts of water, add fiddleheads, and cook for 15 minutes. Strain and place in bowl.

Toast dry coconut along with sesame seeds in dry pan until coconut begins to turn brown, being careful not to burn it.

Add to the cooked fiddleheads along with the rest of the ingredients. Mix well and serve.

Serves 4.

Wilted Spinach Salad

⅓	cup walnuts, halved	1	clove garlic, minced
1	pound spinach	3	tablespoons balsamic vinegar
1	small red onion, thinly sliced	6	ounces feta cheese
3	tablespoons currants (optional)	4	tablespoons olive oil

Roast walnuts in a 350 degree Fahrenheit oven for 5 to 7 minutes or until they smell toasty. Set them aside to cool.

Wash spinach well and remove stems. Cut large leaves in half (the small ones can be left whole). Put the spinach in a big bowl and toss it with the onion, currants (optional), roasted walnuts, garlic, and vinegar. Break up the cheese and crumble over the spinach.

Heat the olive oil in a skillet until it is very hot. Immediately pour over the salad, turning the leaves so that the hot oil coats and wilts as many leaves as possible. Serve immediately.

Serves 4.

Fish

Fresh fish is an excellent source of valuable nutrients that you just can't get from vegetables alone. Buy fish from your local health food store or a reliable market that sells fish from uncontaminated waters.

Fish rich in omega-3 oils include salmon, rainbow trout, tuna, mackerel, halibut, and cod.

Some general notes on fish:

- Three-quarters of a pound provides two generous servings.
- Steaming and oven-roasting are excellent ways to cook fish.
- Herbs and sauces add surprising flavors and nutrients. See Sauces, Dressings, and Spreads (pages 371 to 373).

Skillet Fish

1 pound salmon, or other fish	4 tablespoons olive oil
Flour	½ cup white wine (or water)
1 small bunch scallions, chopped	Salt and pepper
1 tablespoon parsley, finely chopped	1 lemon, quartered, for garnish
Lemon balm, to taste (optional)	

Dip fish lightly in flour and set aside. In a skillet, quickly sauté the scallions, parsley, and lemon balm in the olive oil.

Add the flour-coated fish and brown lightly on one side.

Turn, add wine (or water), and cover in order to steam the fish for the balance of its cooking time. Check for doneness in 5 minutes. Depending on thickness, 10 to 15 minutes' cooking time will suffice.

Season with salt and pepper, if desired.

Serve directly from the skillet, spooning pan juices over each serving. Garnish with lemon wedges.

Serves 3 to 4.

Steamed Salmon and Sage

10 to 12 fresh sage leaves

¾ to 1 pound salmon

Freshly ground pepper, to taste

1 lemon, quartered, for garnish

Arrange sage leaves in steamer basket and place salmon, skin side down, on top of them.

Steam 10 to 15 minutes, until salmon is pale in color and flakes easily.

Remove to serving platter, season with freshly ground pepper, and garnish with lemon wedges.

Serves 3 to 4.

Curried Fish

¼ cup sesame oil

1½ to 2 pounds mahi mahi or sea bass

8 ounces coconut milk

½ cup water

3 cloves garlic, crushed

1 whole bay leaf

2 tablespoons curry powder

¼ cup desiccated coconut

4 ounces pineapple chunks

Salt and pepper, to taste

In skillet, heat sesame oil and brown fish on both sides. Remove fish and set aside.

In same skillet, mix coconut milk, water, garlic, and bay leaf and cook over medium heat for about 10 minutes.

Add curry powder, desiccated coconut, and pineapple chunks and mix well.

Return fish to skillet, add salt and pepper to taste, and continue to cook for 5 to 10 minutes.

Serve with rice.

Serves 4 as a main dish.

Roasted Salmon with Greens

¾ pound salmon

½ pound dark greens (broccoli rabe, dandelions, nettles, chard)

1 bunch scallions, chopped

Olive oil

Salt and pepper

Mustard-Dill Sauce

In a 350 degree Fahrenheit oven, roast the salmon until pale and flaky (about 20 minutes).

Meanwhile, steam the greens until soft and drain.

Sauté the scallions in a little oil and, when translucent, add the drained greens along with salt and pepper to taste. Sauté for 5 minutes.

Remove salmon to serving platter and arrange the greens around the salmon as a border.

Top with Mustard-Dill Sauce (see page 372).

Serves 2 to 3.

Rainbow Trout

2 cloves garlic, minced

1 small onion, chopped finely

2 tomatoes, chopped

1 tablespoon soy sauce

2 tablespoons parsley, minced

Salt and pepper, to taste

2 fresh trout, cleaned and ready for stuffing

Mix all ingredients, except the fish, together in a bowl.

Stuff the trout, wrap in parchment paper, and place on baking sheet in oven.

Bake at 375 degrees Fahrenheit for about 30 minutes.

Serve with rice.

Serves 4.

Soy Foods

Soy foods, including soybeans, tofu, tempeh, miso, soy milk, and soy sauce are all excellent sources of protein, especially for vegetarians. They also happen to be the best source of genistein and other soy isoflavones, which have a particularly beneficial effect on hormonal receptor-type cancers as well as an antiangiogenesis effect on tumors of any kind.

Although soy foods are relatively unfamiliar in American diets, I recommend including them at least three to four times each week. The recipes included here are easy to prepare and are good examples of the diverse ways you can incorporate this important food group into your diet.

Lemon-Broiled Tempeh

1 12-ounce package tempeh

1 sliced onion

2 freshly squeezed lemons

2 tablespoons tamari

2 tablespoons toasted sesame seed oil

2 tablespoons untoasted sesame seed oil

3 medium zucchini, sliced

1 cup shiitake mushrooms, sliced

1 red pepper, cut into bite-size pieces

  Dash of ground pepper

  Splash of white wine (optional)

  Toasted almonds (optional)

Combine all ingredients, except almonds, in a glass baking dish and marinate for several hours or overnight.

Bake in a 400 degree Fahrenheit oven for 30 minutes, stirring occasionally to prevent sticking. After baking, finish by broiling for 10 minutes.

Serve over rice (a combination of basmati and wild rice is good) or grain. Garnish with toasted almond pieces if you wish.

Serves 4.

Tofu Chili

1 onion, finely chopped	3 teaspoons chile powder
2 tablespoons olive oil	½ teaspoon turmeric
½ pound tofu, chopped into 1-inch cubes	Salt and pepper, to taste
1 can organic crushed tomatoes	Topping: plain yogurt, diced onion,
3 cups cooked kidney beans	minced cilantro

Sauté onion in olive oil until translucent. Add tofu and continue to sauté for about 3 minutes. Add tomatoes, beans, and spices and stir well. Cook uncovered over low heat for about 30 minutes, stirring occasionally.

Serve over brown rice and top with yogurt, diced onion, and a sprinkling of minced cilantro.

Serves 4.

Asian Tofu with Bok Choy

1 pound tofu, extra firm, cut into 1-inch slices	3 cloves garlic, minced
	1 pound bok choy, chopped
2 tablespoons toasted sesame oil	1 to 2 tablespoons tamari
1 onion, sliced	1 tablespoon hulled sesame seeds

Sauté tofu in 1 tablespoon sesame oil until lightly browned. Set aside.

Sauté onion, garlic, and bok choy in 1 tablespoon sesame oil until bok choy is soft and wilted, about 10 to 15 minutes.

Return tofu to pan with vegetables, add tamari and sesame seeds, and mix well.

Serve over brown rice.

Serves 4 as a main dish.

Pasta, Rice, Grains

The pasta, rice, and grain family is an important part of a balanced diet. For vegetarians, this food group not only provides the main source of carbohydrates, but it also offers the accompaniment for other necessary nutrients, such as vegetables and legumes.

We prefer using organic pasta or pasta that is imported from Italy and made with semolina flour. There are unlimited ways to sauce your pasta—from the traditional Italian tomato sauce to plain steamed vegetables and a little olive oil. Pasta is truly a comfort food, and it can be used in most diets, no matter how restricted they may be during an illness or convalescence. For those sensitive to wheat, try 100 percent soba noodles, rice noodles, or pasta made from quinoa.

Rice, like pasta, is also a staple in many diets throughout the world and, when combined with beans, offers an important source of protein to those who do not eat meat. Of course, unrefined, long-grain brown rice is best, and once you get used to that flavor, you will eliminate the refined, white gummy-like rice from your pantry forever.

Other grains that are not so well known, such as millet and quinoa, are also good dietary choices. They just haven't had center stage yet in mainstream marketing. Buy them at your health food store.

Shiitake Mushrooms and Pasta

4 cloves garlic, chopped	Salt and pepper, to taste
1 onion, chopped	1 cup pasta water
3 tablespoons olive oil	¼ cup soy milk (optional)
½ pound shiitake mushrooms, sliced	1 pound spiral pasta, cooked
2 tablespoons parsley, chopped	

Sauté garlic and onion in oil until golden.

Add mushrooms, parsley, salt, and pepper. Sauté until tender, about 10 minutes.

Meanwhile, cook pasta according to package directions, reserving 1 cup of the liquid for sauce.

Add reserved pasta water (and soy milk, if desired) to mushrooms, heat thoroughly, and toss over pasta. Serve immediately.

Serves 4.

Vegetable Lasagna

1 pound lasagna (Barilla thin lasagna is recommended)
1 recipe tomato sauce (see page 372)

Cheese mixture:

1 pound tofu (silken texture)	2 eggs
½ pound mozzarella cheese	Parsley, chopped
½ pound ricotta cheese	

Filling mixture (include one of the following):

1 pound spinach, cleaned and steamed	2 medium zucchini, chopped
4 carrots, chopped	1 large onion, chopped
½ head broccoli, chopped	

Sauté these vegetables together until tender.

Mix the filling mixture with the cheese mixture and set aside.

Cover bottom of a large oblong baking pan with a little tomato sauce.

Lay out lasagna sheets (uncooked) over the sauce. Spoon a layer of the filling mixture over the lasagna. Repeat above steps until all ingredients are used.

Cover and bake at 400 degrees Fahrenheit for 45 minutes. Uncover and bake 15 minutes more or until sauce is bubbling.

Serves 4.

Pasta and Vegetables

1 pound pasta (your choice)	Salt and pepper
Sautéed vegetables (again, your choice)	Parmesan cheese
Olive oil	

This recipe may sound a little vague, but it is meant to be unique each time you make it. Check the refrigerator for ideas!

For example, for 4 servings, use about 1 onion, 4 carrots, 2 zucchini, ¼ pound green beans, and about 2 cups of fresh or frozen peas. Sauté all these together in a little olive oil for about 15 to 20 minutes (about as long as it takes to boil the water and cook the pasta).

Drain the pasta, toss with the cooked vegetables, and season with some oil, salt, pepper, and a shaking of Parmesan cheese.

You can use virtually any pasta or any vegetable that suits you. It works every time!

Serves 4.

Black Bean and Rice Burritos

4 cups cooked black beans

1 small onion, diced

1 tablespoon cilantro, finely chopped

1 teaspoon cumin

4 cups cooked brown rice

Chapati bread

Organic salsa

In a skillet, gently heat the cooked beans, add the onion, cilantro, and cumin, and simmer for a few minutes.

Assemble the burritos as follows: Spoon rice onto a chapati, followed by black beans, and top with salsa. Fold into burritos and serve immediately.

Serves 4.

Sauces, Dressings, Spreads

One of the keys to simple cooking is to have a good stockpile of sauce and dressing recipes. Pastas, rice, vegetables, salads, and fish dishes all benefit from a freshly made sauce. The bounty of herbs really shine in this category—they transform simple meals into wonderful taste treats.

Here are a few of our favorites—some are simple and some require a bit of time and patience, but they are all time-tested and really good.

Zennie's Salad Dressing

½ cup balsamic vinegar
½ cup flaxseed oil (keep refrigerated)
½ cup olive oil
1 clove garlic, crushed
½ teaspoon prepared mustard (not dried)

1 celery heart, chopped
Salt and pepper, to taste
1 to 2 teaspoons honey or maple syrup, to taste

Mix all ingredients well and store in the refrigerator in a covered jar. Will keep for a week. Use on salads or vegetables.

Ginger Salad Dressing

½ carrot, chopped
1 tablespoon ginger, grated
2 tablespoons onion, chopped
1 to 2 tablespoons toasted sesame oil

½ cup olive oil
Pinch dry mustard
1 tablespoon mirin (sweet rice-wine marinade)

Mix all ingredients well in blender and store in refrigerator. Use as a dressing on salad or vegetables.

Tofu Marinade

1 tablespoon toasted sesame oil
1 tablespoon regular sesame oil
1 tablespoon plus 1 teaspoon tamari
1 tablespoon plus 2 teaspoons maple syrup

1 tablespoon plus 1 teaspoon brown rice vinegar
1 to 2 tablespoons sesame seeds (optional)

Mix tofu marinade ingredients. Slice tofu into ¼- to ½-inch slices and marinate for several hours, or overnight. Bake in a 375 degree Fahrenheit oven until tofu is lightly browned, about 15 minutes.

Use slices as a snack by themselves, as a sandwich filler, or as part of a vegetable stir-fry. This recipe makes enough marinade for about 2 pounds of tofu. Keeps well in refrigerator.

Teriyaki Marinade

⅓ cup olive oil	1 tablespoon ginger, grated
⅓ cup soy sauce	2 cloves garlic, crushed
2 tablespoons toasted sesame oil	⅛ tablespoon dried mustard powder
½ cup mirin (sweet rice-wine marinade)	

Mix ingredients well and use as a marinade for fish or tofu. Store in refrigerator.

Tomato Sauce

2 to 6 cloves garlic, crushed	2 tablespoons olive oil
1 small onion, chopped	Red wine
2 tablespoons fresh basil	1 28-ounce can organic whole plum tomatoes
Optional: 1 tablespoon fresh rosemary or 1 to 2 tablespoons fresh oregano, finely chopped	

Sauté garlic, onion, and herbs in the olive oil. Add a little red wine and simmer for about 5 minutes. Crush the tomatoes and add to the sauce. Simmer slowly for 20 to 30 minutes.

Mustard-Dill Sauce

2 tablespoons organic Dijon mustard	1 teaspoon organic unrefined mayonnaise
Chopped fresh dill, to taste	

Mix ingredients well and store in refrigerator. An excellent spread for baked salmon.

Sprouted Hummus Spread

2 cups dried chickpeas
Water
1 tomato, chopped
4 stalks celery, chopped
4 cloves garlic, minced
1 teaspoon unrefined salt (or crumbled, dried organic seaweed)

1 to 2 tablespoons tahini
Juice of 1 lemon
1 teaspoon parsley, finely chopped
1 to 2 tablespoons olive oil
Pinch cayenne pepper (optional)

Using a sprouting jar, soak the beans overnight. Rinse daily, and allow the beans to sprout for 1 to 2 days.

When sprouted, mix beans with all other ingredients and place in food processor. Blend until you achieve the consistency you like.

Keep refrigerated and use as a sandwich spread or dip for fresh vegetables.

Variation: Substitute lentils for chickpeas and add ½ teaspoon curry powder.

Soups

Making soup is a wonderful thing to do. As a soup simmers, it fills your home with aromas that stimulate the appetite. Long regarded as basic sustenance, soup seems to bring out the best of each ingredient as the combination of vegetables and herbs blend their nutrients and flavors into a satisfying and hearty meal. Soup is easy to make, economical, and, especially for someone who is ill, an excellent way to take nourishment that is easily digestible.

Seasonal vegetables and herbs can combine to yield delicious health-enhancing brews from mild broths to thick, strongly flavored soups; the addition of beans can result in a hearty meal in and of itself. Included here are a few of our favorites, but don't hesitate to try different combinations, using ingredients you may have on hand. Soup making is an area where experimentation and resourcefulness can produce surprisingly good results.

Immune-Strengthening Soup

Sauté:

2 tablespoons toasted sesame oil	½ to 1 cup cubed tofu
1 chopped onion	2 cups chopped vegetables of choice
3 to 5 sticks astragalus	(carrots, celery, beet greens, cabbage,
3 to 5 cloves garlic	kale, daikon, lotus root, turnips, etc.)
2 to 3 pieces burdock	1 cup chopped mushrooms of choice
1 piece ginger	(shiitake, cordyceps, etc.)
1 to 2 reishi mushrooms, crumbled	½ cup wakame or kombu (seaweed)

Add:

8 cups spring or purified water

Bring to a boil, reduce heat, and simmer, covered, for 15 minutes.

Whisk:

2 to 3 tablespoons miso into small
    amount of soup stock and add to soup

Do not boil soup after miso is added.

Simmer for 1 to 2 hours. *Note:* Soup base may be started with beef bones to strengthen bone marrow, if needed.

Lentil Soup

²⁄₃ cup dried lentils

4 cups water

1 onion, chopped

4 carrots, chopped

2 stalks celery, chopped

Parsley

Thyme

Dill

Tarragon

1 cup tomato purée

Put the washed and drained lentils into a soup pot with the water, onion, carrots, and celery.

Simmer slowly for 1 hour, stirring occasionally and adding more water as needed.

Add herbs to taste, along with the tomato purée, and simmer slowly for 30 minutes more.

This soup is even better the next day.

Serves 4.

Miso Soup

1 onion, thinly sliced

3 carrots, chopped into matchsticks

2 stalks celery, chopped

¹⁄₃ pound tofu, cubed

3 tablespoons sesame oil

4 cups vegetable stock

1 strip kombu or wakame

Fresh juice of 1 small piece of ginger

Splash of tamari

2 to 3 teaspoons miso

1 scallion, chopped

1 squash, cubed (optional)

Sauté onion, carrots, celery, squash, and tofu in sesame oil.

Add stock, kombu, ginger, and tamari, and simmer for 30 minutes or until vegetables are tender. Add miso and stir well.

Garnish with chopped scallions.

Serves 4.

Arugula and Potato Soup

2 potatoes, peeled and cut into
   ½-inch slices

4 cups water

1 large bunch arugula

⅓ cup day-old bread, chopped into
   1-inch cubes

3 cloves garlic, minced

¼ teaspoon crushed red pepper flakes

2 tablespoons olive oil

   Salt and pepper

   Parmesan cheese

Put potatoes and water in a deep saucepan and bring the water to a boil. Reduce heat to medium and cook about 15 minutes, covered.

Wash arugula well, discard any thick stems, and chop. Add to soup pot with bread cubes and simmer for about 10 minutes.

Meanwhile, in small pan, slowly sauté the garlic and red pepper flakes in olive oil for about 2 to 3 minutes. Do not allow to brown. Add to soup pot and season with salt and pepper to taste.

Sprinkle with Parmesan cheese and serve piping hot.

Serves 4.

Baked Desserts

Perhaps because of the pace of life today, perhaps because everyone seems to work outside the home now, or perhaps because we have just gotten a little lazy, somehow baking at home has slipped away as an old-time habit. Try to change that—it will be so worthwhile!

Baking does take a little practice—you have to become familiar with your stove and its temperature fluctuations and the feel of flour and water as it becomes dough—but it's not nearly as complicated or difficult as you might think. It's actually very calming and surprisingly gratifying to turn out something that tastes delicious, is wholesome and nutritious, and makes your house smell fragrantly welcoming.

The first thing to consider is flour. We recommend Arrowhead Mills as the best organic brand; however, our first choice for flour is to buy the whole wheat fresh from your health food store or food cooperative and grind it yourself. We use an Osttiroler Betreidemuhlen wooden flour grinder; it just sits on the counter and we grind what we need when we need it. A grinder such as this is not inexpensive, but it is a one-time purchase that, over a lifetime of baking, surely pays for itself. Economics aside, the taste of freshly ground flour is a bonus. Nutty and sweet, you'll find that when you use it in your baked goods, you'll need very little additional sweetener.

To keep your immune system strong, avoid using sugar in your baked goods. Honey or maple syrup does the job when you need a sweetener, and every cell in your body will thank you for the substitution!

Following are a few of our most frequently used recipes. If you become interested in baking, and we hope that you do, there are many good books on baking out there. Better yet, once you get the feel for baking, perhaps you'll start creating recipes of your own.

Fruit Cobbler

3 cups fresh fruit (apples, peaches, pears, or whatever is in season)	4 tablespoons butter
1 tablespoon cinnamon	1 cup pastry flour
2 to 4 tablespoons maple syrup	1 teaspoon baking powder
	½ cup water

Combine fruit with cinnamon and maple syrup. Mix well and put into baking dish. Dot with 1 tablespoon of the butter.

Combine flour and baking powder in bowl. Cut in remaining 3 tablespoons butter until mixture looks like meal. Stir in water.

Drop by spoonfuls onto fruit. Bake 25 to 30 minutes in a 400 degree Fahrenheit oven, covered for the first 15 minutes. Then remove cover to finish baking. In this way, the top will brown but will not dry out.

This is a seasonal dessert—use whatever fruit is in season because that's when it's at its very best.

Serves 6.

Maple Blueberry Cake

Dry ingredients:

3½ cups freshly ground whole-wheat pastry flour	Pinch salt
1 tablespoon baking powder	Pinch nutmeg
1 teaspoon cinnamon	Pinch lemon peel, freshly ground

Liquid ingredients:

3 eggs, lightly beaten	¼ to ⅓ cup melted butter (or 2 tablespoons melted butter and
1 small container Stoneyfield low-fat organic blueberry yogurt	2 tablespoons organic sunflower oil)
½ to ⅓ cup maple syrup (Grade B is fine)	1 teaspoon vanilla (optional)
½ cup chopped walnuts (optional)	

Mix together dry ingredients and set aside.

When liquid ingredients are well blended, slowly add dry ingredients and mix well.

Add 2 cups fresh blueberries.

Bake at 350 degrees Fahrenheit for 35 to 45 minutes in a buttered 9-inch square baking pan. (You can also make muffins; decrease the baking time by 10 minutes.)

Maple Oat Wheat-Free Cookies

1 cup softened organic butter (or use safflower oil to avoid dairy)

1 cup maple syrup

1 tablespoon vanilla and/or ½ teaspoon almond extract

3 cups organic rolled oats

2 cups barley flour (or whole-wheat pastry flour, if you need to avoid wheat)

Optional additions: 1 tablespoon organic buttermilk powder, 1 teaspoon baking powder, 3 to 4 tablespoons organic chocolate chips, 1 to 3 tablespoons shredded coconut. If you like a super flat and crunchy cookie, omit the baking powder.

Place all ingredients in a large bowl and mix well.

Scoop by the teaspoon or tablespoon and press on cookie sheet pan in whatever size you like.

Bake at 325 degrees Fahrenheit for 15 minutes until done.

These simple cookies are wonderful and taste even better a few days later. The flavor of real maple syrup can't be beat.

Baked Apples

4 pippin or macoun apples

2 tablespoons maple syrup

½ cup raisins or currants

1 tablespoon cinnamon

Core the apples.

Combine the remaining ingredients, mix well, and fill each apple.

Place the stuffed apples in a shallow baking dish and add about ¼ inch of water.

Bake at 350 degrees Fahrenheit, uncovered, for about 40 minutes.

May be served warm, at room temperature, or cold. If you'd like a piping-hot dessert on a cold night, put these in the oven as you sit down to dinner—they'll be ready just in time for dessert.

Serves 4.

Baked Peaches

6 peaches, fresh, ripe, skinned,
    and cut into slices
⅓ cup honey

1 tablespoon cinnamon
¼ teaspoon nutmeg

Mix all ingredients in baking dish and bake for 15 to 20 minutes at 250 degrees Fahrenheit. Peaches will be warm but not overdone.

—Nutritional Smoothies and Other Drinks—

These blender drinks are very helpful for healing. They are easy to digest, their nutrients are immediately absorbable, and they are easy to make. They need to be made fresh daily and can be consumed for breakfast or throughout the day between meals. If you let them sit too long they may get thick, viscous, and mucilaginous because of the glycosaminoglycans and lignans present in the flaxseeds. If this happens, just add water, soy milk, aloe juice, or more fruit or vegetable juice.

The health benefits of these shakes are legion. Most important, they possess broad-spectrum, easily absorbable nutrition and can thus serve as superior options to the sugar-laden weight-gain drinks usually prescribed for cancer patients.

People who regularly drink these shakes for a month or two begin to show improvement in their health. Overall, there is an increase in energy, improved blood work, and high-quality weight gain (muscle-tissue growth). These foods feed and promote the health of the body, not the cancer.

Note: I suggest goat's milk yogurt instead of cow's milk; if it's unavailable, use organic yogurt. If you are allergic to milk products, use soy yogurt. Another option is amasaki, a thick, sweet, milklike drink made with koji rice that is easily digested. Instead of yogurt, fresh goat's milk, coconut milk, or creamed coconut (sugar-free) may be used.

Any fat-soluble supplements that you are taking, such as CoQ10, Beta-Plex, or vitamin E, can be added directly to this shake. The fatty acids in the shake will enhance the absorption of these nutrients.

Morning Smoothie

4 ounces maple or vanilla goat yogurt (optional dairy-free alternatives are sesame, almond, or soy milk)

1 level tablespoon flaxseeds, freshly ground

1 tablespoon SuproProtein 95

1 tablespoon chlorella (or Greens Plus)

1 tablespoon flaxseed oil (or 1 teaspoon Eskimo Oil)

½ cup fresh or frozen fruit of choice

Crushed ice

Mix all ingredients in blender. Blend on high speed for 2 minutes.

Some good fruit additions: blackberries, raspberries, strawberries, papaya, mango, or orange (use one whole orange, quartered, and leave the peel on).

Flaxseed and Chlorella Shake

6 ounces organic yogurt

4 ounces fresh organic juice or whole fruit (orange, papaya, banana, apple, strawberries, or any berries; or use a vegetable juice, such as carrot, beet, dark leafy greens, and asparagus purée)

1 teaspoon to 2 tablespoons flaxseed oil

1 teaspoon to 2 tablespoons chlorella

1 to 2 scoops Protein 95 (or any high quality supro soy protein)

1 tablespoons freshly ground flaxseeds

Mix all ingredients in blender.

Nutritional Smoothie Options

Under the guidance of a health care professional (nutritionist, herbalist, naturopath, or medical doctor), these blender drinks can be customized for specific conditions by using various additives. The options listed here are a few of the many ways to custom-blend nutritional smoothies. Generally, options are intended to be additions to the basic shake with the following exceptions: whey protein replaces soy protein, Greens Plus replaces chlorella, and Eskimo Oil replaces flaxseed oil. When quantities are given as a range (1 teaspoon to 2 tablespoons), start with the lower amount and increase gradually.

Option I: 1 to 4 teaspoons MCP (modified citrus pectin)

Option II: 1 to 2 teaspoons of EPA omega-3 rich oil (use Eskimo Oil by Tyler, see Resources)

Option III: 1 tablespoon MCT (medium-chain triglycerides) oil

Option IV: 1 to 2 tablespoons low-temperature whey protein (Immunocal or Probioplex by Metagenics, see Resources)

Option V: 8 to 10 drops Beta-Plex by Scientific Botanicals

Option VI: 1 to 4 teaspoons glutamine powder

Option VII: Use soy milk or aloe leaf juice in place of yogurt and/or juice.

Option VIII: 1 to 4 capsules of lipase or papaya enzymes, to improve digestibility and assimilation for the very weak or those recovering from intensive surgery.

Option IX: 5 to 10 fresh almonds or 1 teaspoon fresh almond butter or sesame seeds. Soak almonds or sesame seeds overnight before using.

Option X: 1 to 2 tablespoons lecithin.

Cranberry Juice

1 pound cranberries, cleaned
3 quarts water

⅓ to ½ cup honey

Place cranberries and water in large pot. Bring to boil.

Remove from heat and let stand until cool enough to handle.

Pour off and reserve most of the liquid.

Mix the remaining berries and liquid (a little at a time) in a blender and then strain into the reserved liquid.

Add honey, stir, and refrigerate. Will keep for several days.

Sesame Seed Milk

1 pint water
3 heaping tablespoons sesame seeds

1 to 2 tablespoons honey
½ teaspoon vanilla

Boil water in a small pan. Remove from heat and add sesame seeds. Cover and let sit for 1 to 3 hours.

Place in blender and blend at high speed. Add honey and a splash of vanilla and blend again.

Strain and serve. Refrigerate leftovers and use within 3 days.

For those who have trouble digesting cow's milk or soy milk, this is a wonderful alternative.

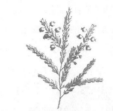

Conclusion

The human body is the universe in miniature. That which cannot be found in the body is not to be found in the universe. Hence the philosopher's formula that the universe within reflects the universe without. It follows therefore that if our knowledge of our own body could be perfect, we would know the universe.

—*Mahatma Gandhi*

Medicine and health care ideally should be an integrated system that encompasses all forms of medical techniques, philosophies, and practices. The World Health Organization has proclaimed:

1. The enjoyment of the highest attainable standard of health is one of the fundamental rights of every human being.

2. Health is more than the absence of illness; it is an active state of physical, emotional, mental, and social well-being.

3. Governments must give adequate importance to the utilization of traditional systems of medicine with appropriate regulations as suited to national health systems.

Unfortunately, a highly polarized situation exists in the United States today that must be resolved if we are to achieve the goals stated by the World Health Organization. Meanwhile, the incidence of cancer, along with the death rates from cancer, continues to rise. The average survival time for people with cancers of the breast, lung, ovary, or prostate has not changed dramatically in the last decade. On a more positive note, progress has been made in treating childhood leukemia, lymphoma, Hodgkin's disease and germ-cell cancers such as testicular cancer, but even here, we still have far to go. The nation's budget for cancer exceeds five billion dollars. The Federal government alone spends almost two billion dollars per year on cancer research.[1] Despite education and prevention, there have been no major changes in the incidence of cancer.

The battling between proponents of different approaches to curing cancer only exacerbates the problem. The cancer establishment has characterized natural adjunctive therapies as the work of quacks, offering questionably "miraculous" cures to desperate and hopeless cancer victims, while the proponents of alternative therapies have depicted established therapies as a "cut, burn, and poison" approach that is completely profit-driven. Although I believe there is some kernel of truth in both these exaggerations, it is unproductive to stereotype either side in this way. Who benefits? Surely not those who have cancer. We need to respect each other. We need to talk with each other. We need to put our resources together. This is what I am striving for.

Adjunctive nutritional therapies aren't simply less invasive options to replace surgery, radiation, or chemotherapy; they can also be used to enhance the effectiveness of these conventional treatments, reduce recurrence of the cancer, improve quality of life, and increase survival.

Conventional therapies focus on the question: "What is the most effective way to kill the cancer?" Holistic medicine, including herbalism and other natural treatments, focuses on the question: "What is the most effective way to enhance the body's ability to fight the cancer?"

Because modern medicine has tried to function solely in a "scientific" way, it has sacrificed compassion. As Larry Dossey writes in one of his early books,

"Without the catalyst of love and caring, medicine becomes a mere manipulation of tissues, an orchestration of chemistry."

Conventional and holistic practitioners must work together in a compassionate way to help those afflicted with cancer, using any effective treatment available. With herbs, proper diet, and lifestyle guidelines to enhance each patient's vitality, we can create the best physical environment for patients to fight their cancers and potentiate their own innate healing abilities.

Quality of life is something rarely studied or even discussed when it comes to conventional cancer therapies and cancer patients. Many times the therapy itself diminishes the qualify of life. I believe it is time to weigh this in the decision-making process, especially with advanced cancer or those cancers for which there is little or no benefit to be derived from any invasive cancer therapy. Quality of life should also be considered when it comes to unnecessary invasive testing. Too often we make the mistake of thinking that modern medicine has all the answers.

When a patient comes to the last days of his physical life in a hospital, he is often drugged out of consciousness while family and loved ones look on helplessly and doctors reassure them that nothing more can be done. I feel strongly that what sick people need is loving care—at home, whenever possible, surrounded by their own families and in their own beds; they need nourishing foods, like homemade soups and fresh juices; most of all, they need compassion. If I were sick and in my last days, this is what I would want rather than a last-ditch surgical procedure, or even worse, an experimental chemotherapy that might keep me alive for another few days so that I can lie in pain in a hospital bed. I think we need to look at the big picture when considering what course to follow. Most of all, we need to feel love for the human being who is ill and dying, and we need to pray. Through loving prayer comes clarity and peace.

I hope that this book will help you or your loved ones. I am thankful to God for giving me the grace to write this book. Works of love are a way to become closer to God; the more we help each other, the more we love God. We who work with cancer must keep in mind that we are only humble instruments and servants of the great Physician, and that love is the greatest healer of all.

Peace be to you.

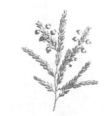

Resources

The resources mentioned throughout this book are listed in the left-hand column below in alphabetical order. To the right of each resource is the name of the company that distributes it. Beginning on page 391, each company is listed alphabetically with its address and phone number.

Products	*Distributor*
Aqueous Liver Extract™	Phyto Pharmica
Arnica-Ginger Gel™	New Chapter
Atomidine™	Heritage Village
Beta-Plex™	Scientific Botanicals
Bio Pro Protein A™	Bio-Nutritional Formulas
Biogestin	AgriGenic Food Corp.
Black Cohosh Extract	Source Naturals
Breast Basics™	New Chapter
Cellular Forte (IP6)™	Phyto Pharmica
Chem-Defense™	Source Naturals
Chlorella	New Chapter
Clinical Nutrients Antioxidant	Phyto Pharmica

Products	*Distributor*
Composition-A	Health Concerns
Cyto-Redoxin™	Tyler Encapsulations
DGL (Rhizinate)	Phyto Pharmica
Earth Salt	Herb Pharm
Eskimo-3™ (Eskimo Oil)	Tyler Encapsulations
Evening Primrose Oil	Source Naturals
Every Man II™	New Chapter
Every Woman II™	New Chapter
FemTone™	Phyto Pharmica
Folirinse™	Scientific Botanicals
Glucosamine Sulfate	Phyto Pharmica
Greens Plus®	Orange Peel Enterprises
Harmonizer	Nutritional Therapeutics
Hepastat™	Botaniclab
Herbal Ed's Salve	Herb Pharm
Herbal Suppositories for vaginal dryness and infection	Earth's Harvest
Hesperidin™	Thorne Research
Hydroxy Folate™	Scientific Botanicals
Lacto Brev™	Source Naturals
Laktoferrin™	Allergy Research Group
Lavender Poke Oil	WellSprings Center for Natural Healing
Maine Coast Seaweeds	Ryan Drum
Marrow Plus™	Health Concerns
Melazepam (Azelaic Acid)	Emerson Ecologics
Modified Citrus Pectin	Source Naturals
Multi-Pure Water Filter	Multi-Pure Corporation
Ocean Herbs™	New Chapter
PB8®	Nutrition Now, Inc.
PC SPES®	Botaniclab
PCO Phytosome™	Phyto Pharmica
Pectasol MCP	Source Naturals
Pregnenolone	Life Link

Probioplex®	Metagenics
Protein 290	Country Life
Protein 95	Nature's Life
Reishi 5™	New Chapter
Resveratrol	Source Naturals
Saccharomyces Boulardii	Allergy Research Group
Selensaff™	Scientific Botanicals
7-Keto (DHEA)	Phyto Pharmica
Soy Power	Nutritional Therapeutics
SP500 (Spleen Extract)™	Phyto Pharmica
SPES®	Botaniclab
SPES I®	Botaniclab
SPES M®	Botaniclab
Super-Tonic™	Pioneer Nutritional Formulas
Throat Care	Nutritional Therapeutics
Tooth and Gum Tonic™	Dental Herb Company
Two Immortals™	Health Concerns
Udo's Choice Oil	Flora
Varicosin™	Phyto Pharmica
Wobenzym®	Marlyn Healthcare Group
Women's Transition	Pioneer Nutritional Formulas
Zinc (Whole Food Complex)	New Chapter

DISTRIBUTORS

AgriGenic Food Corp.
5152 Bolsa Avenue, Suite 101
Huntington Beach, CA 92649
1-800-788-1084

Allergy Research Group
Distributed by Emerson Ecologics, Inc.
18 Lomar Park
Pepperell, MA 01463
1-800-654-4432

Bio-Nutritional Formulas
106 E. Jericho Turnpike
Mineola, NY 11501
1-800-950-8484
Fax: 1-800-321-2573

Botaniclab
2900-B Saturn Street
Brea, CA 92821
1-800-242-5555
Fax: (714) 524-5533

Cardiovascular Research
Distributed by Emerson Ecologics, Inc.
18 Lomar Park
Pepperell, MA 01463
1-800-654-4432

Country Life
101 Corporate Drive
Hauppauge, NY 11788
1-800-645-5768

Dental Herb Company
P.O. Box 687
78 Main Street
Northampton, MA 01061
1-800-747-4372

Earth's Harvest, Inc.
Gresham, OR 97030
1-800-428-3308

Emerson Ecologics, Inc.
18 Lomar Park
Pepperell, MA 01463
1-800-654-4432

Flora, Inc.
P.O. Box 73
805 E. Badger Road
Lynden, WA 98264
(360) 354-2110
Fax: (360) 354-5355

Health Concerns
8001 Capwell Drive
Oakland, CA 94621
(510) 639-0280
Fax: (510) 639-9140

Herb Pharm
P.O. Box 116
20260 Williams Highway
Williams, OR 97544
(541) 846-6262
Fax: (541) 846-6112

Herbalist & Alchemist, Inc. (High Quality Extracts)
51 S. Wandling Avenue
Washington, NJ 07882
(908) 689-9020

Heritage Village
Distributed by Threshold Enterprises, Ltd.
23 Janis Way
Scotts Valley, CA 95066
1-800-777-5677

Life Link
P.O. Box 1299
Grover Beach, CA 93483
1-888-433-5266

Marlyn Healthcare Group
14851 N. Scottsdale Road
Scottsdale, AZ 85254
1-800-4-MARLYN

MediHerb (High Quality Extracts)
P.O. Box 713
Warwick, Queensland 4370
Australia
(61) 7-4661-0788

Metagenics North East
P.O. Box 848
Kingston, NH 03848
1-800-343-3965

Multi-Pure Corporation
P.O. Box 4179
Chatsworth, CA 91313
1-800-622-9206

Nature's Herbs
Quality Drive
American Fork, UT 84003
1-800-437-4372

Nature's Life
MK Healthfood Distribution
7180 Lampson Avenue
Garden Grove, CA 92841
1-800-854-6837

New Chapter
22 High Street
Brattleboro, VT 05301
(802) 257-0018
Fax: (802) 257-0652

Nutrition Now, Inc.
6350 N.E. Campus Drive
Vancouver, WA 98661
1-800-929-0418

Nutritional Therapeutics, Inc.
P.O. Box 5963
Hauppauge, NY 11788
1-800-982-9158
Fax: (516) 979-1572

Orange Peel Enterprises
2183 Ponce deLeon Circle
Vero Beach, FL 32960
1-800-643-1210
Fax: (561) 562-9848

Phyto Pharmica
P.O. Box 174
825 Challenger Drive
Green Bay, WI 54305
1-800-553-2370
Fax: (920) 469-4418
(sold in health food stores under the label Enzymatic Therapy)

Pioneer Nutritional Formulas
304 Shelburne Center Road
Shelburne Falls, MA 01370
(413) 625-8212
Fax: (413) 625-9619

Ryan Drum, Ph.D.
8 Knoway
Waldron Island, WA 98297

Scientific Botanicals Co., Inc.
P.O. Box 31131
Seattle, WA 98103
(206) 527-5521

Source Naturals
Distributed by Threshold Enterprises, Ltd.
23 Janis Way
Scotts Valley, CA 95066
1-800-777-5677

Thorne Research
Distributed by Emerson Ecologics
18 Lomar Park
Pepperell, MA 01463
1-800-654-4432

Tyler Encapsulations
2204-8 NW Birdsdale
Gresham, OR 97030
(503) 661-5401
Fax: (503) 666-4913

WellSprings Center for Natural Healing, Inc. East
2226 Black Rock Turnpike
Fairfield, CT 06432
(203) 333-6007
Fax: (203) 333-6093

WellSprings Center for Natural Healing, Inc. West
1639 Jackson Road
Ashland, OR 97520
(541) 488-3130
Fax: (541) 488-3133

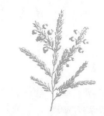

References

INTRODUCTION

1. D. Hever, "The Role of Nutrition in Cancer Prevention and Control," *Oncology* 6 (2 supp): 9–14 (1992).

CHAPTER 2

1. S. Epstein, "Winning the War Against Cancer? . . . Are They Even Fighting It?" *The Ecologist* 28 (2) (March/April 1998).
2. M.B. Sporn, "The War on Cancer," *Lancet* 347 (9012): 1377–81 (1996).
3. National Cancer Institute, *U.S. Bureau of the Census*, 1998.
4. J. Marx, "Oncogenes Reach a Milestone," *Science* 266 (5193): 1942–44 (1994).
5. M.T. Huang, ed., *Food Phytochemicals for Cancer Prevention I, Fruits and Vegetables* (Washington, D.C.: ACA Symposium Series 546), 49–50.
6. W.H. Lewis and M.P.F. Elvin-Lewis, *Medical Botany* (New York: John Wiley & Sons, 1977), 115.

7. A. Ensminger et al., *Foods & Nutrition Encyclopedia, 2d ed.* (Boca Raton, Fla.: CRC Press, 1994), 319–24.

8. D. Forman et al., "Cancer of the Liver and the Use of Oral Contraceptives," *British Medical Journal* 292: 1357–61 (1986).

9. N.C. Lee et al., "A Case-control Study of Breast Cancer and Hormonal Contraception in Costa Rica," *Journal of the National Cancer Institute* 79 (6): 1247–54 (1987).

10. C. Paul et al., "Depo Medroxyprogesterone (Depo-Provera) and Risk of Breast Cancer," *British Medical Journal* 299 (6702): 759–62 (1989).

11. L. Bergkvist et al., "The Risk of Breast Cancer After Estrogen and Estrogen-Progestin Replacement," *New England Journal of Medicine* 321 (5): 293–7 (1989).

12. X.Q. Shan et al., "Glutathione-Dependent Protection Against Oxidative Injury," *Pharmacology Therapeutics* 47 (1): 61–71 (1990).

13. G. Olenschager et al., "Reduced Glutathione and Anthocyans: Redox Cycling and Redox Recycling in Living Systems," *Praxis-Telegramm* 6: 1–20.

14. S. Cascinu et al., "Neuroprotective Effect of Reduced Glutathione on Cisplatin-based Chemotherapy in Advanced Gastric Cancer: A Randomized Double-Blind Placebo-Controlled Trial," *Journal of Clinical Oncology* 13 (1): 26–32 (1995).

15. J.F. Smyth et al., "Glutathione Reduces the Toxicity and Improves Quality of Life of Women Diagnosed with Ovarian Cancer Treated with Cisplatin: Results of a Double-Blind, Randomised Trial," *Annals of Oncology* 8 (6): 569–73 (1997).

16. T.M. Hagen et al., "Glutathione Uptake and Protection Against Oxidative Injury in Isolated Kidney Cells," *Kidney International* 34 (1): 74–81 (1988).

17. K.J. Pienta et al., "Inhibition of Spontaneous Metastasis in a Rat Prostate Cancer Model by Oral Administration of Modified Citrus Pectin," *Journal of the National Cancer Institute* 87 (5): 348–53 (1995).

18. H.I. Robins et al., "Cytotoxic Interactions of Tumor Necrosis Factor, Melphalan and 41.8 Degrees C Hyperthermia," *Cancer Letters* 89 (1): 55–62 (1995).

19. I.B. Shchepotin, "Hyperthermia and Verapamil Inhibit the Growth of Human Colon Cancer Xenografts *in Vivo* Through Apoptosis," *Anticancer Research* 17 (3C): 2213–16 (1997).

CHAPTER 3

1. R.R. Watson and S.I. Mufti, *Nutrition and Cancer Prevention* (Boca Raton, Fla.: CRC Press, Inc., 1996), 6–8.

2. J. Beasley, M.D. and J. Swift, "Impact of Nutrition, Environment and Lifestyle on the Health of Americans," *Kellogg Report, Chapter 3D* (Annandale-on-Hudson, N.Y.: Bard College Center, 1989), 73–81.

3. J.L. Freudenheim et al., "Premenopausal Breast Cancer Risk and Intake of Vegetables, Fruits and Related Nutrients," *Journal of the National Cancer Institute* 88 (6): 340–48 (1996).

4. G. Block et al., "Fruits, Vegetables, and Cancer Prevention: A Review of the Epidemiological Evidence," *Nutrition and Cancer* 18 (1): 1–29 (1992).

5. E. Negri et al., "Vegetable and Fruit Consumption and Cancer Risk," *International Journal of Cancer* 48 (3): 350–54 (1991).

6. S.A. Olivera and M.P. Osborne, "Diet, Breast Cancer, and Case-Controlled Studies," *Lancet* 34 (9012): 1346 (1996).

7. M.A. Morse et al., "Effects of Aromatic Isothiocyanates on Tumorigenicity, 06-Methylguanine Formation, and Metabolism of the Tobacco-Specific Nitrosamine 4-(Methylnitrosamino)-1-(3-Pyridyl)-1-Butanone in A/J Mouse Lung," *Cancer Research* 49 (11): 2894–97 (1989).

8. J.W. Fahey et al., "Broccoli Sprouts: An Exceptionally Rich Source of Inducers of Enzymes that Protect Against Chemical Carcinogens," *Proceedings of the National Academy of Science USA* 94 (19): 10367–72 (1997).

9. J.J. Michnovicz et al., "Changes in Levels of Urinary Estrogen Metabolites After Oral Indole-3-Carbinol Treatment in Humans," *Journal of the National Cancer Institute* 89 (10): 718–23 (1997).

10. J. Heinerman, *Encyclopedia of Fruits, Vegetables and Herbs* (West Nyack, N.Y.: Parker Publishing, 1988), 29–30.

11. J.A. Milner and L.M. Knowles, "Garlic Constituents Alter Cell Progression and Proliferation," *FASEB Journal* 11: A422 (1997).

12. "Garlic Helps Inhibit Cancer," *The Nutrition Report* (January, 1994), 3.

13. J. Raloff, "Aged Garlic Could Slow Prostate Cancer," *Science News Online* (April 19, 1997).

14. Hans A. Nieper, M.D., *New Horizons in Health—Cancer* (Richland Center, Wisc.: A. Keith Brewer Science Library, Admiral Ruge Archives of Bio-Physics and Future Science, 1989), 2–3.

15. E.M. Daniel and G.D. Stoner, "The Effects of Ellagic Acid and 13-Cis-Retinoic Acid on N-Nitrosobenzylmethylamine-induced Esophageal Tumorigenesis in Rats," *Cancer Letters* 56 (2): 117–24 (1991).

16. R.R. Watson and J. Lee, "Cranberry: A Role in Health Promotion," *Nutrients and Foods in Aids* (Boca Raton, Fla.: CRC Press, 1998), 217–22.

17. S.A. Oliveria and M.P. Osborne, "Diet, Breast Cancer and Case-Controlled Studies," op. cit.

18. M.R. Werbach, M.D., "Immunodepression," *Basic and Clinical Immunology, 4th ed.* (Los Altos, Calif.: Lange Publications, 1982).

19. M.F. McCarty, "Fish Oil May Impede Tumor Angiogenesis and Invasiveness by Down-Regulating Protein Kinase C and Modulating Eicosanoid Production," *Medical Hypotheses* 46: 107–15 (1996).

20. A. Biffi et al., "Antiproliferative Effect of Fermented Milk on the Growth of a Human Breast Cancer Cell Line," *Nutrition and Cancer* 28 (1): 93–9 (1997).

21. L. He et al., "Isoprenoids Suppress the Growth of Murine B16 Melanomas *in vitro* and *in vivo*," *Journal of Nutrition* 127: 668–74 (1997).

22. R. Medenica et al., "Antiangiogenic Activity of *Negella Sativa* Plant Extract in Cancer Therapy," *Proceedings of the Annual Meeting of the American Association of Cancer Research* 38: A1377 (1997).

23. T. Ong et al., "Comparative Antimutagenicity of 5 Compounds Against 5 Mutagenic Complex Mixtures in *Salmonella Typhimurium* Strain TA98," *Mutation Research* 222 (1): 19–25 (1989).

24. B. Jenson, *Jewel of the Far East* (Escondido, Calif.: B. Jenson, 1992), 54–56.

25. D.P. Rose and M.A. Hatala, "Dietary Fatty Acids and Breast Cancer Invasion and Metastasis," *Nutrition and Cancer* 21 (2): 103–11 (1994).

26. "Fish Oil May Protect Against Colon Cancer," *Family Practice News* (March 1, 1994), 7.

27. K.P. Cantor et al., "Bladder Cancer, Drinking Water Source, and Tap Water Consumption: A Case-Controlled Study," *Journal of the National Cancer Institute* 79 (6): 1269–79 (1987).

28. R. R. Watson and S. Mufti, *Nutrition and Cancer Prevention* (Boca Raton, Fla.: CRC Press, 1996), 99.

29. L. Kohlmeier et al., "Adipose Tissue Transfatty Acids and Breast Cancer in the European Community Multicenter Study on Antioxidants, Myocardial Infarction and Breast Cancer," *Cancer Epidemiology, Biomarkers and Prevention* 6 (9): 705–10 (1997).

30. P. Greenwald, B.S. Krammer, and D.L. Weed, *Cancer Prevention and Control* (New York: Marcel Dekker, 1995), 353–69.

CHAPTER 4

1. Jinhuang Zhou, M.D. and Ganzhong Liu, M.D., *Recent Advances in Chinese Medicine* (Beijing, China: Science Press, 1991), 236–60.
2. J. Boik, *Cancer and Natural Medicine* (Princeton, Minn.: Oregon Medical Press, 1995), 58–64.
3. W. Zhang et al., "Growth Inhibition and Apoptosis in Human Neuroblastoma SK-N-SH Cells Induced by Hypericin, a Potent Inhibitor of Protein Kinase C," *Cancer Letters* 96 (1): 31–35 (1995).
4. P. deWitte et al., "Inhibition of Epidermal Growth Factor Receptor Tyrosine Kinase Activity by Hypericin," *Biochemical Pharmacology* 46 (11): 1929–36 (1993).
5. E. Turley and D. Moore, "Hyaluronate Binding Proteins Also Bind to Fibronectin, Laminin and Collagen," *Biochemical and Biophysical Research Communications* 121 (3): 808–14 (1984).
6. T.D. Babu et al., "Cytotoxic and Anti-tumor Properties of Certain Taxa of Umbelliferae with Special Reference to Centella Asiatica (L.) Urban," *Journal of Ethnopharmacology* 48 (1): 53–7 (1995).
7. T.K. Yun and S.Y. Choi, "A Case-Control Study of Ginseng Intake and Cancer," *International Journal of Epidemiology* 19 (4): 871–76 (1990).
8. J. Boik, *Cancer and Natural Medicine* (Princeton, Minn.: Oregon Medical Press, 1995), 123.
9. A. Schauss, Ph.D., "Cat's Claw," *Natural Medical Journal* 16–19 (1998).
10. M.M. Taketo, "Cyclooxygenase-2 Inhibitors in Tumorigenesis," *Journal of the National Cancer Institute* 90 (20): 1529–36 (1998).
11. Eric J. Lien and Wen Li, *Anticancer Chinese Drugs* (Taiwan, R.O.C.: Oriental Healing Arts Institute, 1995), 21.
12. M.A. Pereira et al., "Effects of the Phytochemicals, Curcumin and Quercetin, upon Azoxymethane-Induced Colon Cancer and 7,12-Dimethylbenz(a)anthracene-Induced Mammary Cancer in Rats," *Carcinogenesis* 17 (6): 1305–11 (1996).
13. K. Krishnaswamy et al., "Retardation of Experimental Tumorigenesis and Reduction of DNA Adducts by Turmeric and Curcumin," *Nutrition and Cancer* 30 (2): 163–66 (1998).
14. A. Khafif et al., "Quantitation of Chemopreventive Synergism Between (-) epigallocatechin-3 fallate and Curcumin in Normal, Premalignant and Malignant Human Oral Epithelial Cells," *Carcinogenesis* 19 (3)L 419–24 (1998).

15. Sreejayan and M.N. Rao, "Nitric Oxide Scavenging by Curcuminoids," *Journal of Pharmacy and Pharmacology* 49 (1): 105–57 (1997).

16. G. Garcia-Carde and J. Folkman, "Is There a Role for Nitric Oxide in Tumor Angiogenesis?" *Journal of the National Cancer Institute* 90 (8): 560–61 (1998).

17. M.C. Reccio et al., "Anti-inflammatory Activity of Saikosaponins from Hetermorpha Trifoliata," *Journal of Natural Products* 58 (1): 140-44 (1995).

18. Y. Motoo and N. Sawabu, "Antitumor Effects of Saikosaponins, Baicalin and Baicalein and Human Hepatoma Cell Lines," *Cancer Letters* 86 (1): 91–95 (1994).

19. S. Sinclair et al., "Chinese Herbs: A Clinical Review of Astragalus, Ligusticum and Schizandra," *Alternative Medical Review* 3 (5): 338–44 (1998).

20. M. Wahlstrom, "Adaptogens," *Herbal Healthline* (3): 13 (1987).

21. M. Nomura et al., "Gomisin A, a Lignan Component of Schizandra Fruits, Inhibits Development of Preneoplastic Lesions in Rat Liver by 3'-methyl-4-dimethylamino-azobenzene," *Cancer Letters* 76: 11–18 (1994).

22. N. Ahmad et al., "Green Tea Constituent Epigallocatechin-3-gallate and Induction of Apoptosis and Cell Cycle Arrest in Human Carcinoma Cells," *Journal of the National Cancer Institute* 89 (24): 1881–86 (1997).

23. S. Okabe et al., "Mechanisms of Growth Inhibition of Human Lung Cancer Cell Line, PC-9, by Tea Polyphenols," *Japanese Journal of Cancer Research* 88 (7): 639–43 (1997).

24. H.F. Stich, "Teas and Tea Components as Inhibitors of Carcinogen Formation in Model Systems and Man," *Preventive Medicine* 21: 337–84 (1992).

25. S.K. Katiyar et al., "Green Tea in Chemoprevention of Cancer," *Comprehensive Therapies* (10): 3–8 (1992).

26. H. Hibasami et al., "Induction of Apoptosis in Human Stomach Cancer Cells by Green Tea Catechins," *Oncology Report* 5 (2): 527–29 (1998).

27. S.H. Gohla et al., "Mitogenic Activity of High Molecular Polysaccharide Fractions Isolated from the Cupressaceae Thuja Occidentale L.I. Macrophage-dependent Induction of CD-4-positive T-helper (TH+) Lymphocytes," *Leukemia* 2 (8): 528–33 (1988).

28. E. Finley, M.D., *Eclectic Medical Journal* 2 (5): 2–3 (1933).

29. J.L. Poyet and A. Hoeveler, "cDNA Cloning and Expression of Pokeweed Antiviral Protein from Seeds in Escherichia Coli and Its Inhibition of Protein Synthesis *in Vitro*," *FEBS Letters* 406 (1–2): 97–100 (1997).

30. N. E. Tumer et al., "C-terminal Deletion Mutant of Pokeweed Antiviral Protein Inhibits Viral Infection But Does Not Depurinate Host Ribosomes," *Proceedings of the National Academy of Science USA* 94 (8): 3866–71 (1997).

31. H. A. Nieper, M.D., *New Horizons in Health—Cancer* (Richland Center, Wisc.: A. Keith Brewer Science Library, Admiral Ruge Archives of Biophysics and Future Science, 1989), 1–2.

32. K. Umehara et al., "Studies on Differentiation Inducers. VI. Lignan Derivatives from Arctium Fructus (2)," *Chemical Pharmacy Bulletin* 44 (12): 2300–4 (1996).

33. D. Waltregny et al., "Independent Prognostic Value of the 67-kd Laminin Receptor in Human Prostate Cancer," *Journal of the National Cancer Institute* 89 (16): 1224–27 (1997).

34. H.Y. Hsu, "Treating Cancer with Chinese Herbs," *Chemistry of Chinese Herb Drugs* (Taiwan, R.O.C.: Brion Research Institute of Taiwan, 1979), 205–40.

35. E.J. Lien and W. Li, *Anticancer Chinese Drugs* (Taiwan, R.O.C.: Oriental Healing Arts Institute, 1985), 85.

36. Ibid., 71–79.

37. D. Brown, N.D., *Quarterly Review of Natural Medicine* (Winter 1995), 283–87.

38. M.O. Ripple et al., "Prooxidant-Antioxidant Shift Induced by Androgen Treatment of Human Prostate Carcinoma Cells," *Journal of the National Cancer Institute* 89 (1): 40–48 (1997).

39. D. Thornes et al., "Prevention of Early Recurrence of High Risk Malignant Melanoma by Coumarin. Irish Melanoma Group," *European Journal of Surgical Oncology* 15 (5): 431–35 (1989).

40. Y. Arase et al., "The Long Term Efficacy of Glycyrrhizin in Chronic Hepatitis C Patients," *Cancer* 79 (8): 1494–500 (1997).

41. K. Kitamura et al., "Baicalin, an Inhibitor of HIV-1 Production *in Vitro*," *Antiviral Research* 37 (2): 131–40 (1998).

42. I.M. van Loon, N.D., "The Golden Root: Clinical Applications of Scutellaria Baicalensis George Flavonoids as Modulators of the Inflammatory Response," *Alternative Medicine Review* 2 (6): 472–80 (1997).

43. P. Kaufman et al., *Natural Products from Plants* (Boca Raton, Fla.: CRC Press, 1998), 172–73.

44. V. Sodhi, N.D., "Ayurvedic Immune Enhancement and Anti-Aging (Rasayan) Therapies," *Gaia Symposium Proceedings on Naturopathic Herbal Medicine* (1993), 98–99.

45. S. Holt, M.D. and L. Comac, *Miracle Herbs* (Seacaucus, N.J.: Birch Lane Press, 1998), 107–14.

46. P.U. Devi, "Withania Somnifera Dunal (Ashwagandha): Potential Plant Source of a Promising Drug for Cancer Chemotherapy and Radiosensitization," *Indian Journal of Experimental Biology* 34 (10): 927–32 (1996).

47. M. Ziauddin et al., "Studies on the Immunomodulatory Effects of Ashwagandha," *Journal of Ethnopharmacology* 50 (2): 69–76 (1996).

48. S. Sinclair et al., "Chinese Herbs: A Clinical Review of Astragalus, Ligusticum and Schizandra," *Alternative Medical Review* 3 (5): 388–394 (1998).

49. E. Lien and Wen Li, *Anticancer Chinese Drugs* (Taiwan, R.O.C.: Oriental Healing Arts Institute, 1985), 21.

50. Kee Chang Huang, *The Pharmacology of Chinese Herbs, 2d ed.* (Boca Raton, Fla.: CRC Press, 1998), 347.

51. *The Cancer Solution* (Boca Raton, Fla.: Peltec Publishing Co., 1994), 131–32.

52. J.E. Cunnick et al., "Induction of Tumor Cytotoxic Immune Cells Using a Protein from the Bitter Melon (Momordica Charantia)," *Cellular Immunology* 126 (2): 278–89 (1990).

53. H. Shi et al., "Antioxidant Property of Fructus Momordicae Extract," *Biochemistry and Molecular Biology International* 40 (6): 1111–21 (1996).

54. F. Ellingwood, *American Materia Medica, Therapeutics and Pharmacognosy, vol. 2* (Portland, Oreg.: Eclectic Medical Publications, 1983), 145–47.

55. M.D. Faddeeva and T.N. Beliaeva, "Sanguinarine and Ellipticine Cytotoxic Alkaloids Isolated from Well-known Antitumor Plants. Intracellular Targets of Their Action," *Tsitologiia* 39 (2–3): 181–208 (1997).

56. T. Syrovets et al., "Inhibition of Topoisomerase I and II by Boswellic Acids," Naunyn-Schmeidelberg's *Archives of Pharmacology* 357: R11 (1998).

57. M.L. Sharma et al., "Immunomodulatory Activity of Boswellic Acids (Pentacyclic Triterpene Acids) From Boswellia Serrata," *Phytotherapy Research* 10: 107–12 (1996).

58. E.M. Epstein, *Alkaloidal Therapeutics* (Chicago: Clinic Publishing Co., 1904), 74–76.

59. R.F. Weiss, M.D., *Herbal Medicine* (Beaconsfield, England: Beaconsfield Publishers, Ltd., 1988), 212.

60. H.C.A. Vogel, *The Nature Doctor* (Los Angeles: Keats Publishing, 1991), 292.

61. M.L. Colombo and E. Bosisio, "Pharmacological Activities of Chelidonium Majus L. (Papaveraceae)," *Pharmacology Research* 33 (2): 127–34 (1996).

62. D.J. Kim et al., "Potential Preventive Effects of Chelidonium Majis L. (Papaveraceae) Herb Extract on Glandular Stomach Tumor Development in Rats Treated with N-methyl-N'-nitro-N Nitrosoguanidine (MNNG) and Hypertonic Sodium Chloride," *Cancer Letters* 112 (2): 203–8 (1997).

63. E. Pisha et al., "Discovery of Betulinic Acid as a Selective Inhibitor of Human Melanoma that Functions by Induction of Apoptosis," *Natural Medicine* 1 (10): 1046–51 (1995).

64. R. Weiss, M.D., *Herbal Medicine* (Stuttgart, Germany: Hippokrates Verlag Publishers, 1985), 317–18.

65. E. Lien and W. Li, *Anticancer Chinese Drugs* (Taiwan, R.O.C.: Oriental Healing Arts Institute, 1985), 111.

66. M.T. Murray, N.D., *The Healing Power of Herbs* (Rocklin, Calif.: Prima Publishing, 1991), 148–51.

67. K. Hyashi et al., "Antitumor Active Glycosides from Condurango Cortex," *Chemical and Pharmaceutical Bulletin* (Tokyo) 28 (6): 1954–58 (1980).

68. C.C. Benz et al., "Gossypol Effects on Endothelial Cells and Tumor Blood Flow," *Life Science* 49 (12): PL67–72 (1991).

69. V. Band et al., "Antiproliferative Effect of Gossypol and Its Optical Isomers on Human Reproductive Cancer Cell Lines," *Gynecologic Oncology* 32 (3): 273–7 (1989).

70. M.T. Murray, N.D., op. cit., 58–64.

71. D. Orinda et al., "Antiviral Activity of Components of Echinacea Purpurea," *Arzneimittelforschung* 23 (8): 1119–20 (1973).

72. F. Ellingwood, *American Materia Medica, Therapeutics and Pharmacognosy, Volume 2* (Portland, Oreg.: Eclectic Medical Publications, 1983), 358–76.

73. H.W. Felter and J.U. Lloyd, *King's American Dispensatory, 18th ed., vol. 1* (Portland, Oreg.: Eclectic Medical Publications, 1983), 671–77.

74. V. Sodhi, N.D., "Traditional Ayurvedic Herbal Therapies for Common Illnesses," *Gaia Symposium Proceedings on Naturopathic Herbal Medicine* (1993), 100–102.

75. H.C. Wood, M.D. et al., *U.S. Dispensatory, 6th ed.* (Washington, D.C.: H.C. Wood, 1883), 1651.

76. F. Ellingwood, *American Materia Medica, Therapeutics and Pharmacognosy, vol. 2* (Portland, Oreg.: Eclectic Medical Publications, 1983), 673–74.

77. B. Stenkvist et al., "Cardiac Glycosides and Breast Cancer, Revisited," *New England Journal of Medicine* 306 (8): 484 (1982).

78. S.W. Ha et al., "Enhancement of Radiation Effect by Ginkgo Biloba Extract in C3H Mouse Fibrosarcoma," *Radiotherapy and Oncology* 41 (2): 163–67 (1996).

79. R.X. Zhang et al., "Laboratory Studies of Berberine Used Alone and in Combination with 1,3-bis (2-chloroethyl) -1-nitrosourea to Treat Malignant Brain Tumors," *Chinese Medical Journal (English)* 103 (8): 658–65 (1990).

80. R. Weiss, M.D., *Herbal Medicine* (Stuttgart, Germany: Hippokrates Verlag Publishers, 1985), 320–21.

81. H.C. Wood, M.D. et al., *U.S. Dispensatory, 6th ed.* (Washington, D.C.: H.C. Wood, 1883), 728–29.

82. K.C. Huang, *The Pharmacology of Chinese Herbs* (Boca Raton, Fla.: CRC Press, 1998), 155–56.

83. Y. Yamaoka, et al., "A Polysaccharide Fraction of Zizyphi Fructus in Augmenting Natural Killer Activity by Oral Administration," *Biological and Pharmaceutical Bulletin* 19 (7): 936–99 (1996).

84. E.M. McKelvey et al., "Dichloroallyl Lawsone," *Clinical Pharmacology and Therapeutics* 25 (5 Pt 1): 586–90 (1979).

85. D.B. Mowrey, *Herbal Tonic Therapies* (Los Angeles: Keats Publishing, 1993), 74–78.

86. S. Sinclair et al., "Chinese Herbs: A Clinical Review of Astragalus, Ligusticum and Schizandra," *Alternative Medicine Review* 3 (5): 338–44 (1998).

87. D.P. Reid, *Chinese Herbal Medicine* (Boston: Shambhala Publications, Inc., 1990), 553–54.

88. Ibid., 386–87.

89. S.K. Katiyar et al., "Protective Effects of Silymarin Against Photocarcinogenesis in a Mouse Skin Model," *Journal of the National Cancer Institute* 89 (9): 556–66 (1997).

90. J. Gaedeke et al., "Cisplatin Nephrotoxicity and Protection by Silibinin," *Nephrology, Dialysis and Transplantation* 11 (1): 55–62 (1996).

91. G. Scambia et al., "Antiproliferative Effect of Silybin on Gynaecological Malignancies: Synergism with Cisplatin and Doxorubicin," *European Journal of Cancer* 32A (5): 877–82 (1996).

92. X. Zi et al., "Anticarcinogenic Effect of a Flavonoid Antioxidant, Silymarin, in Human Breast Cancer Cells MDA-MB 468: Induction of G1 Arrest Through an Increase in Cip1/p21 Concomitant with a Decrease in Kinase Activity of Cyclin-Dependent Kinases and Associated Cyclins," *Clinical Cancer Research* 4 (4): 1055–64 (1998).

93. C.E. Elson et al., "Anti-carcinogenic Activity of D-limonene During the Initiation and Promotion/Progression Stages of DMBA-induced Rat Mammary Carcinogenesis," *Carcinogenesis* 9 (2): 331–32 (1988).

94. J.A. Elegbede et al., "Regression of Rat Primary Mammary Tumors Following Dietary D-limonene," *Journal of the National Cancer Institute* 76 (2): 323–25 (1986).

95. K.C. Huang, *The Pharmacology of Chinese Herbs* (Boca Raton, Fla.: CRC Press, 1998), 345.

96. P.S. Venkateswaran et al., "Effects of an Extract from Phyllanthus Niruri on Hepatitis B and Woodchuck Hepatitis Viruses: *in Vitro* and *in Vivo* Studies," *Proceedings of the National Academy of Science USA* 84 (1): 274–78 (1987).

97. M.A. El-Ghazaly and M.T. Khayyal, "The Use of Aqueous Propolis Extract Against Radiation-Induced Damage," *Drugs Under Experimental and Clinical Research* 21 (6): 229–36 (1995).

98. J. Boik, *Protocol Journal of Botanical Medicine* 2 (3): 5–9.

99. R.L. Wang, "A Report of 40 Cases of Esophageal Carcinoma Surviving for More Than 5 Years After Treatment with Drugs," *Chung Hua Chung Liu Tsa Chih* 15 (4): 300–2 (1993).

100. K.C. Huang, *The Pharmacology of Chinese Herbs* (Boca Raton, Fla.: CRC Press, 1998), 466–67.

101. Z.G. Gao et al., "Synergistic Effect of Oridonin and Cisplatin on Cytotoxicity and DNA Cross-link Against Mouse Sarcoma S180 Cells in Culture," *Chung Kuo Yao Li Hsueh Pao* 14 (6): 561–64 (1993).

102. C.T. Ho, ed., *Food Phytochemicals for Cancer Prevention II* (Washington, D.C.: American Chemical Society, 1992), 14–15.

103. X. Shen et al., "Effects of Lyophilized Royal Jelly on Experimental Hyperlipidemia and Thrombosis," *Chung Hua Yu Fang I Hsueh Tsa Chih* 29 (1): 27–29 (1995).

104. S.C. Nair et al., "Saffron Chemoprevention in Biology and Medicine: A Review," *Cancer Biotherapy* 10 (4): 257–64 (1995).

105. J. Escribano et al., "Crocin, Safranal and Picrocrocin from Saffron (Crocus Sativus L.) Inhibit the Growth of Human Cancer Cells in Vitro," *Cancer Letters* 100 (1–2): 23–30 (1996).

106. M.T. Murray, N.D., *The Healing Power of Herbs* (Rocklin, Calif.: Prima Publishing, 1991), 148–51.

107. M.T. Huang, ed., *Food Phytochemicals for Cancer Prevention I* (Washington, D.C.: American Chemical Society, 1992), 338.

108. D. Bensky and G.A. Kaptchuk, *Chinese Herbal Medicine* (Seattle, Wash.: Eastland Press, 1986), 217–18.

109. N.F. Chang et al., "Purification and Partial Characterization of an Active Anti-HIV Compound from the Chinese Medicinal Herb, Viola," *Antiviral Research* 10 (123): 107–16 (1988).

110. J.M. Scudder, *Specific Medication* (Cincinnati, Ohio: John M. Scudder, 1880), 88–89.

111. E.M. Epstein, *Alkaloidal Therapeutics* (Chicago: Clinic Publishing Company, 1904), 74–76.

112. E. Lien and W. Li, *Anticancer Chinese Drugs* (Taiwan, R.O.C.: Oriental Healing Arts Institute, 1985), 21.

113. K.C. Huang, *The Pharmacology of Chinese Herbs* (Boca Raton, Fla.: CRC Press, l998), 461–3.

114. S. Zheng et al., "Initial Study on Naturally Occurring Products from Traditional Chinese Herbs and Vegetables for Chemoprevention," *Journal of Cell Biochemistry Supplement* 27: 106–12 (1997).

115. S. Lieberman, *Maitake, King of Mushrooms* (Los Angeles: Keats Publishing, 1991), 16–19.

116. E. Lien and W. Li, *Anticancer Chinese Drugs* (Taiwan, R.O.C.: Oriental Healing Arts Institute, 1985), 116.

117. J. Zhou, M.D. and G. Liu, M.D., *Recent Advances in Chinese Medicine* (Beijing, China: Science Press, 1991), 133–41.

118. M. Suzuki et al., "Antitumor and Immunological Activity of Lentinan in Comparison with LPS," *International Journal of Immunopharmacology* 16 (5–6): 463–68 (1994).

119. T. Kunimoto et al., "Tumor-Regressing Factor Induced by Antitumor Polysaccharide in the Serum of Tumor-bearing Mice," *Human Cell* 3 (2): 124–30 (1990).

120. M. Torisu et al., "Eighteen-Year Experience of Cancer Immuno-therapies—Evaluation of Their Therapeutic Benefits and Future," *Nippon Geka Gakkai Zasshi* 92 (9): 1212–16 (1991).

121. M. Torisu et al., "Significant Prolongation of Disease-free Period Gained by Oral Polysaccharide K (PSK) Administration after Curative Surgical Operation of Colorectal Cancer," *Cancer Immunology and Immunotherapy* 31 (5): 261–68 (1990).

122. H. Kobayashi et al., "Antimetastatic Effects of PSK (Krestin), a Protein-Bound Polysaccharide Obtained from Basidiomycetes: An Overview," *Cancer Epidemiology Biomarkers and Prevention* 4 (3): 275–81 (1995).

123. H. Nakazato et al., "Efficacy of Immunochemotherapy as Adjuvant Treatment after Curative Resection of Gastric Cancer. Study Group of

Immunochemotherapy with PSK for Gastric Cancer," *Lancet* 343 (8906): 1122–26 (1994).

124. K. Hayakawa et al., "Effect of Krestin (PSK) as Adjuvant Treatment on the Prognosis after Radical Radiotherapy in Patients with Non-small Cell Lung Cancer," *Anticancer Research* 13 (5C): 1815–20 (1993).

125. Y. Iino et al., "Immunochemotherapies Versus Chemotherapy as Adjuvant Treatment after Curative Resection of Operable Breast Cancer," *Anticancer Research* 15 (6B): 2907–11 (1995).

126. S. Tsukagoshi et al., "Krestin (PSK)," *Cancer Treatment Review* 11 (2): 131–55 (1984).

127. T. Kaminaga et al., "Inhibitory Effects of Lanostane-type Triterpene Acids, the Components of Poria Cocus, on Tumor Promotion by 12-0-tetradecanoylphorbol-13-acetate in Two-Stage Carcinogenesis in Mouse Skin," *Oncology* 53 (5): 382–5 (1996).

128. U. Erasmus, *Fats and Oils* (Vancouver, B.C.: Alive Books, 1986), 191.

129. X. Wang, S. Chen, and H. Huang, "Anti-cancer Pain—Potency and Mechanism of SPES," *Management of Pain—A World Perspective, International Proceedings Division, World Association of Pain Clinic*, 1996: 411–15.

130. T. Hsieh et al., "Regulation of Androgen Receptor (AR) and Prostate Specific Antigen (PSA) Expression in the Androgen-responsive Human Prostate LNCaP Cells by Ethanolic Extracts of the Chinese Herbal Preparation, PC-SPES," *Biochemistry and Molecular Biology International* 42 (3): 535–44 (1997).

131. A.S. Breathnach, "Melanin Hyperpigmentation of Skin: Melasma, Topical Treatment with Azelaic Acid and Other Therapies," *Cutis* 57 (1 Suppl): 36–45 (1996).

132. P.G. Parsons et al., "Tumor Selectivity and Transcriptional Activation by Azelaic Bishydroxamic Acid in Human Melanocytic Cells," *Biochemical Pharmacology* 53 (11): 1719–24 (1997).

133. L. Lemic-Stojcevic et al., "Effect of Azelaic Acid on Melanoma Cells in Culture," *Experimental Dermatology* 4 (2): 79–81 (1995).

CHAPTER 5

1. A. Lupulescu, "Inhibition of DNA Synthesis and Neoplastic Cell Growth by Vitamin A (Retinol)," *Journal of the National Cancer Institute* 77 (1): 149–56 (1986).

2. H.B. Stahelin, "Vitamins and Cancer," *Recent Results in Cancer Research* 108: 227–34 (1988).

3. W.J. Blot et al., "Nutrition Intervention Trials in Linxian, China: Supplementation with Specific Vitamin/Mineral Combinations, Cancer Incidence, and Disease-specific Mortality in the General Population," *Journal of the National Cancer Institute* 85 (18): 1483–92 (1993).

4. M. Takimoto et al., "Protective Effect of CoQ10 Administration on Cardial Toxicity in FAC Therapy," *Gan To Kagaku Ryoho* 9 (1): 116–21 (1982).

5. E. Seifter et al., "Regression of C3HBA Mouse Tumor Due to X-ray Therapy Combined with Supplemental Beta-carotene or Vitamin A," *Journal of the National Cancer Institute* 71 (2): 409–17 (1983).

6. U. Pastorino et al., "Lung Cancer Chemoprevention with Retinol Palmitate. Preliminary Data from a Randomized Trial on Stage IA Non Small-cell Lung Cancer," *Acta Oncology* 27 (6b): 773–82 (1988).

7. "Vitamin A Reduces Lung Cancer," *The Nutrition Report* (November 1993), 84.

8. U. Pastorino et al., "Adjuvant Treatment of Stage I Lung Cancer with High-Dose Vitamin A," *Journal of Clinical Oncology* 11: 1216–22 (1993).

9. G.W. Comstock et al., "Prediagnostic Serum Levels of Carotenoids and Vitamin E as Related to Subsequent Cancer in Washington County, Maryland," *American Journal of Clinical Nutrition* 53 (1 Suppl): 260-64S (1991).

10. E. Giovannucci et al., "Intake of Carotenoids and Retinol in Relation to Risk of Prostate Cancer," *Journal of the National Cancer Institute* 87 (23): 1767–76 (1995).

11. H.S. Black and M.M. Mathews-Roth, "Protective Role of Butylated Hydroxytoluene and Certain Carotenoids in Photocarcinogenesis," *Photochemistry and Photobiology* 53 (5): 707–16 (1991).

12. L.X. Zhang et al., "Carotenoids Enhance Gap Junctional Communication and Inhibit Lipid Peroxidation in C3H/10T1/2 Cells: Relationship to Their Cancer Chemopreventive Action," *Carcinogenesis* 12 (11): 2109–14 (1991).

13. P.R. Palan et al., "Beta-carotene Levels in Exfoliated Cervicovaginal Epithelial Cells in Cervical Intraepithelial Neoplasia and Cervical Cancer," *American Journal of Obstetrics and Gynecology* 167 (6): 1899–903 (1992).

14. P. Quillan, *Adjuvant Nutrition in Cancer Treatment* (Arlington Heights, Ill.: Cancer Treatment Research Foundation, 1994), 212–23.

15. G.A. Kune et al., "Diet, Alcohol, Smoking, Serum Beta-carotene, and Vitamin A in Male Nonmelanocytic Skin Cancer Patients and Controls," *Nutrition and Cancer* 18 (3): 237–44 (1992).

16. P. Reddanna et al., "The Role of Vitamin E and Selenium on Arachidonic Acid Oxidation By Way of the 5-Lipoxygenase Pathway," *Annals of the New York Academy of Science* 570: 136–45 (1989).

17. M.M. Jacobs, ed., *Vitamins and Minerals in the Prevention and Treatment of Cancer* (Boca Raton, Fla.: CRC Press, 1991), 54–55.

18. I.R. Record et al., "The Influence of Topical and Systemic Vitamin E on Ultraviolet Light-induced Skin Damage in Hairless Mice," *Nutrition and Cancer* 16 (3–4): 219–25 (1991).

19. K.B. Olson and K.J. Pienta, "Vitamins A and E: Further Clues for Prostate Cancer Prevention," *Journal of the National Cancer Institute* 90 (6): 414–15 (1998).

20. "Vitamin E and Colon Cancer," *Cancer Epidemiology, Biomarkers and Prevention* 6: 769–74 (1997).

21. A. Lupulescu, *Hormones and Vitamins in Cancer Treatment* (Boca Raton, Fla.: CRC Press, 1990), 28.

22. R. Watson and S. Mufti, *Nutrition and Cancer Prevention* (Boca Raton, Fla.: CRC Press, 1996), 205–31.

23. D.E. Henson et al., "Ascorbic Acid: Biologic Functions and Relation to Cancer," *Journal of the National Cancer Institute* 83 (8): 547–50 (1991).

24. K. Shimpo et al., "Ascorbic Acid and Adriamycin Toxicity," *American Journal of Clinical Nutrition* 54 (6 Suppl): 1298–301S (1991).

25. G. Block et al., "Vitamin C: A New Look," *Annals of Internal Medicine* 114 (10): 909–10 (1991).

26. M.M. Jacobs, ed., *Vitamins and Minerals in the Prevention and Treatment of Cancer* (Boca Raton, Fla.: CRC Press, 1991), 173–88.

27. P. Quillan, *Adjunct Nutrition in Cancer Treatment* (Arlington Heights, Ill.: Cancer Treatment Research Foundation, 1994).

28. S. Krishnamurthi et al., "Combined Therapy in Buccal Mucosal Cancers," *Radiology* 99 (2): 409–15 (1971).

29. A. Lupulescu, *Hormones and Vitamins in Cancer Treatment* (Boca Raton, Fla.: CRC Press, 1990), 28.

30. D.S. Gridley et al., "Evaluation of Cancer Patient Leukocyte Responses in the Presence of Physiologic and Pharmacologic Pyridoxine and Pyridoxal Levels," *Journal of Clinical Laboratory Analysis* 3 (2): 95–100 (1989).

31. D.M. DiSorbo et al., "*In Vivo* and *in Vitro* Inhibition of B16 Melanoma Growth by Vitamin B6," *Nutrition and Cancer* 7 (1–2): 43–52 (1985).

32. G.S. Kelly, "The Co-enzyme Forms of Vitamin B12: Toward an Understanding of Their Therapeutic Potential," *Alternative Medicine Review* 2 (6): 459–71 (1997).

33. E. Giovannucci et al., "Multivitamin Use, Folate, and Colon Cancer in Women in the Nurses' Health Study," *Annals of Internal Medicine* 129 (7): 517–24 (1998).

34. M.M. Jacobs, ed., *Vitamins and Minerals in the Prevention and Treatment of Cancer* (Boca Raton, Fla.: CRC Press, 1991), 135–55.

35. S.L. Morgan et al., "The Effect of Folic Acid Supplementation on the Toxicity of Low-dose Methotrexate in Patients with Rheumatoid Arthritis," *Arthritis and Rheumatism* 33 (1): 9–18 (1990).

36. M. Saito et al., "Folate and Vitamin B12 Versus Cancer," *The Nutrition Report* (December 1, 1994).

37. J.A. Baron et al., "Folate Intake, Alcohol Consumption, Cigarette Smoking and Risk of Colorectal Adenomas," *Journal of the National Cancer Institute* 90 (1): 57–62 (1998).

38. S.M. Lippman et al., "Cancer Chemoprevention," *Journal of Clinical Oncology* 12 (4): 851–73 (1994).

39. I. Duris et al., "Calcium Chemoprevention in Colorectal Cancer," *Hepatogastroenterology* 43 (7): 152–54 (1996).

40. H.L. Newmark and M.Lipkin, "Calcium, Vitamin D and Colon Cancer," *Cancer Research* 52 (7 Suppl): 2067–70S (1992).

41. I.C. Slob et al., "Calcium Intake and 28-Year Gastrointestinal Cancer Mortality in Dutch Civil Servants," *International Journal of Cancer* 54 (1): 20–25 (1993).

42. "Calcium Influences Gastrointestinal Cancer Risk," *The Nutrition Report* (September 1993), 71.

43. M.M. Jacobs, ed., *Vitamins and Minerals in the Prevention and Treatment of Cancer* (Boca Raton, Fla.: CRC Press, 1991), 240.

44. E.E. Vokes et al., "A Randomised Study Comparing Intermittent to Continuous Administration of Magnesium Aspartate Hydrochloride in Cisplatin-induced Hypomagnesaemia," *British Journal of Cancer* 62 (6): 1015–17 (1990).

45. S.K. Alexsander et al., "Effect of Potassium Iodide on Tumor Growth," *Biulleten Eksperimentalnoi Biologii I Meditsiny* 111 (1): 64–66 (1991).

46. F. Ellingwood, M.D., *American Materia Medica, Therapeutics and Pharmacognosy* (Sandy, Oreg.: Eclectic Medical Publications, 1919), 422–25.

47. B.V. Stadel, "Dietary Iodine and Risk of Breast, Endometrial and Ovarian Cancer," *Lancet* 1 (7965): 890–91 (1976).

48. E.E. Deschner and M.S. Zedick, "Lipid Peroxidation in Liver and Colon of Methylazoxymethanol Treated Rats," *Cancer Biochemistry and Biophysics* 9 (1): 25–29 (1986).

49. L.C. Clark et al., "Effects of Selenium Supplementation for Cancer Prevention in Patients with Carcinoma of the Skin. A Randomised Controlled Trial," *Journal of the American Medical Association* 276 (24): 1957–63 (1996).

50. N. Chidambaram and A. Baradarajan, "Effect of Selenium on Lipids and Some Lipid Metabolising Enzymes in DMBA Induced Mammary Tumor Rats," *Cancer Biochemistry and Biophysics* 15 (1): 41–47 (1995).

51. M.M. Jacobs, ed., *Vitamins and Minerals in the Prevention and Treatment of Cancer* (Boca Raton, Fla.: CRC Press, 1991), 95–111.

52. S. Toma et al., "Selenium Therapy in Patients with Precancerous and Malignant Oral Cavity Lesions: Preliminary Results," *Cancer Detection and Prevention* 15 (6): 491–94 (1991).

53. K.J. Helzlsouer et al., "Prospective Study of Serum Micronutrients and Ovarian Cancer," *Journal of the National Cancer Institute* 88 (1): 32–37 (1996).

54. B. Pence, "Dietary Selenium, Skin Cancer and Antioxidant Enzymes," *The Nutrition Report* (December 1, 1995), 89–96.

55. C. Deffuant et al., "Serum Selenium in Melanoma and Epidermotropic Cutaneous T-cell Lymphoma," *Acta Dermato-Venereologica* 74 (2): 90–92 (1994).

56. B. Yu et al., "The Relationship Between Selenium and Immunity in Large Bowel Cancer," *Chung Hua Wai Ko Tsa Chih* 34 (10): 50–53 (1996).

57. Y.J. Hu et al., "The Protective Role of Selenium on the Toxicity of Cisplatin-Contained Chemotherapy Regimen in Cancer Patients," *Biological Trace Element Research* 56 (3): 331–41 (1997).

58. X.M. Luo et al., "Inhibitory Effects of Molybdenum on Esophageal and Forestomach Carcinogenesis in Rats," *Journal of the National Cancer Institute* 71: 75–80 (1983).

59. C. Fortes et al., "Zinc Supplementation and Plasma Lipid Peroxides in an Elderly Population," *European Journal of Clinical Nutrition* 51 (2): 97–101 (1997).

60. W. Mei et al., "Study of Immune Function of Cancer Patients Influenced by Supplemental Zinc or Selenium-Zinc Combination," *Biological Trace Element Research* 28 (1): 11–19 (1991).

61. C. Ripamonti et al., "A Randomized, Controlled Clinical Trial to Evaluate the Effects of Zinc Sulfate on Cancer Patients with Taste Alterations Caused by Head and Neck Irradiation," *Cancer* 82 (10): 1938–45 (1998).

62. K. Lockwood et al., "Partial and Complete Regression of Breast Cancer in Patients in Relation to Dosage of Coenzyme Q10," *Biochemistry and Biophysics Research Communication* 199 (3): 1504–8 (1994).

63. K. Donsbach and R. Alsleben, *Wholistic Cancer Therapy* (New York: Soho Press, 1993), 49.

64. O. Horakova et al., "The Hepatotropic Effect of Alpha-Lipoic Acid," *Ceska Farmacie* 16 (3): 129–33 (1967).

65. K. Hamilton, ed., *The Experts Speak* (Sacramento, Calif.: I.T. Services, 1996), 124–25.

66. A. Baur et al., "Alpha-lipoic Acid Is an Effective Inhibitor of Human Immunodeficiency Virus (HIV-1) Replication," *Klin Wochenschr* 69 (15): 722–74 (1991).

67. R.A. Passwater, *Lipoic Acid: The Metabolic Antioxidant* (Los Angeles: Keats Publishing, 1995), 24–27.

68. B.M. Berkson, M.D., "Hepatic Necrosis and Thioctic Acid," *New Mexico Supplement to the Western Journal of Medicine* 162 (5): 2 (1995).

69. D. Han et al., "Lipoic Acid Increases de Novo Synthesis of Cellular Glutathione by Improving Cystine Utilization," *Biofactors* 6 (3): 321–38 (1997).

70. K.J. Helzlsouer et al., "Association Between Glutathione S-transferase M1, P1 and T1 Genetic Polymorphisms and Development of Breast Cancer," *Journal of the National Cancer Institute* 90 (7): 512–18 (1998).

71. B. Donnerstag et al., "Reduced Glutathione and S-acetylglutathione as Selective Apoptosis-Inducing Agents in Cancer Therapy," *Cancer Letters* 110 (1–2): 63–70 (1996).

72. D. Trickler et al., "Inhibition of Oral Carcinogenesis by Glutathione," *Nutrition and Cancer* 20 (2): 139–44 (1993).

73. J.F. Smyth et al., "Glutathione Reduces the Toxicity and Improves Quality of Life of Women Diagnosed with Ovarian Cancer Treated with Cisplatin: Results of a Double-blind, Randomised Trial," *Annals of Oncology* 8 (6): 569–73 (1997).

74. M. Tedeschi et al., "Glutathione and Detoxification," *Cancer Treatment Review* 17 (2–3): 203–8 (1990).

75. N. DeVries and S. DeFlora, "N-acetyl-l-cysteine," *Journal of Cellular Biochemistry Supplement* 17F: 270–77 (1993).

76. C.Y. Yim et al., "Use of N-acetyl cysteine to Increase Intracellular Glutathione During the Induction of Antitumor Responses by IL-2," *Journal of Immunology* 152 (12): 5796–805 (1994).

77. B.J.M. Braakhuis, "Antioxidant-Related Parameters in Patients Treated for Cancer Chemoprevention with N-acetyl cysteine," *European Journal of Cancer* 31A (6): 921–23 (1995).

78. V. Bongers et al., "Antioxidant-Related Parameters in Patients Treated for Cancer Chemoprevention with N-acetyl cysteine," *European Journal of Cancer* 31A (6): 921–23 (1995).

79. J.A. Timbrell et al., "The *in Vivo* and *in Vitro* Protective Properties of Taurine," *General Pharmacology* 26 (3): 453–62 (1995).

80. L.R. Bucci, *Nutrition Applied to Injury Rehabilitation and Sports Medicine* (Boca Raton, Fla.: CRC Press, 1995), 37–39.

81. "Glutamine," *P.A. Practice* 12 (2): 14–16 (1993).

82. R. Denno et al., "Glutamine-Enriched Total Parenteral Nutrition Enhances Plasma Glutathione in the Resting State," *Journal of Surgical Research* 61 (1): 35–38 (1996).

83. R.D. Griffiths et al., "Six-Month Outcome of Critically Ill Patients Given Glutamine-supplemented Parenteral Nutrition," *Nutrition* 13 (4): 295–302 (1997).

84. V.S. Klimberg et al., "Effect of Supplemental Dietary Glutamine on Methotrexate Concentrations in Tumors," *Archives of Surgery* 127 (11): 1317–20 (1992).

85. V.S. Klimberg et al., "Oral Glutamine Accelerates Healing of the Small Intestine and Improves Outcome After Whole Abdominal Radiation," *Archives of Surgery* 125 (8): 1040–45 (1990).

86. M. Muscaritoli et al., "Oral Glutamine in the Prevention of Chemotherapy-induced Gastrointestinal Toxicity," *European Journal of Cancer* 33 (2): 319–20 (1997).

87. Z. Walaszek, "Potential Use of D-glucaric Acid Derivatives in Cancer Prevention," *Cancer Letters* 54 (1–2): 1–8 (1990).

88. A.S. Heerdt et al., "Calcium Glucarate as a Chemopreventive Agent in Breast Cancer," *Israel Journal of Medical Sciences* 31 (2–3): 101–5 (1995).

89. J. Boik, *Cancer and Natural Medicine* (Princeton, Minn.: Oregon Medical Press, 1995), 150.

90. G. Pratesi et al., "Differential Efficacy of Flavone Acetic Acid Against Liver Versus Lung Metastases in a Human Tumor Xenograft," *British Journal of Cancer* 63 (1): 71–74 (1991).

91. M.C. Bibby et al., "Anti-tumor Activity of Flavone Acetic Acid (NSC 347512) in Mice—Influence of Immune Status," *British Journal of Cancer* 63 (1): 57–62 (1991).

92. D.J. Kerr et al., "Phase I and Pharmacokinetic Study of Flavone Acetic Acid," *Cancer Research* 47 (24 Pt 1): 6776–81 (1987).

93. R.L. Hornung et al., "Augmentation of Natural Killer Activity, Induction of IFN and Development of Tumor Immunity During the Successful Treatment of Established Murine Renal Cancer Using Flavone Acetic Acid and IL-2," *Journal of Immunology* 141 (10): 3671–79 (1988).

94. R.H. Wiltrout et al., "Flavone-8-acetic Acid Augments Systemic Natural Killer Cell Activity and Synergizes with IL-2 for Treatment of Murine Renal Cancer," *Journal of Immunology* 140 (9): 3261–65 (1988).

95. G. Pratesi et al., "Role of T Cells and Tumor Necrosis Factor in Antitumor Activity and Toxicity of Flavone Acetic Acid," *European Journal of Cancer* 26 (10): 1079–83 (1990).

96. J. Boik, *Cancer and Natural Medicine* (Princeton, Minn.: Oregon Medical Press, 1995), 152–54.

97. J. Masquelier, *OPCs in Practice* (Rome, Italy: Alpha Omega Editrice, 1995), 118–20.

98. J.P. Boissin et al., "Chorioretinal Circulation and Dazzling Use of Procyanidol Oligomers," *Bulletin Société d'Opthalmologie Fr* 88 (173–74): 177–79 (1988).

99. L.M. Larocca et al., "Growth-Inhibitory Effect of Quercetin and Presence of Type II Estrogen Binding Sites in Primary Human Transitional Cell Carcinomas," *Journal of Urology* 152 (3): 1029–33 (1994).

100. F.O. Ranelletti et al., "Growth-Inhibitory Effect of Quercetin and Presence of Type II Estrogen Binding Sites in Human Colon Cancer Cell Lines and Primary Colorectal Tumors," *International Journal of Cancer* 50 (3): 486–92 (1992).

101. M. Yoshida et al., "The Effect of Quercetin on Cell Cycle Progression and Growth of Human Gastric Cancer Cells," *FEBS Letters* 260 (1): 10–13 (1990).

102. N. Kioka et al., "Quercetin, a Bioflavonoid, Inhibits the Increase of Human Multidrug Resistance Gene (MDR1) Expression Caused By Arsenite," *FEBS Letters* 301 (3): 307–9 (1992).

103. G. Elia and M.G. Santoro, "Regulation of Heat Shock Protein Synthesis by Quercetin in Human Erythroleukemia Cells," *Biochemical Journal* 300 (Pt. 1): 201–9 (1994).

104. M. Koishi et al., "Quercetin, an Inhibitor of Heat Shock Protein Synthesis, Inhibits the Acquisition of Thermotolerance in a Human Colon Carcinoma Cell Line," *Japanese Journal of Cancer Research* 83 (11): 1216–22 (1992).

105. G. Scambia et al., "Quercetin Potentiates the Effect of Adriamycin in a Multidrug-resistant MCF-7 Human Breast Cancer Cell Line: P-glyco-protein As a Possible Target," *Cancer Chemotherapy and Pharmacology* 34 (6): 459–64 (1994).

106. M. Piantelli et al., "Tamoxifen and Quercetin Interact with Type II Estrogen Binding Sites and Inhibit the Growth of Human Melanoma Cells," *Journal of Investigative Dermatology* 105 (2): 248–53 (1995).

107. J. Boik, *Cancer and Natural Medicine* (Princeton, Minn.: Oregon Medical Press, 1995), 151–53.

108. H. Wei et al., "Inhibitory Effects of Apigenin, a Plant Flavonoid, on Epidermal Ornithine Decarboxylase and Skin Tumor Promotion in Mice," *Cancer Research* 50 (3): 499–502 (1990).

109. D.F. Birt et al., "Anti-mutagenesis and Anti-promotion by Apigenin, Robinetin and Indole-3-carbinol," *Carcinogenesis* 7 (6): 959–63 (1986).

110. M. Hertog et al., "Intake of Potentially Anticarcinogenic Flavonoids and Their Determinants in Adults in the Netherlands," *Nutrition and Cancer* 20 (1): 21–29 (1993).

111. M.E. Begin et al., "Differential Killing of Human Carcinoma Cells Supplemented with n-3 and n-6 Polyunsaturated Fatty Acids," *Journal of the National Cancer Institute* 77 (5): 1053–62 (1986).

112. C.F. van der Merwe et al., "Oral Gamma-Linolenic Acid in 21 Patients with Untreatable Malignancy. An Ongoing Pilot Open Clinical Trial," *British Journal of Clinical Practice* 41 (9): 907–15 (1987).

113. M.E. Begin et al., "Selective Killing of Human Cancer Cells by Polyunsaturated Fatty Acids," *Prostaglandin and Leukotriene Medicine* 19 (2): 177–86 (1985).

114. M. Nakagawa et al., "Potentiation by Squalene of the Cytotoxicity of Anticancer Agents Against Cultured Mammalian Cells and Murine Tumor," *Japanese Journal of Cancer Research* 76 (4): 315–20 (1985).

115. A.K. Sills, Jr. et al., "Squalamine Inhibits Angiogenesis and Solid Tumor Growth *in Vivo* and Perturbs Embryonic Vasculature," *Cancer Research* 58 (13): 2784–92 (1998).

116. A. Brohult et al., "Effect of Alkoxyglycerols on the Frequency of Injuries Following Radiation Therapy for Carcinoma of the Uterine Cervix," *Acta Obstetricia et Gynecologica Scandinavica* 56 (4): 441–48 (1977).

117. D.J. Canty and S.H. Zeisel, "Lecithin and Choline in Human Health and Disease," *Nutrition Review* 52 (10): 327–39 (1994).

118. J.V. Wright, "Butyrate Determination and Colon Cancer," *International Clinical Nutrition Review* 9 (2): 66–67 (1989).

119. H.K. Hagopian et al., "Effect of N-Butyrate on DNA Synthesis in Chick Fibroblasts and HeLa Cells," *Cell* 12 (3): 855–60 (1977).

120. K.N. Prasad, "Butyric Acid: A Small Fatty Acid with Diverse Biological Functions," *Life Science* 27 (15): 1351–58 (1980).

121. T. Taki et al., "Effect of Butyrate on Glycolipid Metabolism of Two Cell Types of Rat Ascites Hepatomas with Different Ganglioside Biosynthesis," *Journal of Biochemistry (Tokyo)* 86 (5): 1395–402 (1979).

122. J. Leavitt and R. Moyzis, "Changes in Gene Expression Accompanying Neoplastic Transformation of Syrian Hamster Cells," *Journal of Biological Chemistry* 253 (8): 2497–500 (1978).

123. E. Borenfreund et al., "Constitutive Aggregates of Intermediate-sized Filaments of the Vimentin and Cytokeratin Type in Cultured Hepatoma Cells and Their Dispersal by Butyrate," *Experimental Cell Research* 127 (1): 215–35 (1980).

124. C. Ip et al., "Conjugated Linoleic Acid Suppresses Mammary Carcinogenesis and Proliferative Activity of the Mammary Gland in the Rat," *Cancer Research* 54 (5): 1212–15 (1994).

125. L. Desser and A. Rehberger, "Induction of Tumor Necrosis Factor in Human Peripheral-blood Mononuclear Cells by Proteolytic Enzymes," *Oncology* 47 (6): 475–77 (1990).

126. P. Quillan, *Adjuvant Nutrition in Cancer Treatment* (Arlington Heights, Ill.: Cancer Treatment Research Foundation, 1994), 253–66.

127. S. Batkin et al., "Modulation of Pulmonary Metastasis (Lewis Lung Carcinoma) by Bromelain, an Extract of the Pineapple Stem (Ananas Comosus)," *Cancer Investigation* 6 (2): 241–42 (1988).

128. H.R. Maurer et al., "Bromelain Induces the Differentiation of Leukemic Cells in Vitro: An Explanation for Its Cytostatic Effects," *Planta Medica* 54 (5): 377–81 (1988).

129. S. Batkin et al., "Antimetastatic Effect of Bromelain With or Without Its Proteolytic and Anticoagulant Activity," *Journal of Cancer Research and Clinical Oncology* 114 (5): 507–8 (1988).

130. M.T. Murray, "The Therapeutic Uses of Spleen Extracts," *American Journal of Natural Medicine* 2 (6): 6–7 (1995).

131. Y. Watanabe and T. Iwa, "Clinical Value of Immunotherapy for Lung Cancer by the Streptococcal Preparation OK-432," *Cancer* 53 (2): 248–53 (1984).

132. K. Tanaka et al., "Oral Administration of Chlorella Vulgaris Augments Concomitant Antitumor Immunity," *Immunopharmacology and Immunotoxicology* 12 (2): 277–91 (1990).

133. K. Tanaka et al., "Augmentation of Antitumor Resistance by a Strain of Unicellular Green Algae, Chlorella Vulgaris," *Cancer Immunology and Immunotherapy* 17 (2): 90–94 (1984).

134. Kanazawa Medical College, Department of Serology, *Scientific Reports on Chlorella in Japan* (Kyoto, Japan: Silpaque Publishing, 1992), 59–60.

135. Y. Miyazawa et al., "Immunomodulation by a Unicellular Green Algae (Chlorella Pyrenoidosa) in Tumor-Bearing Mice," *Journal of Ethnopharmacology* 24 (2–3): 135–46 (1988).

136. R.E. Merchant et al., "Dietary Chlorella for Patients with Malignant Glioma: Effects of Immunocompetence, Quality of Life and Survival," *Phytotherapy Research* 4: 220–31 (1990).

137. A.M. Shamsuddin et al., "IP6: A Novel Anti-cancer Agent," *Life Science* 61 (4): 343–54 (1997).

138. I. Vucenik et al., "Comparison of Pure Inositol Hexaphosphate and High-bran Diet in the Prevention of DMBA-Induced Rat Mammary Carcinogenesis," *Nutrition and Cancer* 28 (1): 7–13 (1997).

139. I. Vucenik et al., "Inositol Hexaphosphate and Inositol Inhibit DMBA-Induced Rat Mammary Cancer," *Carcinogenesis* 16 (5): 1055–58 (1995).

140. A. Challa et al., "Interactive Suppression of Aberrant Crypt Foci Induced by Azoxymethane in Rat Colon by Phytic Acid and Green Tea," *Carcinogenesis* 18 (10): 2023–26 (1997).

141. I. Vucenik et al., "Antitumor Activity of Phytic Acid (Inositol Hexaphosphate) in Murine Transplanted and Metastatic Fibrosarcoma, a Pilot Study," *Cancer Letters* 65 (1): 9–13 (1992).

142. A. Baten et al., "Inositol Phosphate-Induced Enhancement of Natural Killer Cell Activity Correlates with Tumor Suppression," *Carcinogenesis* 10 (9): 1595–98 (1989).

143. I. Vucenik and A.M. Shamsuddin, "3H Inositol Hexaphosphate (Phytic Acid) Is Rapidly Absorbed and Metabolised by Murine and Human Malignant Cells *in Vitro*," *Journal of Nutrition* 124 (6): 861–68 (1994).

144. A.M. Shamsuddin and A. Ullah, "Inositol Hexaphosphate Inhibits Large Intestinal Cancer in F344 Rats 5 Months After Induction by Azoxymethane," *Carcinogenesis* 10 (3): 625–26 (1989).

145. A. Kishi et al., "Effect of the Oral Administration of Lactobacillus Brevis Subsp. Coagulans on Interferon-Alpha Producing Capacity in Humans," *Journal of the American College of Nutrition* 15 (4): 408–12 (1996).

146. G. Abel and J.K. Czop, "Stimulation of Human Monocyte Beta-glucan Receptors by Glucan Particles Induces Production of TNF-alpha and IL-1 Beta," *International Journal of Immunopharmacology* 14 (8): 1363–73 (1992).

147. D.D. Poutsiaka et al., "Cross-linking of the Beta-glucan Receptor on Human Monocytes Results in Interleukin-1 Receptor Antagonist But Not Interleukin-1 Production," *Blood* 82 (12): 3695–700 (1993).

148. M. Jang et al., "Cancer Chemopreventive Activity of Resveratrol, a Natural Product Derived from Grapes," *Science* 275 (5297): 218–20 (1997).

149. N. Kawada et al., "Effect of Antioxidants, Resveratrol, Quercetin and N-acetylcystein, on the Functions of Cultured Rat Hepatic Stellate Cells and Kupffer Cells," *Hepatology* 27 (5): 1265–74 (1998).

150. H. Naik et al., "Inhibition of *in Vitro* Tumor Cell Endothelial Adhesion by Modified Citrus Pectin: A Ph-modified Natural Complex Carbohydrate," *Proceedings of the Annual Meeting of the American Association of Cancer Research* 36: A377 (1995).

151. K.J. Pienta et al., "Inhibition of Spontaneous Metastasis in a Rat Prostate Cancer Model by Oral Administration of Modified Citrus Pectin," *Journal of the National Cancer Institute* 87 (5): 348–53 (1995).

152. H.G. Zhu et al., "Enhancement of MHC-unrestricted Cytotoxic Activity of Human CD56+ CD3- Natural Killer (NK)Cells and CD3+ T Cells by Rhamnogalacturonan: Target Cell Specificity and Activity Against NK-Insensitive Targets," *Journal of Cancer Research and Clinical Oncology* 120 (7): 383–88 (1994).

153. I.V. Gmoshinski et al., "The Effect of a Protein Concentrate from Milk Whey and Its Fractions on the Macromolecular Permeability of the Intestinal Barrier in Rats with Experimental Food Anaphylaxis," *Voprosy Pitaniia* (1): 3–6 (1996).

154. R.G. Stevens et al., "Body Iron Stores and the Risk of Cancer," *New England Journal of Medicine* 319 (16): 1047–52 (1988).

155. L.J. Lu et al., "Effects of Soya Consumption for One Month on Steroid Hormones in Premenopausal Women: Implications for Breast Cancer Risk Reduction," *Cancer Epidemiology, Biomarkers and Prevention* 5 (1): 63–70 (1996).

156. A. Moltini et al., "*In Vitro* Hormonal Effects of Soybean Isoflavones," *Journal of Nutrition* 125 (3 Suppl): 751–756S (1995).

157. E. Kyle et al., "Genistein-induced Apoptosis of Prostate Cancer Cells Is Preceded by a Specific Decrease in Focal Adhesion Kinase Activity," *Molecular Pharmacology* 51 (2): 193–200 (1997).

158. D.M. Walker, "Bovine and Shark Cartilage," *Townsend Newsletter* (June 1989).

159. J. Boik, *Cancer and Natural Medicine* (Princeton, Minn.: Oregon Medical Press, 1995), 163.

160. "Shark Cartilage Flunks Cancer Test," *Townsend Letter for Doctors and Patients* (1987), 26.

161. J.F. Dorgan et al., "Relationship of Serum DHEA, DHEA Sulfate and 5-Androstene 3-Beta, 17-Betadiol to Risk of Breast Cancer in Postmenopausal Women," *Cancer Epidemiology, Biomarkers and Prevention* 6: 177–81 (1997).

162. M.H. Davidson et al., "Safety and Endocrine Effects of 3-Acetyl-7-oxo-DHEA (7-Keto DHEA)," Chicago Center for Clinical Research, Chicago, Ill. 60610. Accepted for Presentation at Experimental Biology 98, April 19, 1998, San Francisco, Calif.

163. R. Sahelian, *Pregnenolone: Nature's Feel Good Hormone* (Garden City Park, N.Y.: Avery Publishing Group, Inc., 1997).

164. L. Tamarkin et al., "Decreased Nocturnal Plasma Melatonin Peak in Patients with Estrogen Receptor Positive Breast Cancer," *Science* 216 (4549): 1003–5 (1982).

165. P. Lissoni et al., "A Randomized Study of Neuroimmunotherapy with Low-dose Subcutaneous Interleukin-2 Plus Melatonin Compared to Supportive Care Alone in Patients with Untreatable Metastatic Solid Tumor," *Supportive Care in Cancer* 3 (3): 194–97 (1995).

166. J. Boik, *Cancer and Natural Medicine* (Princeton, Minn.: Oregon Medical Press, 1995), 75.

167. P. Montilla et al., "Hyperlipidemic Nephropathy Induced by Adriamycin: Effect of Melatonin Administration," *Nephron* 76 (3): 345–50 (1997).

168. P. Lissoni et al., "Reversal of Clinical Resistance to LHRH Analogue in Metastatic Prostate Cancer by the Pineal Hormone Melatonin: Efficacy of LHRH Analogue Plus Melatonin in Patients Progressing on LHRH Analogue Alone," *European Urology* 31 (2): 178–81 (1997).
169. R. Reiter and J. Robinson, *Melatonin, Your Body's Natural Wonder Drug* (New York: Bantam Books, 1995).
170. J. Boik, *Cancer and Natural Medicine* (Princeton, Minn.: Oregon Medical Press, 1995), 161–62.
171. R. Moss, *The Cancer Industry* (New York: Equinox Press, 1996), 192–93.

CHAPTER 6

1. "Faith May Lower Blood Pressure," *Preventive Medicine* 27: 545–52 (1998).
2. D.A. Mathews, M.D., *The Faith Factor* (New York: Viking Penguin, 1998), 201.
3. P. Knekt et al., "Elevated Lung Cancer Risk Among Persons with Depressed Mood," *American Journal of Epidemiology* 144 (12): 1096–103 (1996).

CHAPTER 7

1. J. Schmidt et al., "Molecular Effects of Vitamin D on Cell Cycle and Oncogenesis," *Ugeskr Laeger* 160 (30): 4411–14 (1998).
2. R.S. Pritchard et al., "Dietary Calcium, Vitamin D, and the Risk of Colorectal Cancer in Stockholm, Sweden," *Cancer Epidemiology, Biomarkers and Prevention* 5 (11): 897–900 (1996).
3. R.V. Brenner et al., "The Antiproliferative Effect of Vitamin D Analogs on MCF-7 Human Breast Cancer Cells," *Cancer Letters* 92 (1): 77–82 (1995).
4. "Sunlight Prevents Ovarian Cancer," *The Nutrition Report* (April 1995), 13 (4): 19.
5. C. Molina et al., "Pineal Functioning (Melatonin Levels) in Healthy Children of Different Ages. An Update and the Value of Pineal Gland Study in Pediatrics," *Anales Españoles de Pediatria* 45 (1): 33–44 (1996).
6. C.D. Hutter and P. Laing, "Multiple Sclerosis: Sunlight, Diet, Immunology and Aetiology," *Medical Hypotheses* 46 (2): 67–74 (1996).
7. C.F. Garland et al., "Rising Trends in Melanoma. An Hypothesis Concerning Sunscreen Effectiveness," *Annals of Epidemiology* 3 (1): 103–10 (1993).

8. M.B. Veierod, "Diet and Risk of Cutaneous Malignant Melanoma: A Prospective Study of 50,757 Norwegian Men and Women," *Internal Journal of Cancer* 71 (4): 600–4 (1997).

9. L.E. Rhodes et al., "Dietary Fish Oil Reduces Basal and Ultraviolet B-generated PGE2 Levels in Skin and Increases the Threshold to Provocation of Polymorphic Light Eruption," *Journal of Investigative Dermatology* 105 (4): 532–35 (1995).

10. J.F. Ashton and R.S. Laura, "Environmental Factors and the Etiology of Melanoma," *Cancer Causes and Control* 4 (1): 59–62 (1993).

11. C. Bain et al., "Diet and Melanoma. An Exploratory Case-control Study," *Annals of Epidemiology* 3 (3): 235–38 (1993).

12. I.M. Lee, "Exercise and Physical Health: Cancer and Immune Function," *Research Quarterly for Exercise and Sport* 66 (4): 286–91 (1995).

13. K. Duncan et al., "Running Exercise May Reduce Risk for Lung and Liver Cancer by Inducing Activity of Antioxidant and Phase II Enzymes," *Cancer Letters* 116 (2): 151–58 (1997).

14. "Pesticide Usage," *Nutrition Week* (May 26, 1995), 25 (20): 7.

15. "Hormone-Disrupting Chemicals," *Center for Medical Consumers HealthFacts* 23 (11): 4 (1998).

CHAPTER 8

1. S. Kneipp, *My Water Cure* (Kempton, Bavaria: Joseph Koesel Publishers, 1892).

2. P.K. Sneed, M.D., "Hyperthermia," *Everyone's Guide to Cancer Therapy* (New York: Andrews and McMeel Publishers, 1991), 74.

3. C.C. Vernon et al., "Radiotherapy With or Without Hyperthermia in the Treatment of Superficial Localized Breast Cancer," *International Journal of Radiation, Oncology, Biology and Physics* 35 (4): 731–44 (1996).

4. F.F. Buell et al., "Synergistic Effect and Possible Mechanisms of Tumor Necrosis Factor and Cisplatin Cytotoxicity Under Moderate Hyperthermia Against Gastric Cancer Cells," *Annals of Surgical Oncology* 4 (2): 141–48 (1997).

5. M. Hiraoka et al., "Site-specific Phase I, II Trials of Hyperthermia at Kyoto University," *International Journal of Hyperthermia* 10 (3): 403–10 (1994).

6. M. Kakehi et al., "Multi-institutional Clinical Studies on Hyperthermia Combined with Radiotherapy or Chemotherapy in Advanced Cancer of

Deep-seated Organs," *International Journal of Hyperthermia* 6 (4): 719–40 (1990).

7. K.S. Bisht et al., "Hyperthermia in Cancer Research: Current Status," *Indian Journal of Experimental Biology* 34 (12): 1183–89 (1996).

8. H.M. Sharma et al., "Effect of Different Sounds on Growth of Human Cancer Cell Lines *in Vitro*," *Alternative Therapies in Clinical Practice* 3 (4): 25–32 (1996).

9. W. Andritzky, "Medical Students and Alternative Medicine—A Survey," *Gesundheitswesen* 57 (6): 345–8 (1995).

10. M.F. Cunningham et al., "Introducing a Music Program in the Perioperative Area," *AORN Journal* 66 (4): 674–82 (1997).

11. B. Wu, "Effect of Acupuncture on the Regulation of Cell-Mediated Immunity in Patients with Malignant Tumors," *Chen Tzu Yen Chiu* 20 (3): 67–71 (1995).

CHAPTER 9

1. M. Buyse et al., "Adjunctive Therapies of Colorectal Cancers: Why We Still Don't Know," *Journal of the American Medical Association* 259 (24): 3571–78 (1988).

2. D. Drum, *Making the Chemotherapy Decision* (Los Angeles: Lowell House, 1996), 96–113.

3. E. Gilboa et al., "Immunotherapy of Cancer With Dendritic-cell-based Vaccines," *Cancer Immunology and Immunotherapy* 46 (2): 82–87 (1998).

4. J. Groopman, "Dr. Fair's Tumor," *The New Yorker* (October 26, 1998), 78–106.

5. A. Luenig et al., "Fibroblast Growth Factor (b-FGF) in Serum and Urine of Patients with Head-Neck Malignancies," *Laryngorhinootologie* 76 (7): 421–24 (1997).

6. J.H. Mydlo et al., "Preliminary Results Comparing the Recovery of Basic Fibroblast Growth Factor (FGF-2) in Adipose Tissue and Benign and Malignant Renal Tissue," *Journal of Urology* 159 (6): 2159–63 (1998).

CHAPTER 10

1. M. Baum, "Does Surgery Disseminate or Accelerate Cancer?" *Lancet* 347 (8996): 260 (1996).

2. P.H. Wiernick et al., "Adjuvant Radiotherapy for Breast Cancer as a Risk Factor for the Development of Lung Cancer," *Medical Oncology* 11 (3–4): 121–25 (1994).

3. M. Morrow, M.D., "Second Opinions Help Cancer Patients," Presentation at the San Antonio Breast Cancer Symposium, December 13, 1998.

4. E.L. McGarvey et al., "Evidence of Acute Stress Disorder After Diagnosis of Cancer," *Southern Medical Journal* 91 (9): 864–66 (1998).

CHAPTER 11

1. T. Okusaka et al., "Prognosis of Advanced Pancreatic Cancer Patients with Reference to Calorie Intake," *Nutrition and Cancer* 32 (1): 55–58 (1998).

2. F. Damrau, M.D., "The Value of Bentonite for Diarrhea," *Medical Annals of the District of Columbia* 30 (6): 326 (1961).

3. Ibid., 327–28.

CHAPTER 12

1. S.L. Parker et al., "Cancer Statistics, 1997," *CA: A Cancer Journal for Clinicians* 47 (1): 5–27 (1997).

2. B.C. Pence and D.M. Dunn, M.D., *Nutrition and Women's Cancers* (Boca Raton, Fla.: CRC Press, 1998), 14.

3. B. Liebman, "Fighting Cancer Without Fat," *Nutrition Action Health Letter* (June, 1993), 8–9.

4. B.A. Muller et al., "Cancer Statistics Review, 1973–89," *DHEW Publication Number (NIH) 92-2789* (Bethesda, Md.: National Cancer Institute, 1992).

5. A.G. Glass and R.N. Hoover, "Rising Incidence of Breast Cancer: Relationship to Stage and Receptor Status," *Journal of the National Cancer Institute* 82 (8): 693–96 (1990).

6. E. White et al., "Evaluation of the Increase in Breast Cancer Incidence in Relation to Mammography Use," *Journal of the National Cancer Institute* 82 (19): 1546–52 (1990).

7. M.P. Longnecker et al., "Risk Factors for *in Situ* Breast Cancer," *Cancer Epidemiology, Biomarkers and Prevention* 5 (12): 961–65 (1996).

8. V.L. Ernster and J. Barclay, "Increases in Ductal Carcinoma *in Situ* (DCIS) of the Breast in Relation to Mammography: A Dilemma," *Journal of the National Cancer Institute Monographs* (22): 151–56 (1997).

9. B.C. Pence and D.M. Dunn, M.D., *Nutrition and Women's Cancers*, op. cit.

10. G. Cowley, "Cancer and Diet," *Newsweek* (November 30, 1998), 60–66.

11. "Breast Cancer Screening in Women Under 50," *Lancet* 337 (8757): 1575–6 (1991).

12. D. Gillett et al., "Breast Cancer in Young Women," *Australia/New Zealand Journal of Surgery* 67 (11): 761–64 (1997).

13. B.C. Pence and D.M. Dunn, M.D., *Nutrition and Women's Cancers*, op. cit., 16–17.

14. M. King et al., "Inherited Breast and Ovarian Cancer. What Are the Risks? What Are the Choices?" *Journal of the American Medical Association* 269: 1975 (1993).

15. D.E. Anderson, "Genetic Study of Breast Cancer: Identification of a High-risk Group," *Cancer* 34 (4): 1090–97 (1974).

16. D.B. Berman et al., "A Common Mutation in BRCA 2 that Predisposes to a Variety of Cancers Is Found in Both Jewish Ashkenazi and non-Jewish Individuals," *Cancer Research* 56 (15): 3409–14 (1996).

17. A. Wolk et al., "A Prospective Study of Association of Monounsaturated Fat and Other Types of Fat with Risk of Breast Cancer," *Archives of Internal Medicine* 158 (1): 41–45 (1998).

18. E. Barrett-Connor and N.J. Friedlander, "Dietary Fat, Calories and the Risk of Breast Cancer in Postmenopausal Women: A Prospective Population-Based Study," *Journal of the American College of Nutrition* 12 (4): 390–99 (1993).

19. J.L. Freudenheim et al., "Premenopausal Breast Cancer Risk and Intake of Vegetables, Fruits and Related Nutrients," *Journal of the National Cancer Institute* 88 (6): 340–8 (1996).

20. N. Ito et al., "A New Colon and Mammary Carcinogen in Cooked Food, 2-amino-1-methyl-6-phenylimidazo(4,5-b)pyridine (PhIP)," *Carcinogenesis* 12 (8): 1503–6 (1991).

21. E. DeStefani et al., "Meat Intake, Heterocyclic Amines, and the Risk of Breast Cancer: A Case Control Study in Uruguay," *Cancer Epidemiology, Biomarkers and Prevention* 6 (8): 573 (1997).

22. W.C. Willett et al., "Moderate Alcohol Consumption and the Risk of Breast Cancer," *New England Journal of Medicine* 316 (19): 1174–80 (1987).

23. M.P. Longnecker et al., "Risk of Breast Cancer in Relation to Lifetime Alcohol Consumption," *Journal of the National Cancer Institute* 87 (12): 923–29 (1995).

24. G.A. Colditz, "Relationship Between Estrogen Levels, Use of Hormone Replacement Therapy, and Breast Cancer," *Journal of the National Cancer Institute* 90 (11): 814–23 (1998).

25. G. Williams et al., "Oral Contraceptive (OCP) Use Increases Proliferation and Decreases Estrogen Receptor Content of Epithelial Cells in the Normal Human Breast," *International Journal of Cancer* 48 (2): 206–10 (1991).

26. B.C. Pence and D.M. Dunn, M.D., *Nutrition and Women's Cancers*, op. cit., 17.

27. D. Hurley, "Breast-feeding May Lower the Risk of Early-Age Cancer," *Medical Tribune* (July 22, 1993), 10.

28. B.E. Henderson et al., *Cancer Epidemiology and Prevention, 2d ed. (Breast Cancer)* (New York: Oxford University Press, 1996), 1022.

29. R.G. Stevens et al., "Electric Power, Pineal Function and the Risk of Breast Cancer," *FASEB Journal* 6 (3): 853–60 (1992).

30. M.S. Wolff et al., "Blood Levels of Organochlorine Residues and Risk of Breast Cancer," *Journal of the National Cancer Institute* 85: 648 (1993).

31. D. Milne, "Toxins Play Role in Breast Cancer: 50% to 60% Higher Levels of PCBs Were Found in Women with Malignant Tumors," *Medical Tribune* (May 7, 1992), 4.

32. C. Dees et al., "DDT Mimics Estradiol Stimulation of Breast Cancer Cells to Enter the Cell Cycle," *Molecular Carcinogenesis* 18 (2): 107–14 (1997).

33. F. Falck, Jr. et al., "Pesticides and Polychlorinated Biphenyl Residues in Human Breast Lipids and Their Relation to Breast Cancer," *Archives of Environmental Health* 47 (2): 143–46 (1992).

34. "Nuclear Reactors and Breast Cancer," *Townsend Letter for Doctors* (July, 1996), 144: 58–67.

35. J.G. Schmidt, "The Epidemiology of Mass Breast Cancer Screening—a Plea for a Valid Measure of Benefit," *Journal of Clinical Epidemiology* 43 (3): 215–25 (1990).

36. S.W. Fletcher et al., "Report of the International Workshop on Screening for Breast Cancer," *Journal of the National Cancer Institute* 85 (20): 1644–56 (1993).

37. N.F. Boyd et al., "Quantitative Classification of Mammographic Densities and Breast Cancer Risk: Results from the Canadian National Breast Screening Study," *Journal of the National Cancer Institute* 87 (9): 670–75 (1995).

38. C. Byrne, "Studying Mammographic Density: Implications for Understanding Breast Cancer," *Journal of the National Cancer Institute* 89 (8): 531–33 (1997).

39. F.C. Garland et al., "Geographic Variation in Breast Cancer Mortality in the United States; a Hypothesis Involving Exposure to Solar Radiation," *Preventive Medicine* 19 (6): 614–22 (1990).

40. E.D. Gorham et al., "Sunlight and Breast Cancer Incidence in the USSR," *International Journal of Epidemiology* 19 (4): 820–24 (1990).

41. B. Davanzo et al., "Physical Activity and Breast Cancer Risk," *Cancer Epidemiology, Biomarkers and Prevention* 5 (3): 155–60 (1996).

42. L. Bernstein et al., "Physical Exercise and Reduced Risk of Breast Cancer in Young Women," *Journal of the National Cancer Institute* 86 (18): 1403–8 (1994).

43. B.C. Pence and D.M. Dunn, M.D., *Nutrition and Women's Cancers*, op. cit., 18–19.

44. B.S. Thomas et al., "Thyroid Function and the Incidence of Breast Cancer in Hawaiian, British and Japanese Women," *International Journal of Cancer* 38 (3): 325–29 (1986).

45. S.G. Shering et al., "Thyroid Disorders and Breast Cancer," *European Journal of Cancer Prevention* 5 (6): 504–6 (1996).

46. P.M. Ravdin et al., "Prediction of Axillary Lymph Node Status in Breast Cancer Patients by Use of Prognostic Indicators," *Journal of the Naitonal Cancer Institute* 86 (23): 1771–75 (1994).

47. V.L. Ernster et al., "Incidence of and Treatment for Ductal Carcinoma *in Situ* of the Breast," *Journal of the American Medical Association* 275 (12): 913–18.

48. R. Silvestrini et al., "Expression of p53, Glutathione S-transferase-pi, and Bcl-2 Proteins and Benefit from Adjuvant Radiotherapy in Breast Cancer," *Journal of the National Cancer Institute* 89 (9): 639–45 (1997).

49. A. Lupulescu, M.D., *Hormones and Vitamins in Cancer Treatment* (Boca Raton, Fla.: CRC Press, 1990), 140–41.

50. "Late Cycle Mastectomies May Reduce Recurrences," *Medical Tribune* (May 7, 1992), 3.

51. "Sector Resection with or without Postoperative Radiotherapy for Stage I Breast Cancer: A Randomized Trial. Uppsala-Orebro Breast Cancer Study Group," *Journal of the National Cancer Institute* 82 (4): 277–82 (1990).

52. R.M. Clark et al., "Randomized Clinical Trial of Breast Irradiation Following Lumpectomy and Axillary Dissection for Node-negative Breast Cancer: An Update. Ontario Clinical Oncology Group," *Journal of the National Cancer Institute* 88 (22): 1659–64 (1996).

53. "Early Stage Breast Cancer," *National Institute of Health Consensus Development Conference on Treatment of Early Stage Breast Cancer Consensus Statement* (June 18–21, 1990) 8 (6): 1–19.

54. A. Nawa et al., "Testing Histologically Negative Lymph Nodes for Papillomavirus When Evaluating Metastasis in Cervical Cancer," *Lancet* 339 (8803): 1231 (1992).

55. J. Ralof, "Tamoxifen Quandary: Promising Cancer Drug May Hide a Troubling Dark Side," *Science News* 141: 266–69 (1992).

56. N.A. Pavlidis et al., "Clear Evidence that Long-Term, Low-Dose Tamoxifen Treatment Can Induce Ocular Toxicity. A Prospective Study of 63 Patients," *Cancer* 69 (12): 2961–64 (1992).

57. R.R. Love et al., "Effects of Tamoxifen on Bone Mineral Density in Postmenopausal Women with Breast Cancer," *New England Journal of Medicine* 326 (13): 852–56 (1992).

58. G.B. Anker et al., "Thyroid Function in Postmenopausal Breast Cancer Patients Treated with Tamoxifen," *Scandinavian Journal of Clinical Laboratory Investigation* 58 (2): 103–7 (1998).

59. S. Langdon, W. Miller, and A. Berchuck, *Biology of Female Cancers* (Boca Raton, Fla.: CRC Press, 1997), 82.

60. R.L. Barbieri and K.J. Ryan, "Danazol: Endocrine Pharmacology and Therapeutic Applications," *American Journal of Obstetrics and Gynecology* 141 (4): 453–63 (1981).

61. E. Rochelle et al., "Solid Cancers after Bone Marrow Transplantation," *New England Journal of Medicine* 336 (13): 897–904 (1997).

CHAPTER 13

1. M.C. Bosland et al., "Dietary Fat, Calories, and Prostate Cancer Risk," *Journal of the National Cancer Institute* 91 (6): 489–91 (1999).

2. I.J. Powell, "Early Detection Issues of Prostate Cancer in African-American Men," *In Vivo* 8 (3): 451–52 (1994).

3. G.C. Steinberg et al., "Family History and Risk of Prostate Cancer," *Prostate* 17 (4): 337–47 (1990).

4. L. Rosenberg et al., "Vasectomy and the Risk of Prostate Cancer," *American Journal of Epidemiology* 132 (6): 1051–55 (1990).

5. C. Mettlin et al., "Vasectomy and Prostate Cancer Risk," *American Journal of Epidemiology* 132 (6): 1056–61 (1990).

6. R. Steele et al., "Sexual Factors in the Epidemiology of Cancer of the Prostate," *Journal of Chronic Diseases* 24 (1): 29–37 (1971).

7. D.P. Rose, "Dietary Fatty Acids and Cancer," *American Journal of Clinical Nutrition* 66 (4 Supp): 998–1003S (1997).

8. E. Giovanucci, "How Is Individual Risk for Prostate Cancer Assessed?" *Hematology/Oncology Clinicians of North America* 10 (3): 537–48 (1996).

9. J.R. Hebert et al., "Nutritional and Socioeconomic Factors in Relation to Prostate Cancer Mortality: A Cross-National Study," *Journal of the National Cancer Institute* 90 (21): 1637–47 (1998).

10. E. Giovanucci and S.K. Clinton, "Tomatoes, Lycopene and Prostate Cancer," *Proceedings of the Society for Experimental Biology and Medicine* 218 (2): 129–39 (1998).

11. K. Israel et al., "RRR-alpha-tocopherol Succinate Inhibits the Proliferation of Human Prostatic Tumor Cells with Defective Cell Cycle/Differentiation Pathways," *Nutrition and Cancer* 24 (2): 161–69 (1995).

12. J.M. Turley et al., "RRR-a-tocopherol Succinate Modulation of Human Promyelocytic Leukemia (HL-60) Cell Proliferation and Differentiation," *Nutrition and Cancer* 18: 201–213 (1992).

13. O.P. Heinonen et al., "Prostate Cancer and Supplementation with A-tocopherol and B-carotene: Incidence and Mortality in a Controlled Trial," *Journal of the National Cancer Institute* 90: 440–46 (1998).

14. K.J. Pienta et al., "Inhibition of Spontaneous Metastasis in a Rat Prostate Cancer Model by Oral Administration of Modified Citrus Pectin," *Journal of the National Cancer Institute* 87 (5): 348–53 (1995).

15. M.D. Krahn et al., "Screening for Prostate Cancer: A Decision Analytic View," *Journal of the American Medical Association* 272 (10): 773–80 (1994).

16. J.K. Gohagan, Early Detection Branch, DCP, National Cancer Institute and National Institute of Health, "A 16-Year Randomized Screening Trial for Prostate, Lung, Colorectal and Ovarian Cancer-PLCO Trial," (Summary Last Modified 12/96), PLCO-1, Clinical Trial, Active, 11/16/93.

17. M.L. Schiebler et al., "MR Imaging in Adenocarcinoma of the Prostate: Interobserver Variation and Efficacy for Determining Stage C Disease," *American Journal of Roentgenology* 158 (3): 559–62 (1992).

18. "Prostate." In *American Joint Committee on Cancer: AJCC Cancer Staging Manual* (Philadelphia, Pa.: Lippincott-Raven Publishers, 5th ed. 1997), 219–224.

19. D. Kaltenbach, *Prostate Cancer: A Survivor's Guide* (New Port Richey, Fla..: Seneca House Press, 1995), 78–79.

20. J.A. Connolly et al., "Should Cryosurgery Be Considered a Therapeutic Option in Localized Prostate Cancer?" *Urologic Clinics of North America* 23 (4): 623–31 (1996).

21. H.P. Schmid and A. Bitton, "Therapeutic Options in Advanced Cancer of the Prostate," *Schweizerische Rundschau fur Medizin Praxis* 86 (44): 1734–39 (1997).

22. R.S. DiPaola et al., "Clinical and Biologic Activity of an Estrogenic Herbal Combination (PC-SPES) in Prostate Cancer," *New England Journal of Medicine* 339 (12): 785–91 (1998).

CONCLUSION

1. R.K. Oldham, M.D., "The War on Cancer: New Battle Plan Needed," *Cancer Biotherapy* 9 (4): 289–90, 1994.

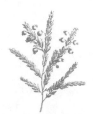

Index

(‘b’ indicates boxed material; ‘i’ indicates an illustration; ‘t’ indicates a table)